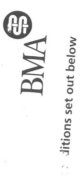

BMA

...ition

...ditions set out below

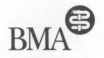
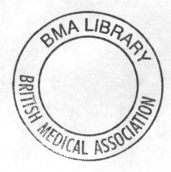

Head, Neck, and Dental Emergencies

Edited by

Mike Perry FRCS, FDS, BSc

Consultant Maxillofacial Surgeon
The Royal Group of Hospitals
Belfast
Northern Ireland

formerly

Consultant Maxillofacial Surgeon and Trauma Team Leader
University Hospital of North Staffordshire
Stoke on Trent

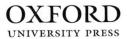

OXFORD
UNIVERSITY PRESS

OXFORD
UNIVERSITY PRESS

Great Clarendon Street, Oxford OX2 6DP

Oxford University Press is a department of the University of Oxford.
It furthers the University's objective of excellence in research, scholarship,
and education by publishing worldwide in

Oxford New York

Auckland Cape Town Dar es Salaam Hong Kong Karachi
Kuala Lumpur Madrid Melbourne Mexico City Nairobi
New Delhi Shanghai Taipei Toronto

With offices in

Argentina Austria Brazil Chile Czech Republic France Greece
Guatemala Hungary Italy Japan Poland Portugal Singapore
South Korea Switzerland Thailand Turkey Ukraine Vietnam

Oxford is a registered trade mark of Oxford University Press
in the UK and in certain other countries

Published in the United States
by Oxford University Press, Inc., New York

A catalogue record for this title is available from the British Library

Library of Congress Cataloging in Publication Data

(Data available)

ISBN 0-19-852910-4

10 9 8 7 6 5 4 3 2 1

Typeset by Newgen Imaging Systems (P) Ltd., Chennai, India
Printed in Italy
on acid-free paper by Legoprint S.p.A.

Preface

This book has been written in an attempt to identify and outline the management of those diseases, injuries or complaints, which may occur above the collar bones, presenting to an accident and emergency department. As such, many of the subjects covered here are not *true* emergencies (although some patients may feel otherwise!). In its strictest sense an emergency condition may be argued as one that requires *immediate* recognition or treatment in order to salvage life, sight, or limb; for instance, airway obstruction, ruptured aortic aneurism, retrobulbar haemorrhage, or traumatic amputation. These patients clearly need to be processed as quickly as possible in the A&E department and, where necessary, will jump the queue for theatre.

Strictly applying this principle to the head and neck would result in a book only a few pages in size, as very few *true* emergencies exist. These are, of course, covered in the text. However, it is hoped that at least 90% of problems in this anatomical region, which regularly attend a casualty department, will be in here somewhere.

This book is therefore aimed primarily at any health professional or undergraduate who has to assess or treat patients in an accident and emergency department setting. However, due to the variety of conditions covered, health professionals in related fields may also find it useful. The book is therefore aimed at:

- doctors in accident and emergency medicine, anaesthetics, neurosurgery, maxillofacial surgery, ENT, ophthalmology, and general plastic surgery;
- surgical trainees;
- medical/dental students;
- allied health professions.

In many cases, even to the inexperienced, the degree of urgency of a problem soon becomes very apparent within a few minutes of assessment. This becomes easier the more experienced you get. Unfortunately, prioritizing head and neck problems is not always straightforward, and (as with all acute problems) a *high index of suspicion* is always required to ensure pathology and complications are not missed. Very often what appears initially to be a trivial problem, turns out to be much worse; sometimes the opposite occurs. Patients, therefore, need to be *frequently re-assessed* until their condition has been fully defined and treatment well underway. This is commonly seen in patients with head injuries (minor or major), headache (minor, subarachnoid haemorrhage, or meningitis), neck swellings (lymph node, Ludwig's angina), and facial trauma (minor, major, multisystem).

In an attempt to try and address this dilemma, a coding system has been applied. This is by no means fool-proof and should only be used as a guide. It must be remembered that *priorities can rapidly change* as co-existing problems are identified, and this will only be picked up with regular re-assessment. For instance, a minor facial injury may become a real problem if a drunk patient is left supine unsupervised and then vomits. Similarly, neck and floor of mouth swellings can rapidly develop, compromising the airway, as can facial burns. Deterioration in vision may also upgrade priorities. Conversely, initial concerns may subside in head injuries as the GCS improves or the CT scan shows no abnormality. Needless to say these are only a few examples. The codes therefore are:

:☻: —A true emergency, as outlined above. Memorizing these conditions may help, rather than referring to this book when the patient is in the department! Call for immediate senior help. Try to remain calm and quickly assess the ABCs. Once the problem has been dealt with, remember to re-assess—other problems may have been forgotten or missed in the heat of the moment.

:☺: —These patients still need to be assessed very quickly, but you do not need to drop everything and run (so long as their ABCs have been managed). These patients can quickly shift into the emergency category if not sorted soon. Consider senior help/advise.

① —The majority of patients will fall into this and the last category. Although they do not need to be seen straight away, make sure you assess them thoroughly—fractured mandibles can still bleed a lot and patients can inhale loose teeth (especially if they are obtunded). Think carefully of potential complications that may develop, such as loss of sight with orbital trauma or hypovolaemia with epistaxis. Most headaches are in this group, but subarachnoid bleeds and meningitis will need to be reprioritised. Liaise with specialist help, if necessary.

② —These are non urgent conditions and general points of interest. Many of these patients, strictly speaking, should not come to casualty in the first place.

The format of this book is mostly concise text and note form, drawing on the current literature and multidisciplinary experiences of many senior clinicians. Established principles of care are therefore emphasized, together with top-tips gained from personal experiences. There is a minor degree of repetition in some chapters, but this is really to minimize annoying cross-referencing and to help revision. Topics are grouped into anatomical and pathological categories to help find them easily—patients may present with a 'head' problem, 'neck' problem, infection or following facial trauma.

MP
March 2004

Contents

Contributors

Howard Brydon FRCS,
Consultant neurosurgeon,
University Hospital of North
Staffordshire.

Anne Dancey MRCS,
Specialist registrar in plastic
surgery,
West Midlands Rotation.

Nick Grew FRCS, FDS.
Consultant maxillofacial surgeon,
Wolverhampton.

Manoli Heliotis FRCS, FDS,
Specialist registrar in maxillofacial
surgery,
South Thames Rotation.

Ian Holland FRCS, FDS,
Consultant maxillofacial surgeon,
West of Scotland.

William Kisku FRCS,
Staff grade in burns and plastic
surgery,
University Hospital of North
Staffordshire.

**Professor Nick Maffulli BSc.,
PhD., MBBS, MD., FRCS,**
Consultant orthopaedic surgeon,
University Hospital of North
Staffordshire.

**Kamiar Mireskandari
FRCOpth,**
Specialist registrar in
ophthalmology,
Moorefields Eye Hospital.

Jehanzeb Mughal FDS,
Maxillofacial Unit,
University Hospital of North
Staffordshire.

Mike Perry FRCS, FDS, BSc,
Consultant maxillofacial surgeon
and trauma team leader,
University Hospital of North
Staffordshire.

**Mr Philip Roberts MBBS,
FRCS,**
Specialist registrar orthopaedic
and trauma surgery,
University Hospital of North
Staffordshire.

Mr Mike Shelly FRCS, FDS,
Specialist registrar in maxillofacial
surgery,
South Thames Rotation.

**Richard T Walker RD, BDS,
PhD, MSc, FDS RCS, FDS
RCPS,**
Formerly Centre Director,
International Centre for
Excellence in Dentistry,
Eastman Dental Institute for
Oral Health Sciences,
University College London.

**Lt Col. Mike Williams,
FRCS, FDS,**
Specialist registrar in maxillofacial
surgery,
South Thames Rotation.

Chapter 1

General assessment and preliminary assessment following injuries

⑦ History taking and physical examination

Introduction

In a busy A&E department taking a *full* medical and social history and carrying out a *full* examination on every patient is generally not possible nor practical. That is not to say, these elements are unimportant—the importance of a good history and examination cannot be over-stressed. Indeed, it is often stated that around 90% of the diagnosis comes from the history alone. Therefore a *relevant* detailed history is essential to arrive at a diagnosis for the complaint(s) with which patients may present. Although still time-consuming, this information is necessary in subsequent treatment.

Medico-legal

Medico-legally, a detailed history and physical examination is required prior to commencing treatment. The skill in rapidly processing patients in a busy emergency setting comes from targeting relevant questions (but at the same time not putting words in the patients' mouths) and carrying out a relevant examination, looking out for key signs. This can only come with practice.

In order to recognize the abnormal, you must first be able to recognize what is 'normal'. Practice your examination techniques until you are comfortable with them, this way you will be slick and minimize your chances of missing something.

History taking is the first stage in diagnosis. Even though this is an arduous task, repeated every day, one must not lose sight of the fact that for the patient this may be a sensitive issue. He or she may be asked questions that may be personal and not normally shared, even with their close contacts. Therefore be sensitive to this. Introduce yourself and any member of your team present. Take time and be clear in the introductions. From this point on, start the process of developing a relationship that will be based on confidence and trust.

Try not to interrupt patients when they are talking—not everyone is able to express themselves clearly in few words. Know how to contact interpreters if the patient is having problems in communicating or expressing themselves in English. Remain in control of this question–answer session.

Setting and privacy

These are important and can be difficult in an A&E department. Make sure that you have enough space to be able to create a comfortable environment. Limit the presence of intimidating items such as sharp instruments, needles, etc., especially with children. Try to eliminate empty and distracting space between yourself and the patient, at the same time keeping a respectable distance. For patients accompanied by a carer or member of their family, ask them to join in, as they might be able to provide additional information. However, only include them if the patient consents to this, unless, of course, the patient is of non-consenting age or deemed mentally unable to give consent.

Sometimes your patient may wish to talk in private. In such a situation make sure that necessary precautions to safeguard yourself are taken; include a member of staff as a chaperon. If this is not possible, then leave the door or curtains of the consultation area partially open. Document everyone present in the notes.

Documentation and handwriting

These should be clear enough for all future use. Many 'alleged assaults' that present in or via A&E will result in criminal proceedings, and you or your seniors may be called upon to write a report up to a year later. Try and note as much detail as you can of what is told to you, this may avoid the patient having to repeat potentially embarrassing information to another colleague. Highlight important information with a different coloured pen or a sticker, i.e. allergies, HIV, Hep C status, and sensitive areas (where the patient does not want others to know).

What is written in the notes is accepted as an accurate account of events, anything more is inadmissible unless a chaperon testifies in your favour. It is difficult to defend oneself in a court of law on the basis of memory, and the law favours the patient in this regard. It is argued that since a doctor performs the process of history taking many times a day on many patients, memory of the event cannot be taken for fact, unless it is documented. For the patient, however, this was a unique event and so their testimony of events is deemed more accurate (although some research may indicate otherwise). On a more professional note, colleagues who continue the patient's care will always appreciate being able to actually read the notes!

Photography

This is a bit of a minefield, medico-legally. 'A picture speaks a thousand words' and photographs of injuries to the face are often helpful in assessment, for subsequent medical reports, and for teaching purposes. The problem arises in the unconscious patient, where consent is not possible. In these cases it is best to follow hospital protocol. If you are fortunate enough to work somewhere where this is allowed, always strive to seek consent from the patient at a later date.

History taking

Presenting complaint

This is best recorded briefly and, if possible, in the **patient's own words**. The **most common complaint is pain** and it is important to be able to differentiate the different origins of pain in the oro-facial region. This is covered elsewhere.

A number of complaints tend to be common for certain age groups, and this trend becomes more recognized with the experience of regular history taking. **Be warned not to make a diagnosis at this early stage** without a complete history. It is tempting to do just that and miss what might be a rare or unusual condition.

Patients may also present with a whole host of other problems that may or may not be associated with pain. There are, of course, many presenting complaints and the list below gives an idea of the more common ones. These will be covered in more detail in the relevant sections:

- pain
- stiffness
- injuries
- infections
- lumps or swellings
- bleeding
- rashes, patches, and ulcers
- altered sensation or weakness
- facial asymmetry
- trismus
- abnormal function (e.g. vision, bite)
- social problems.

History of presenting complaint

Consider the following in your history

- Pain:
  - Site of pain—this must be documented with reference to trigger points and/or referred pain. Use a body diagram and date each assessment to determine changes.
  - Description of pain—Terms include constant, intermittent, dull, aching, throbbing, sharp, burning, or shooting. Comparison to previous experience, e.g. like a knife, is helpful.
  - Periodicity—speed of onset, duration, frequency, seasonally.
  - Influences—does anything affect the pain, e.g. movement, heat, or cold. Does the pain fluctuate during the 24-h period?
  - Associated symptoms—swelling, jaw dysfunction, numbness or dysaethesia, pain anywhere else.
  - Previous therapies—has anything to date influenced the pain (analgesics, position, movement, time).
- Stiffness:
  - Which joint?
  - Any preceding cause?
  - When is it most stiff (in the morning/evening)?
  - Does movement improve the stiffness ('rusty gate')?
  - Are other joints affected?
  - Is there associated swelling or pain?
  - Any neurological symptoms (especially with neck stiffness)?
  - Any symptoms to suggest a connective tissue disease (CTD)?
  - Any family history?
- Assaults/injuries:
  - Place of the assault.
  - Time of the assault.
  - Whether the patient was on their own.
  - Does the patient know the attacker?
  - How many assailants were there.
  - Where any weapons used?
  - Any loss of consciousness?
  - Where did the patient go after the assault, e.g. A&E or home, and how did they get there, e.g. ambulance or personal transport?
  - Any other injuries apart from the face?
  - Are the police involved?
  - Any previous injuries (the broken nose may be old)?

- Infections:
  - How long?
  - Any obvious cause (bite/toothache/URTI, etc.)?
  - Is it getting worse?
  - Any signs of systemic upset?
- Lumps or swellings:
  - How long?
  - Is it growing?
  - Is it related to mealtimes (salivary obstruction)?
  - Is it painful (infected or rapid growth)?
  - Any obvious cause (e.g. lymphadenopathy)?
- Bleeding:
  - How long?
  - Where from?
  - Underlying cause?
  - Predisposing history or medication?
  - Symptoms of hypovolaemia?
- Rashes, patches, and ulcers:
  - Dermatological history
  - Associated with vesicles/blisters?
  - Any ocular/genital/joint symptoms?
  - Drug history?
- Altered sensation or weakness:
  - Where—is it anatomical?
  - Any underlying cause (e.g. head injury, MS)
  - Any associated swellings/ulcers (possible tumours)?
  - Assess cranial nerves fully
- Facial asymmetry:
  - Is it progressive?
  - If so how quickly?
- Trismus:
  - Look for associated infections or possible tumours.
  - Can the patient swallow/stick out their tongue?
  - Any signs of systemic upset?
- Abnormal bite:
  - When did it change?
  - Is it painful?

Systems review
Document the patient's general health. This will assess the fitness of the patient, warn of potential complications, decide on the type of anaethesia required, and may modify the treatment. There is no real indication to listen to the chest of a medically fit and healthy 18-year-old who complains of pain from a wisdom tooth.

Medication and allergies
Any medication currently in use must be recorded, as well as allergies to medication and any other substances. This will ensure appropriate risk free drug prescriptions.

Social history

Occupation, family situation, living conditions, smoking, alcohol consumption, employment, hobbies.

Religious convictions

Ask about these. **Jehovah's Witnesses**, for instance, will not accept blood transfusions. This is another potential minefield medico-legally, especially in the unconscious patient (where relatives have been known to be wrong!). Seek help in these cases, preferably find out local protocols before the situation arises.

Physical examination

This compliments the history by providing information leading to appropriate investigations and a diagnosis.

   Remember anatomical variations and age-related changes (especially when examining radiographs)

⑦ The significance of the past medical, social, and drug history in assessing emergencies and admissions

In *all* patients requiring admission, or an anaesthetic, a full medical, social, and drug history should eventually be taken. This will establish the diagnosis, determine the need for treatment, and assess the patient's general health in relation to possible treatments. However, when dealing with emergency or urgent cases, often this is not possible in the early stages of assessment. This is seen particularly in the management of the multiple-injured patient. In these cases it is essential to rapidly identify those factors that may have an *immediate* impact on either establishing the diagnosis or managing the clinical problem. How findings relate to management is outlined below.

Age
Although not a medical condition, the elderly have a decreased physiological reserve and need to be closely monitored. This is particularly so following blood loss (epistaxis, multiple injuries), where prompt fluid replacement is necessary. Care is also required not to overload their cardiovascular system. Elderly patients are also often on a variety of medications, each with their potential for problems from withholding, or drug interactions.

Pregnancy
Ask this in all women of childbearing age. In trauma, the best treatment for the foetus is to treat the mother first. Get the obstetricians involved early. For other emergencies pregnancy may influence the choice of local anaesthesia and other medications. Certain drugs are potentially teratogenic and may affect foetal maturation (e.g. closure of ductus arteriosus) or the onset of delivery. If in doubt **refer to the BNF**. In reality, radiographs (and even CTs) of the face carry very little risk to the foetus, but by and large most units will restrict or minimize these to those regarded as essential.

Ischaemic heart disease
This increases the risks of using general anaesthesia and local anaesthesia with adrenaline. In addition, cardiac pain can occasionally present as discomfort in the neck, mandible, or even 'toothache'. It should therefore be considered in the differential diagnosis. Pain on exertion, which is relieved by rest or GTN spray, is highly suggestive.

Hypertension
This increases the risks of general anaesthesia and local anaesthesia. Hypertensive 'crises', where the blood pressure is extremely high, can present with headaches and drowsiness, and therefore must be part of the differential diagnosis for these conditions.

Rheumatic fever, artificial valves, and endocarditis

Not all abscesses need antibiotics if adequately drained (e.g. dental abscess, boils). However, patients with a history of rheumatic fever, prosthetic heart valves or previous endocarditis are at risk from bacteraemia and in these cases antibiotics may be necessary.

Chronic obstructive airways disease (COAD)

Do not give oxygen over 28%. The exception to this rule is in the multiple-injured patient with life-threatening injuries. Here the 'lesser of two evils' has to be chosen.

Asthma

Avoid aspirin and other NSAIDs

Diabetes

Consider a hypoglycaemic attack in all confused or aggressive head-injured (and non-head-injured) patients, even if they appear to be intoxicated. Diabetics are at risk of infections, which can spread rapidly (notably dental). Occasionally a severe infection may be the presenting feature of diabetes. All patients with facial abscesses should be screened for this.

Hepatitis

Risks of cross-infection. Check LFTs and clotting.

Epilepsy

Fitting can occur after head injuries, especially in children. In epileptics this makes the assessment of head injuries difficult. Status epilepticus aggravates severe head injuries as a result of the fluctuations in blood pressure and hypoxia. Intubation and ventilation may be required.

Blood dyscrasias

Clotting disorders (haemophilia, platelet disorders, etc.) predispose to the same problems as anticoagulants. Leukaemic patients are also at increased risks of severe infections. Sickle cell disease requires care with general anaesthesia and can present acutely with severe pain in the mandible.

Previous injuries

Untreated or poorly treated facial fractures (e.g. nose, zygoma, or mandible) may make it difficult to decide whether a new injury is a new fracture or just bruising. Acute chest injuries preclude the use of entonox, which is particularly helpful in reducing dislocations of the mandibular condyle.

Tetanus status

This is relevant to all lacerations, bites and abrasions. Wounds can be classified as tetanus prone or non-tetanus prone and, depending on the immunization status, a booster course or immunoglobulin may be required.

Drug interactions

Commonly prescribed drugs include opiates, antibiotics, NSAIDs, and sedatives. Each has the potential to interact with other commonly prescribed medications from the patients GP. Remember also **herbal medicines** (e.g. St Johns Wort)—they can also interact.

Anticoagulants

For example, warfarin and aspirin. Reduced clotting may have an impact following trauma in several ways. Head injuries are at an increased risk of intra-cranial bleeding and may require admission for observation. Similarly, retrobulbar haemorrhage and bleeding into easily distensible tissues (floor of mouth, upper airway and eye) are more likely to occur following trauma to these sites. Pan-facial injuries may even require airway protection. Some authorities recommend avoidance of ID nerve blocks. Bleeding into large body cavities (chest, abdomen, pelvis) around fractures (limbs, retro-peritoneum) and externally can rapidly result in haemorrhagic shock. Check clotting and, if necessary, reverse the anticoagulant.

Steroids

Significant infections and trauma may require steroid supplementation. Chronic steroid use predisposes the patient to the risks of infection, poor wound healing, osteoporosis, and a diabetic potential, each with their own attendant problems.

Alcohol intake

Acute alcohol intoxication can result in agitation, unconsciousness, with loss of protective airway reflexes, and vomiting. In the head-injured patient this always makes assessment difficult. Never assume that the drowsy state is simply due to too much booze. Chronic alcoholics are often malnourished and self-neglected and at an increased risk of infections. If it is anticipated that the patient will not be able to drink alcohol for some time, get help in setting up an appropriate withdrawal protocol.

Home circumstances

One of the criteria for discharge of head-injured patients is *appropriate* home support. This involves regular observations for at least 24h by a responsible adult who can either bring the patient back to casualty or phone for an ambulance. If the patient lives in a remote area it might be better to consider overnight observation.

Allergies

Notably with antibiotics used to treat facial infections.

Family history

This may sometimes indicate potential risks from anaesthesia and patients should be asked about a history of **malignant hyperpyrexia, porphyria**, and, if of non-European decent, **sickle cell** disease.

People in certain occupations may be exposed to hazards that can produce respiratory disease. These include cancers (e.g. asbestos workers), infections (e.g. bird breeders), asthma (e.g. painters), pneumoconiosis (e.g. coal miners), allergic alveolitis (e.g. farmers).

⑦ Assessment of patients undergoing surgery

Consider the relevance of:
- age
- smoking
- alcohol abuse
- ischaemic heart disease
- respiratory disease (e.g. chronic obstructive airway disease)
- diabetes
- malnutrition
- blood disorders (haemophilia, sickle cell anaemia)
- head/facial injury
- cervical spine injury.

Assessment/management considerations:
- medical conditions
- deep vein thrombosis (DVT) prophylaxis
- antibiotic cover (ABC)
- steroid cover
- nutritional support
- effective pain relief
- stress ulcer prophylaxis
- early participation of physiotherapists, dieticians, speech therapists and social services.

Emergency surgery

Whereas patients undergoing elective surgery can be pre-assessed in good time, those requiring emergency surgery do not have this luxury and can only be rendered as fit as possible within the time allowed, depending on the degree of urgency. **Relatively few emergencies need *immediate* intervention** (such as airway obstruction, extra-dural haematoma, retrobulbar haemorrhage, etc.) and most can be delayed at least a few hours so that medical optimization is possible. In selected cases, some patients may benefit from a brief period of intensive management on a high-dependency unit (HDU) or intensive care unit (ICU). In all cases, *early* anaesthetist input is essential, particularly in those patients with potential airway hazards.

Principles of assessment

- History taking.
- Clinical examination.
- Special investigations.
- Clinical history:
  - presenting complaint history of presenting complaint
  - past medical/surgical history
  - drug history
  - allergies
  - systems enquiry
  - social/family history
  - pregnancy.

Cardiorespiratory assessment

Symptoms of cardiorespiratory disease:
- chest pain
- angina
- shortness of breath associated with exercise, cold, or after eating
- orthopnoea
- paroxysmal nocturnal dyspnoea (sudden shortness of breath at night-time)
- nocturnal cough
- ankle swelling
- claudication (calf pain on walking, relieved by rest)
- sputum production
- wheeze.

Risk factors for cardiac disease:
- smoking
- diabetes mellitus
- hyperlipidaemia and obesity
- hypertension
- male sex
- family history of cardiac disease.

Thorough assessment of the cardiovascular and respiratory systems is particularly important in patients undergoing surgery. Ischaemic heart disease (myocardial infarction, heart failure, angina), hypertension, asthma, chronic obstructive airways disease, chest injuries, and chest infections all significantly increase the risks of anaesthesia. Where non-urgent surgery is planned, deferral until the patient's condition has been improved is advisable.

Myocardial infarction within the preceding six months is a recognized major risk factor to further infarction and perioperative death. When possible, surgery should be postponed until after this period; some authorities suggest a minimum of one year. Patients with a past history of **rheumatic fever** are predisposed to valvular heart disease, which can lead to heart failure and infection of the valves (infective endocarditis). Intra-oral procedures, especially those involving the teeth (e.g. removal) are well-recognized as high-risk procedures for this. These patients should ideally be seen by a cardiologist, who can assess cardiac function and advise about any risks of endocarditis. Patients at risk may require antibiotic cover, depending on the surgical procedure. Similarly, some types of **congenital heart disease** and all patients with **artificial heart valves** will require appropriate antibiotic cover (ABC) given just before surgery.

Chronic obstructive airways disease

Predisposes to post-operative chest infections and hypoxia. Cessation of smoking, pre-operative physiotherapy, and surgery carried out in the summer months, will all significantly improve post-operative recovery.

Pre-operative measures to reduce post-operative chest infection:
- being aware of high risk patients;
- forbidding smoking for *at least* a few days before surgery;
- timing elective surgery for summer months;

- improving lung function in asthmatics with nebulised beta antagonists and steroids pre-operatively;
- physiotherapy;
- reserving beds in the high dependency or intensive care unit for patients who are particularly at high risk.

Tuberculosis is still seen, even in developed countries, especially among the homeless and deprived inner city areas where poverty and over-crowding contribute to its incidence.

Diabetes mellitus

Death and post-operative complications are more common in diabetic patients. This is due partly to controllable factors such as blood glucose, but also due to unavoidable complications such as ischaemic heart disease and infection, both of which are more common in these patients.

Risks to surgery in diabetic patients:

- acute hypoglycaemia
- ketoacidosis
- ischaemic heart disease
- hypertension (renal disease)
- increased risk of infections (chest, urinary, wound)
- predisposed to pressure sores.

The problems with diabetic patients undergoing major surgery are related to the enforced period of starvation (nil by mouth) and the metabolic effects secondary to the surgery itself. The main source of nutrition to the brain is glucose, yet persistantly high blood sugar predisposes to infections, poor wound healing, and ketoacidosis. The aim of management is therefore to minimize gross variations in blood sugar by ensuring an adequate glucose, calorie, and insulin intake. Blood glucose needs to be within normal limits pre-operatively and maintained until normal feeding is resumed following surgery. For many patients, normal feeding may be delayed many days, especially following major resections for head and neck cancer. Pre-operative blood glucose control can be determined by urinalysis or a random blood sugar. Blood urea and electrolyte concentrations should also be checked to exclude renal disease. Pre-operatively, it is important to determine:

- the type of diabetes;
- the adequacy of blood glucose control;
- the treatment regime (diet, oral hypoglycaemic agent, or insulin);
- established complications (e.g. cardiovascular, renal);
- planned surgery;
- the likely delay in resumption of oral feeding.

Many regimes exist for stabilizing diabetic patients in the pre-operative period.

General principles in diabetic management include:

- getting expert help—liaise *early* with the anaesthetist, if the patient need an operation;
- establish good control of blood sugar long before surgery is planned;
- avoid long-acting insulin preparations or oral hypoglycaemic agents 12–24 h pre-operatively, to prevent hypoglycaemia;

- regularly monitor blood sugar;
- fast from midnight (if on morning list);
- place patient first on the list;
- control blood sugar on the day of surgery using intravenous short-acting insulin and intravenous dextrose (many regimes exist);
- check potassium and supplement if necessary;
- post-operatively, continued use of a sliding scale until an adequate oral diet is re-established and then restart normal regime.

In **acute cases** blood glucose may be grossly abnormal secondary to infection, trauma, or reduced oral intake. Patients are often hyperglycaemic, which can lead to diuresis, dehydration, and ketoacidosis. These patients require intravenous rehydration, correction of sodium depletion, potassium supplementation, and infusion of short-acting soluble insulin. Regular monitoring of blood glucose, sodium, potassium, and acid–base balance is essential. When rehydration is underway and some correction of acidosis and hyperglycaemia has been achieved, emergency surgery may then be carried out continuing management during and after surgery.

Sliding scales involve the continuous infusion (sometimes subcutaneously) of a short-acting insulin, using a syringe pump. The rate of infusion varies according to the patient's blood glucose, which is checked regularly (e.g. hourly, depending on its stability). The higher the blood glucose, the more insulin given. In this way, hyperglycaemia can be controlled without risking profound hypoglycaemia. Sliding scales should be **reviewed constantly** and adjusted to achieve a relatively steady infusion rate. The aim is to establish a steady blood glucose rather than constantly oscillating below a low and high insulin infusion rate.

Bleeding disorders

The presence of blood dyscrasias and other causes of delayed clotting must be considered, especially when there is prolonged bleeding following minor oral surgery. The commoner problems include haemophilia A, haemophilia B, Von Willebrand's disease, liver disease, and patients on anticoagulants. Patients with known or suspected bleeding problems need to be fully assessed by an appropriate specialist, ideally in the out-patient clinic prior to admission. With appropriate prophylactic measures (e.g. local measures, tranexamic acid, DDAVP, factor replacement or adjustment of warfarin doses) surgery can be safely carried out, although the patient may need overnight admission. Patients on warfarin need careful assessment, as they may require adjustment of the dose until the INR is at an acceptable level. Opinions vary considerably as to what is 'acceptable', as reducing the dose of warfarin in itself is not without risks to the patient (inducing a hyperthrombotic state). Most maxillofacial units will, however, have established guidelines, which should be adhered to.

Thyroid surgery

Patients undergoing thyroid surgery for hyperthyroidism must be clinically and biochemically euthyroid before surgery is undertaken. Close co-operation with an endocrinologist is essential to optimize thyroid function prior to surgery.

Deep vein thrombosis (DVT)

Deep vein thrombosis, DVT, is generally uncommon following head and neck trauma or surgery. However, it is a potentially life-threatening condition (pulmonary embolism, PE) and is preventable. Diagnosis is often difficult and it has been estimated that around half of patients with extensive thrombosis have no clinical findings. Such 'silent' thrombi are a particular risk where the condition may remain unrecognized until fatal pulmonary embolism has occurred. It is therefore important that patients are assessed for risk factors and appropriate preventive measures taken.

Risk factors for DVT include:

- previous history of dvt or pulmonary embolism
- age
- myocardial infarction
- obesity
- extensive trauma
- infection
- congestive heart failure
- malignancy
- diabetes mellitus
- length and type of operation
- prolonged immobilization.

Other risk factors include:
- oral contraceptives
- smoking
- sex
- race
- occupation
- type of anaesthetic
- pregnancy and the puerperium
- varicose veins
- drugs.

DVT prophylaxis

Currently, prevention is directed towards elimination of stasis in the veins, or reducing the tendency to clot in the patient. Measures include:
- full length anti-embolism stockings
- physiotherapy
- intermittent pneumatic calf compression
- low voltage electrical calf stimulation
- early mobilization
- heparin.

Other prophylactic measures include intravenous low molecular weight dextrans, oral warfarin.

Heparin is currently available as 'fractionated heparin' and 'low molecular weight', which are reported to be more effective but are more expensive. Low-dose subcutaneous heparin significantly reduces the incidence of DVT in general surgical and orthopaedic patients. Low molecular weight heparins may be given once daily, which is more convenient for staff and patient.

Steroids in surgery 'steroid cover'

Patients on long-term or high-dose steroids, for whatever reason (asthma, rheumatoid arthritis, inflammatory bowel disease), are at risk of adrenocortical suppression. Following surgery, trauma, and infections they are unable to mount a normal 'stress response', which can lead to metabolic disturbances and, occasionally, collapse. Steroid supplementation may be required in the peri-operative period, commencing on induction of anaesthesia and continued post-operatively with a reducing dose. For an 'average' nil by mouth (NBM) patient, one regime might be (protocols vary depending on patient and procedure):

- major surgery—hydrocortisone 100 mg IM or IV with the pre-medication and then four times daily for three days, after which return to previous medication;
- minor surgery—prepare as for major surgery, except that hydrocortisone is given for 24 h only.

Stress ulceration

This occurs in patients after prolonged physiological stresses and is classically seen following extensive burns, major trauma, and multi-organ failure. Patients undergoing surgery for head and neck cancer may similarly be 'stressed' post-operatively, particularly if their recovery is complicated. This can result in fatal gastro-intestinal haemorrhage and in such patients prophylaxis is necessary. Current measures include H_2 receptor blockade and sucralfate.

⑦ **Assessing the elderly**

This can be particularly challenging. Although the principles of assessment in the elderly are no different than in the younger population, some specific points are worth highlighting.

- Chronological age *per se* is no indication of relative risk; careful assessment is still necessary. Contrary to general belief, most old people are fit. A better indication is the 'biological age', i.e. how old the patient looks.
- Hypertension, ischaemic heart disease, and congestive cardiac failure are all common in the elderly and often undiagnosed.
- Several diseases or problems may coexist.
- Elderly patients are often taking one or more different drugs. These should generally be continued throughout the peri-operative period. The potential for drug interactions must always be considered during anaesthesia or drug prescribing. Many exist.
- Patients may have impaired metabolism and excretion of drugs.
- One problem (e.g. poor mobility) may have several causes, each requiring attention.
- Complications are relatively common and may present non-specifically, with absence of typical symptoms (e.g. myocardial infarction without chest pain or a urinary tract infection without dysuria). Rapid deterioration can occur if these are not recognized and treated.
- Incontinence, instability, immobility, hypothermia, and confusion are common problems in the elderly. However, they may be early symptoms of underlying treatable disease, e.g. UTI.
- More time is required for recovery.
- Many elderly people live alone and their social circumstances need evaluating. Early involvement of social services may prevent delayed discharge in patients who go on to become 'social' admissions.

For major surgery routine, pre-operative FBC, biochemistry, blood gases, and chest X-ray, are useful as a baseline against which post-operative investigations can be compared. This is essential in patients with long-standing medical problems and associated biochemical abnormalities. In patients undergoing surgery for malignancy, a chest X-ray is also important to exclude metastasis. A pre-operative ECG is mandatory in all elderly patients, as asymptomatic heart disease may be detected.

Physical examination of the head and neck needs to be tailored according to the individual requirement of the patient.

☠ Primary survey—airway

- Airway—is it patent? Is it secure? Is there any danger of losing it?
- **Speak to the patient**, if they reply in a clear manner, then they have an airway that is patent and have the capacity to use it. A **horse voice** may suggest airway injury.
- Are there **gurgling/stridorous noises** indicating partial obstruction? This must be cleared immediately. Common causes are blood/saliva or the base of the tongue falling back against the pharynx. Other causes of obstruction may relate to swelling in the neck from bleeding or direct trauma to the airway (larynx/hyoid).
- **High flow suction** should be used and the mandible manipulated forward to lift the tongue base **(chin lift/jaw thrust)**. If it re-obstructs on release then an oro-pharyngeal, naso-pharyngeal or a definitive airway will be required. If patients require an oro- or naso-pharyngeal airway for more than a short while, they probably require a definitive airway.
- If the **airway is silent**, it is either completely occluded or the patient is not breathing. In the former, movement of the chest will be apparent and the patient will be in distress. Immediate relief of obstruction is essential. In severe facial/neck trauma this may require a surgical airway.
- **The anterior neck**. This is often a forgotten site and requires careful examination. It should be regarded as a watershed between 'airway' and 'breathing' during the primary survey. Life-threatening problems ~~ar~~ising in both can manifest clinical signs here. Fractures of the larynx ~~an~~d hyoid may lead to substantial glottic swelling. A **horse voice,** ~~h~~**emoptysis, and crepitus** in the neck are highly suggestive of these ~~injur~~ies. Carefully palpate the hyoid and larynx.

~~If the pa~~tient is not breathing, they require ventilating with oxygen either ~~by ba~~nd mask or a definitive airway. This is usually achieved by oro-~~in~~tubation or via a surgical cricothyroidotomy. **Naso-tracheal** ~~intubation~~ **is contraindicated in mid-facial trauma or head** ~~injury.~~

~~Conside~~r the risk to the cervical spine, which must be presumed ~~injured. It m~~ust be stabilized using a correctly fitting collar, 'sandbags' ~~if~~ available stabilise manually.
~~Th~~e patient who has a patent airway and is breathing also ~~require~~s an airway to protect the airway in the event of vomiting.

~~Risk facto~~rs
~~Sign of~~ actual or potential obstruction.
~~Abn~~ormal secretions.

~~Reduced consc~~iousness (may be secondary to alcohol, drugs or ~~lesio~~ns).
~~Haemorrh~~age.

~~Burn~~s/gross swelling.

~~Inju~~ry.
~~Cricothyroido~~tomy.

⑦ Physical examination

If at all possible, document clinical findings (notably injuries) photographically. Not only is this useful from a medico-legal perspective, but wounds, etc., can then be dressed and repeated examinations avoided. If photography is unavailable, use diagrams.

Extra oral examination

Inspection

Standing at a distance form the patient, take a general look at the head and neck. Note any asymmetry, lumps, trauma, discolouration, and muscular neuronal deficit. **Remember the cranial nerves (especially II, V and VII)**

Function

Check eye movements (blowout fractures), vision (ocular trauma), cranial nerves, swallowing, hearing, and jaw movements, where appropriate.

Palpation of the face

Depending on the presenting complaint, a thorough palpation of any visual findings is performed. This includes all surfaces that form the head and neck:

- scalp
- forehead
- supra-orbital ridges
- zygomatico-frontal sutures (lateral orbital margins)
- infra-orbital ridges
- nasal bridge
- maxilla
- zygomatic body and arch.
- temperomandibular joints
- mandibular ramus, body, and lower border
- mandibular range of movement, i.e. opening and lateral excursions
- surface of the neck down to the clavicle, cervical spine, and occiput.

Feel for tenderness, fluctuation, steps in bony continuity, and enlarged lymph nodes in the neck.

Auscultation

Can be considered for vascularized lumps (e.g. haemangioma, AVM, thyroid) or following trauma to the neck (carotid bruit).

Intra-Oral Examination

Occlusion (the bite)

Note whether this is deranged before asking the patient to open. If uncertain, then ask the patient to close their teeth together and retract the cheeks to see if there is contact at the back and front on either side. Ask the patient if the 'bite' feels normal. Be mindful of artificial teeth that can alter the occlusion without underlying bony trauma.

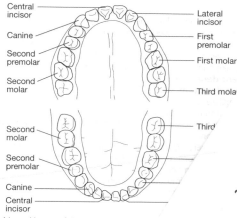

Central incisor — Lateral incisor
Canine — First premolar
Second premolar — First molar
Second molar — Third molar

Second molar — Third
Second premolar —
Canine —
Central incisor —

Fig. 1.1 Normal layout of the adult dentition.

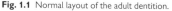

If the pa...
via bag a...
tracheal i...
intubatio...
injuries
Rememb...
injured. This...
and tape. If no...
The **comato**...
requires a defin...

Airway risk fac...
- Physical findings o...
- Inability to handle...
- Foreign bodies...
- Altered level of cons...
- some medical conditi...
- Uncontrolled haemor...
- Surgical emphysema...
- Adjacent soft tissue inju...
- Burns...
- Hyoid/laryngeal/tracheal in...
- Disrupted mid/lower face a...

Beware the patient who keeps trying to sit up—they may be trying to clear their airway. If no spinal injury, let them sit up; if unsure, either lay them on their side or tip the table head down. This is at variance with ATLS guidelines but facial bleeding will continue unrecognized in the supine position until the patient vomits and possibly aspirates. **If the patient vomits, tip them head down and apply wide-bore suction**—in practice there are usually not enough people *immediately* to hand to carry out a safe and co-ordinated log roll. Call for help.

Maxillofacial (trauma) emergencies—airway
Obstruction can be caused by dentures/teeth or severe fractures of the mandible or mid-face. The commonest cause is bleeding and/or saliva, notably when the patient is intoxicated or supine.

Mid-face fractures may displace downwards and backwards along the skull base, impinging on the posterior pharyngeal wall and resulting in obstruction. Bilateral anterior ('bucket handle') or comminuted mandibular fractures can similarly displace backwards allowing the base of the tongue to fall back. Both of these are much more likely when patients are supine and there is alteration in the conscious level. Both can be dealt with by pulling the fractured part forward to relieve the obstruction. This provides only temporary relief and a definitive airway will probably be required.

Saliva and blood should be cleared by suction. If the bleeding is ongoing from an identifiable source that can be stopped, it should be. However, it is usually generalized from multiple sites. Displaced fractures should be manually reduced, as this often helps slow the bleeding. Nasal packs may be necessary (remember the possibility of skull base #). If bleeding continues, the airway should be protected with a definitive airway.

Direct trauma to the airway will probably require a definitive airway to be placed.

Beware the patient who keeps trying to sit up—they may be trying to clear their airway

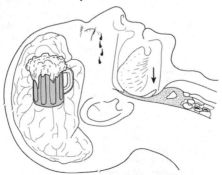

Fig. 1.6 The commonest cause of airway obstruction following probably a mixture of concussion, alcohol, and foreign bodies the back of the mouth—do not leave patients unsupervized

Airway with control of cervical spine

As in all trauma patients, the first priority is to assess the airway **while protecting the cervical spine**. Initial assessment often simply requires a verbal response from the patient—'what happened?' followed by direct inspection of the mouth and pharynx for signs of potential obstruction. The cervical spine should be immobilized along the usual lines, unless the patient is highly agitated and thrashing around.

Remember 'airway' is not just the mouth and obstruction may occur at any point from the lips and nostrils to the carina. It may arise from foreign bodies (dentures), teeth, blood, secretions, or displaced/swollen tissues. The most common foreign bodies encountered in facial injuries are blood and vomit.

The risk of obstruction by the pooling of blood and secretions, is present in almost all patients with injuries to the face. This is made worse with displaced or comminuted fractures of the mandible, where swallowing may be painful. Early signs may be easily missed, particularly when dealing with patients who are intoxicated or have a significant head injury. Not only are they at risk of vomiting, but coma predisposes to loss of protective airway reflexes and care must be taken if these patients are positioned supine, as indicated in the ATLS approach.

If the patient has sustained major facial injuries **be cautious and maintain an index of suspicion if he/she wishes to sit up**. This may indicate concealed mid-face bleeding and awake patients may prefer to sit forwards and drool, allowing the blood and secretions to drain from the mouth, rather than lie supine according to ATLS principles. A judgement call is unfortunately required when positioning the patient with an isolated injury. When multisystem injury is suspected, special care is necessary. **Patients should never be forced or restrained onto their backs, as this is more likely to compromise both the airway and any occult cervical spine injury**.

Loss of tongue support may occur with bilateral (so called 'bucket handle') or comminuted anterior mandibular fractures. However, in the awake patient, airway control may still be possible. It is in the supine, head injured, or intoxicated patient, that loss of tongue control and other protective reflexes may become a problem. **Comminuted, and therefore high energy fractures**, of the mandible carry a greater risk as there is very little tongue support. In addition significant soft tissue swelling and intra-oral bleeding may be associated.

Occasionally **displaced facial fractures** may cause airway problems. Severe injuries to the middle-third of the face may result in comminuted ▪ctures that are displaced backwards and down the inclined surface of ▪skull base. This can result in impaction of the posterior face (notably ▪) on to the pharynx. Combined mandibular and middle-third facial ▪s are indicative of major trauma and, therefore, predispose to ▪oblems. These patients commonly have an associated head ▪ compounds the problem. They also have a tendency to bleed ▪ suffer from severe soft tissue swelling.

▪welling inevitably occurs with these major injuries, often ▪onged intubation or an *elective* tracheostomy. However, ▪lso occur in the absence of any fracture, as occasionally seen in patients taking anticoagulants, or those with clotting abnormalities. Patients with cervical spine fractures may develop posterior pharyngeal swelling contributing to an obstructed airway. Penetrating and blunt (e.g. strangulation/hanging) neck trauma may also be associated with pharyngeal oedema and bleeding. It is important to appreciate that swelling from whatever cause can take several hours to develop. Be wary

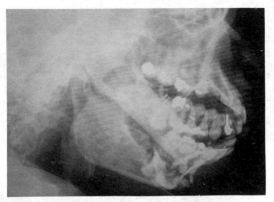

Fig. 1.7 Comminuted fractures place the airway at risk. Comminution implies a high transfer of energy—think about soft tissue swelling.

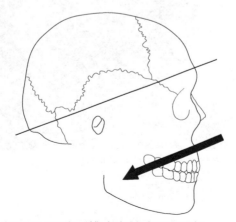

Fig. 1.8 Severe injuries to the middle-third of the face may result in tures that are displaced backwards and down the inclined surface

and regularly re-examine the patient. Of particular concern are those patients who have suffered facial burns. These are frequently associated with inhalation injuries, which can lead to rapid swelling that is not appreciated on initial examination **Stridor is a particularly worrying sign and often necessitates early intubation**.

The anterior neck

This is often a forgotten site and requires careful examination. It should be regarded as a watershed between 'airway' and 'breathing' during the primary survey as life-threatening problems in both can manifest clinical signs here. Pouiselle's law dictates that even a small change in the diameter of a tube can result in a significant change in flow through it. Although strictly applicable to fluid dynamics, this equation highlights the potential for problems to arise with swelling in the larynx and trachea. Although unusual, fractures of the larynx and hyoid do occur and may lead to substantial glottic swelling. **Motorcycle helmet wearers, strangulation**, and **contact-sports injuries** are important clues from the history. A **hoarse voice, haemoptysis**, and **crepitus in the neck** are highly suggestive of these injuries and should be actively sought after. Carefully palpate the hyoid and larynx for signs of injury, and look for external swelling, which may reflect swelling internally.

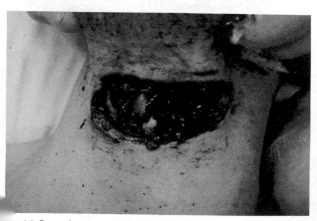

1.9 Do not forget to assess the front of the neck!

Airway maintenance techniques

Control of the airway can be easily lost and may be very difficult to secure following facial trauma and burns. **All trauma patients should receive oxygen**. Often early assistance from an experienced anaesthetist is required and should be anticipated well in advance of signs of impending obstruction. Occasionally an immediate surgical airway is required, notably when there is gross swelling in pan facial injuries. Members of the trauma team should be competent in performing this.

Airway maintenance techniques include:
- suction
- jaw thrust
- chin lift
- oro-/naso-pharyngeal airways
- tongue suture
- laryngeal mask.

Several techniques exist for 'maintaining' an airway. However, it is important to appreciate these are not the same as 'securing' the airway and their **effectiveness may be lost**. High-volume suction using a wide-bore soft plastic sucker should be readily available to clear the mouth, nose, and pharynx of blood and secretions, taking care not to induce vomiting. Loss of the protective gag reflex should prompt consideration of an oro-pharyngeal airway or even intubation.

The jaw thrust and chin lift techniques are commonly used techniques but are occasionally not effective in the presence of severely comminuted mandibular fractures. In these cases it may be useful to use a tongue suture or even a pointed towel clip to initially control an obstructing tongue. Oro-pharyngeal airway (Guedel), naso-pharyngeal airway, and laryngeal mask airways (LMA) are all useful additional techniques available for maintaining an airway. However, it should be remembered that LMA can often induce vomiting and that none provide a definitive and secure airway. **The use of a naso-pharyngeal airway (and naso-tracheal tube) is usually contraindicated in mid-face injuries or suspected basal skull fracture**. Basal skull fracture should be suspected in the presence of periorbital ecchymosis (racoon eyes), mastoid ecchymosis (Battle's sign), VIIth nerve palsy, and CSF leaks.

Posteriorly displaced middle third fractures may be disimpacted to improve the airway. Grasping the maxilla and pulling it anteriorly achieve this. It may be necessary to support this with a mouth prop, provided the patient has an intact lower jaw. This has the additional benefit of controlling haemorrhage from middle-third facial fractures.

Definitive airways
- Oro-endotracheal intubation.
- Naso-endotracheal intubation.
- Surgical cricothyroidotomy.

A definitive airway may be defined as a **cuffed tube in the tra** may be required if there is any doubt about the patient's ability their own airway immediately or in the near future. In the situation, it is important that the technique used is one w clinician is most confident; the trauma setting is not the t unfamiliar procedures.

(a)

(b)

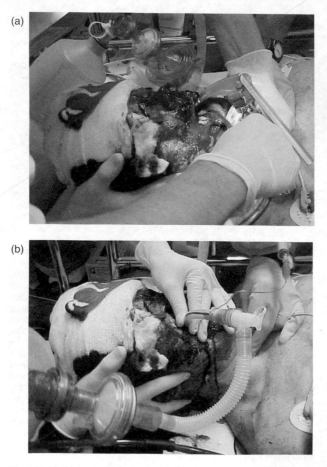

Fig. 1.10 (a)–(c) demonstrate several important principles in securing an airway following serious facial injuries: organization, team-work, c spine immobilization during and after intubation and cricoid pressure (patient was also pre-oxygenated).

(c)

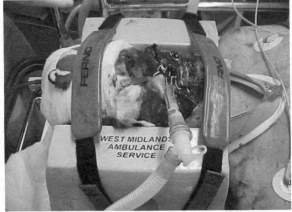

Oro-tracheal intubation with in-line cervical immobilization is usually the technique of choice in the majority of cases. In the absence of mid-facial or cranio-facial fractures, alternative techniques include blind naso-tracheal intubation or fibre-optic assisted oro- and naso-tracheal intubation. Together with surgical airways, these techniques have been shown to be associated with less manipulation of the injured cervical spine. However, they require extensive training. **Naso-tracheal intubation is potentially dangerous—the anterior cranial base can be inadvertently 'intubated' through an unrecognized fracture**. The use of fibre-optic assistance is usually limited, as the view is often obscured by blood. Retrograde intubation avoids cervical spine manipulation but its use is not well established in the trauma setting.

The only indication for creating a surgical airway is failure to secure the airway by any other way. Surgical airways include needle cricothyroidotomy and surgical cricothyroidotomy. **Tracheostomy is now generally regarded as obsolete in the trauma setting** as it is too time-consuming to perform and potentially unsafe. The key factor in performing a needle or surgical cricothyroidotomy is identification of the cricothyroid membrane, which should be possible, provided the anterior neck is not too oedematous. A needle cricothyroidotomy may be used to provide oxygenation while preparing for surgical cricothyroidotomy. It is not secure but may be used in extremis while a definitive (surgical cricothyroidotomy) airway is secured.

Emergency surgical airways

In less emergent cases, an airway can usually be secured by other measures. This depends upon the particular circumstances and includes the use of:

- suction
- tongue suture
- chin lift/jaw thrust
- nasopharyngeal/oropharyngeal airway
- nasotracheal/orotracheal intubation
- cricothyroidotomy
- tracheostomy.

Which method is used depends on:

- type of obstruction
- urgency of airway
- conscious level
- presence or suspicion of cervical spine injury
- experience and skills of clinician.

Indications for urgent surgical airways include:

- actual or potential obstruction
- laryngeal fractures
- upper tracheal injury (if unable to intubate)
- in all cases supplemental inspired oxygen is necessary.

Most authorites generally agree that the most appropriate *emergency* surgical airway for upper airway obstruction is through the **cricothyroid membrane rather than a tracheostomy**. If time allows, a stab incision is made through which a small cuffed tracheostomy or endotracheal tube is passed. Formal tracheostomy takes longer to perform, is more difficult, and has potentially more serious complications. However, fractures of the larynx may make cricothyroidotomy impossible, in which case a tra*cheotomy* should be undertaken. In *extreme* conditions access can be established by passing a brown or grey venflon through the cricothyroid membrane. This can then be connected this to oxygen via a 'Y' shaped cannula. It is however only a temporary measure.

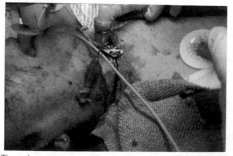

These demonstrate several important principles in securing an airway rious facial injuries: organization, team-work, c spine immobilization ter intubation and cricoid pressure (patient was also pre-oxygenated).

Full c-spine immobilization includes not just the neck but **immobilization of the entire spine**. Movement lower down the spine will result in a degree of movement in the neck. Furthermore injuries of the c-spine may be associated with spinal injuries elsewhere. These also need to be protected.

Following significant injuries most patients arrive supine with

- **spinal board** (solid inflexible plastic board the length and width of the patient with straps that hold the patient rigid across the chest, pelvis and legs);
- **blocks** (usually foam filled rubber coated blocks about the size of a shoe box, on both sides of their head, preventing the neck from rotating, radiolucent to allow radiographic examination of the spine);
- **tape** (often simple elastoplast tape but more commonly two purpose-made straps, one across the mandible, the other across the forehead, holding the head down on to the spinal board);
- **hard collar** (stiff plastic neck collar that holds the cervical spine more stable by reducing flexion, extension, and lateral flexion of the neck).

Go to your A&E department, and ask to see these items, be familiar with how they are applied and taken off. Better to learn now than have to learn during the real thing!

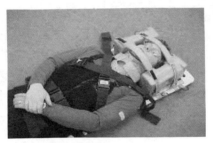

Fig. 1.12 Correct spinal immobilization.

☠ Primary survey—breathing

All patients must be given 100% oxygen.

- Is the patient **breathing adequately**? Speak to them. Can air be heard entering the lungs? If not, determine and treat the cause (pneumothorax/haemothorax, etc.).
- **Comatose patients (head injury/drugs/alcohol may be hypoventilating**. Attach a **pulse oximeter** and get some **blood gases**.

Conditions affecting ventilation

If you are a member of the 'ATLS Fan Club' you will remember life-threatening 'B' problems:

- **A**irway:
  - **foreign bodies** in the chest—emergency bronchoscopy;
  - **aspiration**—supportive care;
  - **inhalation injury**—supportive care.
- **T**ension pnuemothorax—needle decompression and formal chest drain.
- **L**arge (massive) haemothorax—volume replacement and chest drain.
- **S**ucking chest wound (open pneumothorax)—three-sided dressing initially then chest drain.
- **F**lail chest—analgesia, monitoring, and ventilatory support.
- **C**ardiac tamponade—aspirate pericardial blood

In the context of maxillo-facial injuries, breathing problems may occur following **aspiration of teeth, dentures, and other foreign bodies**. If teeth or dentures have been lost and the whereabouts unknown, a chest and neck radiograph should be taken to exclude their presence in the pharynx or lower airway. Unfortunately acrylic, from which 'plastic' dentures are made, is not very obvious on a radiograph and a careful search is necessary. All foreign bodies need to be removed.

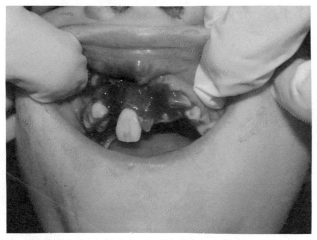

Fig. 1.13 Apparent minor injuries can result in major complications—always consider a CXR when lost teeth cannot be accounted for.

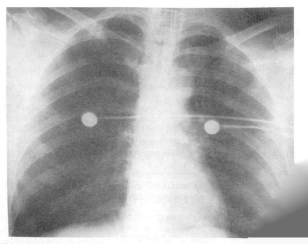

Fig. 1.14 Apparent minor injuries can result in major complications—consider a CXR when lost teeth cannot be accounted for.

☠ Primary survey—circulation

The commonest cause of preventable death following trauma is shock, usually hypovolaemic. This results in inadequate perfusion of the tissues. 'Any patient that is cool and tachycardic is in shock until proven otherwise.' This may be due to blood loss, or the pump (heart) is not working properly. Other less common causes are also recognized.

Assess:
- pulse
- capillary refill
- presence of cool clammy peripheries
- mental status
- respiratory rate
- bood pressure
- urinary output.

Remember—blood pressure does not drop until late in the development of shock.

All trauma patients should have good intravenous access and blood taken for cross match. Initially warmed crystalloid (this varies in different units) should be infused and the patient's response reassessed. The source of blood loss must be identified and further stopped—'putting the plug in the bath'.

Sources of major blood loss:
- external wounds
- chest
- abdomen
- retroperitoneum
- pelvis
- limbs.

Life-threatening haemorrhage **from head and neck injuries** is uncommon but does occur. Consider:
- **epistaxis**—if supine this may go unnoticed as the blood is swallowed;
- **mid-face/displaced mandible fractures;**
- **lacerations** to the neck and scalp;
- **blood loss** in children is more significant.

The chest, pelvis, and limbs can be assessed clinically and radiographically, the abdomen cannot be reliably assessed clinically, especially in the unconscious patient, and may require further investigations (peritoneal lavage, ultrasound or CT). Immobilization of limb/pelvic fractures and a laparotomy for bleeding should be regarded as part of 'C' and not delayed.

In transient responses and non-responders to the fluid challenge, especially in injuries above the diaphragm, other causes should be considered—iogenic, tension pneumothorax, cardiac tamponade, spinal, or septic.

ildren, the elderly, athletes, and patients with pacemakers eta-blockers may respond differently to blood loss.

cial (trauma) emergencies—bleeding

n maxillofacial injury is common but not usually life-threatening.
t is in shock, look for another cause. Actively consider
s supine patients will be swallowing blood which will go

If significant and obvious, bleeding is controlled in the primary survey by **pressure**. Bleeding from lacerations can usually be controlled by pressure applied either with a swab (care with scalps if risk of skull fracture) or by placement of **sutures** to close lacerations. They are used to apply pressure and not intended as definitive closure.

Mid-face bleeding can be troublesome. Bleeding arises from multiple sites within comminuted bones and torn mucosa. Pressure can be applied to the nose with anterior and posterior nasal packs. **Displaced/mobile mid-face fractures should be reduced**. Gentle pressure can be applied antero-superiorly on the maxilla and maintained by placing mouth props bilaterally against an intact mandible. Surprisingly this is not as painful as one might think. In selected cases, use of external fixators applied to the skull and maxilla may be necessary, but this requires transfer to an operating theatre and considerably more time.

Bleeding from a 'hole' (e.g. following a gunshot) can sometimes be stemmed by placing a **urinary catheter** in the hole and inflating it. Obviously be careful and think what may be in the depths of the hole!

If local pressure is not sufficient to stop haemorrhage from either soft or hard tissue injury the use of **angiography and embolisation, or ligation of external carotids should be considered**. This is rare.

Circulation—with control of haemorrhage

'Any cold and tachycardic patient should be considered to be in hypovolaemic shock until proven otherwise' (ATLS).

When shock is present, **facial injuries are unlikely to be the sole cause**. Look carefully for occult bleeding elsewhere (consider chest, abdomen, pelvis, retroperitoneum, limbs, and on the floor). However life-threatening, facial haemorrhage has been reported to occur in up to 10% of serious facial injuries. Blood loss from the scalp, face, and neck can be profuse. This is difficult to control due to the extensive collateral blood supply derived from the internal and external carotid arteries, bilaterally. Bleeding may be either **revealed or concealed**. Bleeding from comminuted fracture sites and soft tissue injuries can contribute to hypovolaemia and should be considered in all mid-face injuries. In such patients the bleeding is usually from multiple sites rather than from a named vessel, making control problematic. Concealed bleeding may occur in the supine patient, and is worth remembering as its contribution to persisting shock may not be recognized until the patient vomits and aspirates. **Arterial blood gases are particularly useful in the evaluation of haemorrhagic shock**. A raised base excess and lactate often represents lactic acidosis and is an indication of tissue hypoperfusion.

Shock management

The first priority is to **stop obvious and significant blood loss** followed by **good intravenous access** through which fluids may be delivered quickly. **Direct pressure, sutures, haemostatic clips, and diathermy** may all be used to control obvious visible bleeding, for example, from the scalp. However, these techniques only have a limited application in facial injuries as bleeding often comes from deep within the nasal and oral cavity. Manual reduction of mid-face fractures is frequently effective in controlling bleeding, although it may be unsuccessful if severely comminuted. This is comparable to the reduction of a displaced femoral fracture limiting haemorrhage. This is surprisingly not as painful as one might think. In selected cases use of external fixators may be necessary but this requires transfer to an operating theatre and considerably more time.

Oral bleeding

This may be controlled with dental gauze packs and manual reduction of obviously displaced jaw fractures. The amount of blood loss is often over estimated as the patient often salivates profusely.

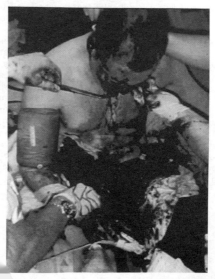

l reduction of midface fractures is frequently effective in
ₑ (why is this patient sitting up?).

Epistaxis

This may be controlled using nasal balloons or packs. If the source of nasal bleeding is high in the posterior nasopharynx, **Foley catheters** can be passed via both nostrils into the post-nasal space and then inflated with 10–20 ml of saline. Again, a judgement call is required with pan-facial injuries due to the **risk of cranial intubation**. Furthermore, inflation of the balloons may distract cranio-facial fractures, thereby increasing blood loss. Temporary stabilization of the fractures using a mouth prop may be necessary before these manoeuvres are attempted. Once inflated, gentle traction can then be applied 'wedging' the balloons in the naso-pharynx. Light anterior nasal packs can then be placed. There is an increased risk of sinusitis and the patient should be commenced on appropriate antibiotics. If CSF leakage is also present there is a risk of brain abscess.

If local pressure is not sufficient to stop haemorrhage from either soft or hard tissue injury the use of angiography and embolisation, or ligation of external carotids should be considered. This is rare.

Surgical intervention

If control of bleeding is not possible, it is important to consider a coagulation screen, prior to surgical control. Surgery may involve ligation of the external carotid via the neck and ethmoidal arteries via the orbits. However, to do so requires a general anaesthetic and, because of extensive collateral supply, may be necessary on both sides. Alternatively, endoscopic techniques such as transantral and intra-nasal approaches may be used. These are of limited use in pan-facial fractures, where multiple bleeding points may be present both in bone and soft tissues. These techniques are best used in localized nasal injuries resulting in uncontrollable epistaxis. Given that the face has a very rich blood supply, the more distal a clip or tie is applied, the more effective the treatment becomes.

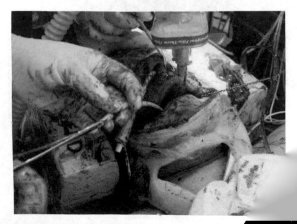

Fig. 1.16 If the source of nasal bleeding is high in the posterior nasal [...] Foley catheters can be passed via both nostrils into the post-nasal [...] inflated, followed by anterior packs.

Supra-selective embolization

The use of supra-selective embolization in trauma is controversial but has been reported to be very successful and has certain advantages over surgery. It is increasingly used in extremity trauma and bleeding secondary to pelvic fractures. Catheter-guided angiography is used to first identify and then occlude the bleeding point or points. This involves the use of balloons, stents, coils or poly vinyl alcohol (PVA).

Supra-selective embolization can be performed without the need for a general anaesthetic and in experienced hands is relatively quick. Its value, therefore, is seen in the unstable patient. Multiple bleeding points can be precisely identified and the technique is repeatable. However, immediate access to facilities and on-site expertise are essential. Complications include intolerance to the iodine and, following extensive embolization, end-organ ischaemia and subsequent necrosis. Stroke and blindness have also been reported.

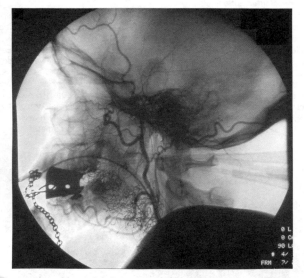

Fig. 1.17 Lateral face and skull view following digital subtraction angiography, r to embolization.

☠ Primary survey—disability

Head injury is a common cause of morbidity and mortality after trauma because of the resulting injury to the brain. The injury may be **primary**, occurring **at the time** of the traumatic episode. Other than preventive measures, there is little that can be done about this. **Secondary** injury occurs later and can be due to reduced perfusion, inadequate oxygenation, and raised ICP—all of which we can do something about.

Assessment is made using the **Glasgow Coma Scale (or AVPU) and pupillary responses. The GCS cannot be accurately interpreted until A, B, and C are optimized. Changes in the GCS with time are more significant than an individual reading. A decrease by 2 points (and the development of a dilated pupil, deviated laterally and downward) indicates a critical head injury**. After Airway Breathing and Circulation have been addressed, this requires emergent neurosurgical evaluation.

CT scanning is often used to assess head-injured patients. Patients must be stable prior to transfer to CT—'the doughnut of death'(!)

Remember—all facial injuries are technically head injuries, which take priority in assessment. Potential complications include:
- associated cspine injury
- reduced airway protection
- profuse bleeding
- blindness.

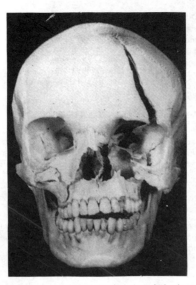

Fig. 1.18 All facial injuries are technically head injuries, which take priority in assessment.

Visual disability

Following trauma vision can be threatened anywhere along the visual pathway from globe to cortex. The main (potentially treatable) causes to consider are:

- direct globe injury
- retrobulbar haemorrhage
- optic nerve compression
- loss of eyelids.

Direct injury to the globe requires urgent ophthalmic referral.

Retrobulbar haemorrhage

Bleeding behind the globe is a form of compartment syndrome. **This is a surgical emergency**. It can lead to an increase in pressure that results eventually in irreversible ischaemia of the retina and optic nerve. Key symptoms are:

- severe pain and progressive loss of vision;
- the eye becomes proptosed with ophthalmoplegia and development of a fixed dilated pupil as the vision deteriorates.

Treatment requires immediate relief of pressure. In the emergency department the following should be given intravenously:

- acetazolamide
- mannitol
- steroids,

during which arrangements are made for surgery. Under LA a lateral canthotomy may be possible but these measures really only buy time while preparation for surgery is made. Deffinitive treatment involves drainage of the haematoma. Decompression should lead to an improvement in visual acuity if undertaken early enough.

Traumatic optic neuropathy

Traumatic optic neuropathy occurs when there is disruption around the optic canal resulting in either compression of the optic nerve, shearing forces to the nerve as it passes through the canal, or haematoma formation within the nerve itself. Untreated it can render the patient blind and the diagnosis needs to be made early to allow the best chance of visual recovery. The signs that suggest an optic nerve injury include **poorly reactive pupil, afferent papillary defect, and decreased colour vision, decreased visual acuity with relatively normal ocular examination**. This is an ophthalmic emergency and should be referred accordingly.

Treatment of optic nerve compression is controversial and again may be ~~either~~ medical or surgical. The options include observation, IV corticosteroids, and optic nerve decompression. The latter option is carried out ~~either~~ a craniotomy approach or lateral facial approach.

~~A st~~eroid regime is:

~~~~ prednisolone 30 mg/kg STAT, followed by
~~~~ prednisolone 15 mg/kg every 6 h.

~~Othe~~rs exist.

~~Tim~~e essence, best results are obtained if steroids are ~~given~~ of the injury.

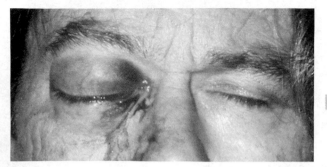

Fig. 1.19 Retrobulbar haemorrhage.

⑦ Primary survey—initial investigations

- During 'A'—clinical assessment.
- During 'B'—clinical assessment + O_2 saturation.
- During 'C'—clinical assessment + ABGs, FBC, U&E, RBS, coagulation screen, cross match (type specific) and, if possible, pregnancy test in females.
- After 'D' and 'E'—chest, pelvic and c-spine X-ray (the latter is not mandatory as long as the c-spine is immobilized).
- Urinary catheterisation.
- Oro-gastric or naso-gastric (if no risk of # skull base) tube placement.
- **Often serial investigations are necessary (ABGs, CXR)— remember these only reflect the condition of the patient *at the time* they were taken.**
- **Facial X-rays can wait**.

CSF leaks

Facial fractures that extend into the base of the skull (e.g. Le Fort II, Le Fort III, naso-ethmoidal and occasionally fractures involving the mandibular condyle), can tear the dural lining and allow cerebral spinal fluid (CSF) to leak from the nose (rhinorrhoea) or from the ear (otorrhoea). Clear CSF tends to mix with blood and presents as a heavily blood-stained, watery discharge. This trickles down the side of the face, where peripherally the blood tends to clot while the non-clotted blood in the centre is washed away by CSF. This creates two parallel lines referred to as **'tramlining'**. One test for CSF is the 'ring test' (allow drops to fall on blotting paper, blood clots centrally, the CSF diffusing outwards to form a target sign). Other tests include examining for eosinophils and sugar. This is helpful in distinguishing between CSF and mucous. More sensitive indicators include B2 transferrin and tau protein, although practically it is easier to simply assume that a leak is present. **Tell the patient not to blow their nose for three weeks (see Head injuries)**.

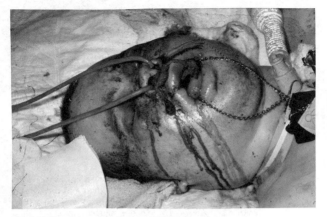

Fig. 1.20 Tramlining—an indication of CSF leakage.

⑦ Primary survey—re-assessment

This should be an ongoing part of the initial management of the trauma patient. All interventions that are undertaken should be reviewed—the condition of the patient should improve! If at any point during resuscitation the patient deteriorates reassess, starting with the airway.

At the end of the primary survey, review the patient along with any results of investigations to ensure they are stable and life threatening problems have been dealt with. Only then can a complete secondary survey examination be undertaken and attention to the face be drawn.

At some point the patient will need to be 'log rolled' to allow inspection of the back. Timing depends on liklyhood of certain injuries—it may be necessary during 'B' if a penetrating injury is suspected (open pneumothorax).

Antibiotics, steroids, and tetanus prophylaxis

Protocols may vary between different units. Antibiotics are usually given for fractures, which are compound (open) into the mouth or through the skin (e.g. mandible). Oral bacteria of a mixed anaerobic type and a combination of a penicillin and metronidazole is one suitable choice.

Prophylactic antibiotics when there is CFS leakage is controversial and the opinion of a neurosurgeon should be sought. At the time of writing, the current advice of the Infection in Neurosurgery Working Party is not to use them—they do not prevent meningitis as they penetrate poorly into the CSF in the absence of infection, but kill of the normal flora. You are thus more likely to get meningitis by a multi-resistant organism.

Tetanus prophylaxis should be considered especially in mucky wounds, which should be thoroughly cleaned as soon as possible. Steroids, e.g. dexamethasone/methylprednisolone are often given to reduce facial swelling.

Chapter 2

First-aid measures

⑦ General principles

Very often patients require some kind of first aid while they wait for further assessment or definitive treatment. Some of these measures are covered elsewhere in the relevant sections, but consider the following options.

The mechanism of injury

Can the patient 'go round for an X-ray' or should they stay in resuscitation? Can they be left unsupervised or do they need frequent observation?— beware leaving patients alone supine if they have facial or head injuries.

Dirty wounds/burns

These need to be irrigated as soon as possible. A bag of saline, giving set and venflon can provide continuous flow if necessary. **Remember tetanus prophylaxis.**

Tacking sutures

Gaping wounds should be loosely approximated either with steristrips or a few sutures. The choice of suture is not crucial, as it will eventually be replaced. Take reasonable size bites, rather than try to cosmetically close the wound, the purpose of the suture is to realign the tissues, stop bleeding, aid perfusion, and protect the underlying tissues. Ensure tags of tissue are not twisted or kinked on their pedicle—if left they may become necrotic.

Dressings

Light saline- or antiseptic-soaked dressings are useful to keep wounds moist, reduce further contamination, and allow relatives to see the patient without fainting! If possible, take some photos—this helps reduce the number of times the wound needs to be inspected. If tissue has been lost (e.g. dog bite to the lip), irrigate the wound and loosely dress.

Pain control

There are many ways to provide effective pain relief, which can be tailored to each circumstance. **Resist the temptation to automatically give opiates to everyone who complains of pain**—it may not be the best analgesic, you may loose your ability to assess their head injury, they may vomit and you may then need to commit them (in many units) to admission or a CT scan. Alternatives include **nerve blocks** (good for facial pain, dental pain, and injuries). '**Bridal wires**' are the maxillofacial equivalent of a backslab in limb fractures. These are passed around the teeth either side of a mandibular fracture and used to support it. However, it requires a certain level of skill and is not without risks (to the teeth).

‸ety control

‸ows the usual protocols with the exception that care is required ‸ting head injuries. In the absence of head injuries, oral or intra- ‸ation may be useful. Entonox has the advantage of being rapidly ‸rwards, so the patient can go home. It is particularly useful in ‸nt of dislocated condyles.

Bleeding from the mouth

Most cases need only simple reassurance and getting the patient to bite
firmly on a clean handkerchief over the wound for at least 20 min. In th~
vast majority of cases, bleeding settles with no further actio~
other than care of the airway, if necessary using gentl~
persists, rinse the mouth out to clear any cl~
site. This can be dealt with by furth~
surgicel. Other measures ~
acid. Patients ra~

If all ~

Local anaesthesia (LA)

Case selection is very important. Child~
a patient for local anaesthesia. Similarly, confus~
and it is potentially to anaesthetize. Surprising, pat~
case of accidental to anaesthetist. Surprising, pa~
also be difficult to anaesthetize, with careful explanation, pa~
incidences where, with careful explanation, can be obtained in those patien~
local anaesthesia can be obtained in those patien~
ered unlikely.

Surgery under local anaesthesia carries a num~
minor treatment can be dealt with quicker and disc~
patients may be offered there and th~
it avoids admission for general anaesthes~
risks and side-effects of general anaesthesia t~
many patients prefer local anaesthesia to~
it is more cost-effective than admission a~

Local anaesthesia can be very useful in th~
blocks (inferior alveolar, infra-orbital, ~
can be used as a diagnostic test for trige~
pain thought to be primarily due~
sultant pain

⑦ Local anaesthesia—general considerations

The ability to produce effective local anaesthesia (LA) in the head and neck, including the oral cavity, is a useful skill allowing out-patient care. It also means that patients with head injuries can have other injuries treated and still be observed. When necessary, local anaesthesia can be supplemented with sedation administered orally, intravenously, or by inhalation. This is particularly useful in anxious patients or in children. However, it be appreciated that sedation by itself is not a substitute for good anaesthetic technique.

With experience and a good technique, anaesthesia almost anywhere in the scalp, and oral cavity can be obtained. **Nerve blocks** placed where large nerve trunks emerge into accessible sites (e.g. infe-

Commonly used techniques include:

- **Inferior alveolar (inferior dental) nerve block**—this is the method of choice for all mandibular teeth, although the more anterior ones are usually supplemented by local infiltration. Local anaesthesia is placed around the inferior alveolar nerve as it enters the mandible approximately 1 cm above and behind the wisdom tooth.
- **Lingual nerve block**—the lingual nerve runs in close proximity to the inferior alveolar nerve in the region of the third molar. This is often anaesthetized at the same time as the inferior alveolar nerve producing anaesthesia to the lining of the floor of the mouth and the tongue on the same side.
- **Mental nerve block**—the mental nerve is a continuation of the inferior alveolar nerve as it leaves the mandible in the region of the first and second premolars and enters the lip. Bilateral blocks can anaesthetize the entire lower lip.
- **Nasopalatine block**—anaesthesia to the palatal aspects of the upper anterior teeth can be obtained by injecting local anaesthetic in the incisive papilla. This is however extremely painful to give.
- **Infra-orbital nerve block**—the infra-orbital nerve emerges through the cheek bone about 1 cm below the orbital rim, in line with the pupil. This can be infiltrated either directly through the overlying skin or by passing the need intra-orally, which tends to be less painful.
- Other named blocks include **trigeminal nerve block, long buccal block, sublingual nerve block, posterior, superior alveolar nerve block,** and **intra-ligamentary analgesia** (for individual teeth).

⑦ Complications of local anaesthesia

- **Incorrect placement.** Injection of local anaesthetic within the parotid fascia (e.g. when attempting to anaesthetize upper third molars), can result in temporary facial weakness. Although quite alarming, no permanent damage occurs and the patient should make a full recovery. An eye patch may be required until normal eyelid closure returns.
- **Muscle injury** (e.g. medial pterygoid during inferior alveolar nerve injection) may result in painful muscle spasm (trismus). This usually resolves spontaneously.
- **Adjacent vascular structures** may be injured, resulting in local haematoma. This may be seen following inferior alveolar nerve injection as the corresponding artery runs close by. Bleeding results in trismus.
- **Toxic symptoms.** Local anaesthetic may be injected directly into the circulation. This may lead to rapid onset of toxic symptoms, which can result in collapse and cardiorespiratory arrest. Rapid injection into tissues by itself may also lead to toxicity.
- **Infected tissues.** Local anaesthetic should not be injected into inflamed or infected tissues. The hyperdynamic circulation locally may lead to rapid absorption of the anaesthetic. In addition, the acid environment associated with infection, reduces the effectiveness of anaesthesia.
- **Hypersensitivity-type** reactions can occur with some anaesthetics.
- **Needle track infection** is extremely rare.
- **Post-injection problems**. It is important to tell the patient to avoid smoking, drinking hot liquids, or biting the lip or cheek until sensation is fully returned.

Infections

⚠ Sinusitis

Sinusitis may present in many ways. **It may be confused with atypical facial pain, dental infections, orbital infections, osteomyelitis, or a tumour**. The majority of infections are related to an initial rhinitis, but some can arise secondarily to dental infections. Untreated sinusitis can spread to involve all four sinuses (maxillary, ethmoid, frontal, and sphenoid)—pansinusitis. This is a **potentially life- and sight-threatening condition**.

Sinusitis often arises following an upper respiratory tract infection. Blockage of the ostia, paralysis of the cilia, and stagnation of secretions predisposes to superadded infection. Any sinus can be affected, but the maxillary and ethmoids are the more common.

Acute maxillary sinusitis

This is commonly caused by viral infections, although upper respiratory commensuals (pneumococci, staphylococci, streptococci, and anaerobes) can infect secondarily. There is often predisposing obstruction to the opening of the middle meatus, draining the sinus, which results in stagnation and then infection. Clinically there is:

- systemic upset;
- severe pain, worse on bending;
- swelling over the cheek;
- numbness of the cheek;
- mobile upper teeth, which are tender to percussion (in severe cases);
- radiographically there may be a radiopacity of the involved sinus on an occipitomental view;
- **closure of the eyelids from swelling should be taken seriously**—the eye should be assessed and the patient often needs to be admitted.

Recurrent sinusitis is sometimes associated with an underlying dental infection.

Chronic maxillary sinusitis

An underlying cause should be considered (cystic fibrosis or Kartagener's syndrome). Symptoms are similar to the acute infection but much less in severity. CT and MRI scans are useful diagnostic tests, although a high percentage of asymptomatic people have similar radiological findings. Diagnosis and treatment is therefore on clinical grounds.

Acute frontal sinusitis

This is potentially serious due to the risk of intra-cranial infection. Patients complain of frontal headache, which is tender to percussion. Untreated, the infection can spread intra-cranially or involve the orbit.

Acute ethmoid sinusitis

This usually occurs in association with other sinus infections. Patients complain of deep-seated pain and throbbing. The medial orbital walls are very thin, so orbital cellulitis can rapidly develop.

Treatment of sinusitis

Antibiotics and, in some cases, sinus washout with opening of the middle meatus, using functional endoscopic sinus surgery. Ephedrine nasal drops and menthol inhalations may help reduce congestion and improve sinus drainage.

Fungal sinusitis

The most common fungus is aspergillus. Mucosporidium can also infect the sinuses. This may occur in otherwise healthy individuals; however, look for underlying causes of immunosupression. It is seen as an opacity on X-ray or CT. A Caldwell–Luc antrostomy with clearing of the sinus may be required.

ⓘ The swollen face—general considerations

This is usually due to a localized or spreading bacterial infection in the fascial spaces of the head and neck. **Most often the underlying cause is a dental infection**. However, be thorough and exclude all other possible causes. **Untreated, these can rapidly progress and become life-threatening**.

Pathways of spread from the teeth

Spread of infection depends on the local anatomy, particularly which tooth the infection originates in, and in which jaw. Virulence of the organism and host resistance are also important factors.

The face has a very rich blood supply from branches of both the external and internal carotid arteries. This helps in resistance to infection. Whereas an open fracture of the tibia or femur runs a high risk of osteomyelitis, fractures of the mandible do not. The maxilla is even more resistant, as its relative blood supply is even richer. However, **the rich venous drainage of the face communicates with the cavernous sinus, potentially draining infections intra-cranially**. These veins are often valveless, allowing infection to pass in a retrograde direction. The communications are mostly around the orbit, the most important being between the angular veins on the face and ophthalmic veins. These then pass through the orbit into the cavernous sinus. **Infected emboli can therefore lead to cavernous sinus thrombosis with intra-cranial abscesses**.

Lymph nodes

These are arranged in recognized patterns, thus partly determining the spread of infection. Involvement of a specific group may therefore give a hint to the source of the infection. These include:

- buccal or facial
- parotid
- occipital
- submental
- submandibular
- jugulodiagastric
- supra-omohyoid
- infra-omohyoid
- posterior triangle.

The jugulodiagastric, supra-omohyoid, and infra-omohyoid groups lie in a chain alongside the jugular vein, beneath the sternocleidomastoid muscle.

Swelling of the upper lip and canine fossa

This is usually dental in origin, arising from the upper incisor and canine teeth. The differential diagnosis includes trauma, allergic reactions, and infected radicular and nasopalatine cysts. Check the vitality of the teeth and, if possible, obtain dental X-rays of them. Non-dental causes of swelling may be secondary to skin infections, e.g. carbuncle. If bilateral consider an allergic reaction. Also remember sinusitis and nasolacrimal dacrocystitis.

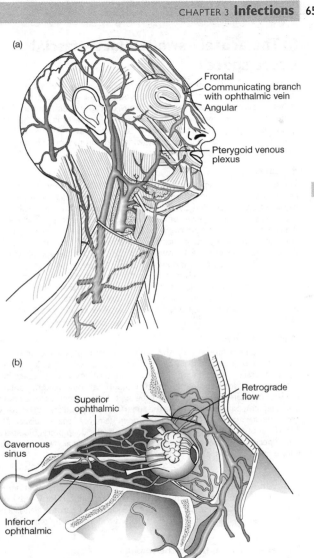

(a)

Frontal
Communicating branch
with ophthalmic vein
Angular

Pterygoid venous
plexus

(b)

Retrograde
flow

Superior
ophthalmic

Cavernous
sinus

Inferior
ophthalmic

Fig. 3.1 (a) and (b) Veins drain into the neck and intra-cranially—infection can therefore spread to the cavernous sinus.

⑦ The acutely swollen face—fascial tissue spaces

Fascial tissue 'spaces' in the head and neck, as elsewhere, are not real spaces. They are *potential* spaces between fibrous and muscular tissue planes that can fill up with serous fluid, pus, blood, or even tumour. These planes open up relatively easily by blunt dissection. Bacteria can therefore spread quickly by lysis of the friable connective tissue between them. The 'spaces' are interconnected, allowing infection to spread widely, but are divided for description, as follows.

Buccal space

This is the most commonly affected space and often presents to casualty as a 'fat face'. Infections can spread into it from the mandibular and maxillary teeth. It is bounded by the buccinator muscle anteromedially, and the masseter muscle posteromedially. Laterally is the deep fascia from the parotid capsule and the overlying platysma. The inferior boundry is the insertion of the deep fascia into the mandible, and its superior boundry the zygomatic process of the maxilla. Its contents are the buccal fat pad, a syssarcosis. Posteriorly it is continuous with the pterygoid space.

Surgical access is usually obtained low inside the cheek. Following a mucosal incision, a sinus forcep should be passed through the buccinator. A drain should be placed. The offending tooth extracted. If the abscess points onto the skin, an incision can be made externally, but a scar will result.

Masticator space

This is bounded laterally by the temporalis facia, zygomatic arch, and masseter muscle, and medially by the medial and lateral pterygoid muscles. The temporalis muscle and mandibular ramus further divide the space into superficial and deep compartments. The superficial compartment contains the submasseteric space below and the superficial temporal space above. The deep compartment contains the superficial pterygoid space (or pterygomandibular space) below and the deep temporal space above. The superficial pterygoid space communicates with the deep pterygoid space. The superficial and deep temporal spaces together are also known as the infratemporal fossa space.

Parotid space

This contains the parotid gland, the parotid lymph nodes, the facial nerve, the external carotid artery, and retromandibular vein. It is formed by the splitting of the deep cervical fascia, to enclose the parotid gland. The fascial covering is generally thin, but thickens to form the stylomandibular ligament.

Fascial spaces related to the maxilla

Upper lip

Cellulitis and pus can create severe swelling of the upper lip, usually deep to orbicularis oris, pointing in the vestibule. It is usually secondary to periapical infections of the incisors.

Canine fossa

This is bounded by the muscles of facial expression around orbicularis oris (levator labii superioris, levator anguli oris, zygomaticus minor and major) and the overlying skin. Infections usually originate from the canine or first premolar teeth. Depending on the length of their roots and their inclination, infections can spread either between these muscles, or it can track to the buccal vestibule within the mouth. Potentially infection can spread superiorly and via the ophthalmic veins intra-cranially (see Cavernous sinus thrombosis).

⑦ Clinical features of fascial space infections and indicators of severity

Symptoms and signs depend on the severity of the infection. This is determined by the health of the patient, the virulence of the micro-organism, antibiotic sensitivity, and the fascial space or spaces involved.

Patients usually present because of a localized or, more commonly, diffuse **swelling** on the face or neck. There is also usually **pain, redness, and warmth** over the swollen area—making four of the five cardinal signs of inflammation. **Pyrexia, tachycardia and generalized malaise** are often present.

There may be **loss of ability to swallow, with drooling, or difficulty breathing and stridor (inspiratory wheeze)**. The latter signs are indicative of a life-threatening airway emergency. Collectively these later signs demonstrate a loss of function, which is the fifth of the cardinal signs of inflammation.

Untreated, these infections may lead to generalized bacteraemia and septicaemia. The latter can lead to septic shock, multi-organ failure and death, if the patient is not resuscitated.

Usually the **full blood count** will show an increased white cell count (leucocytosis). When there is a relatively normal lymphocyte count, but increased neutrophil count, this suggests acute infection. If there has been a chronic abscess, for example, secondary to tuberculosis, you may find an increased lymphocyte count but a normal neutrphil count. Both may occur.

Blood cultures and a raised **ESR** may indicate the presence of bacteraemia or septicaemia.

If the patient is very ill and dehydrated secondary to an inability to swallow fluids, the **haematocrit** will be raised. If dehydrated enough, the **urea and creatinin** will be elevated indicating pre-renal failure.

Never forget to take a random serum glucose sample—the patient may be an undiagnosed diabetic.

⑦ Basic principles in the management of fascial space infections

Treatment depends on the extent of the infection, its location, the patient's general health, and the response to previous treatments. Presentation varies from the ambulant patient with mild cellulitis, to the severely ill, toxic, and bed-bound individual who may have a threatened airway. Judgement and experience are needed as how to proceed with the scenarios between these two extremes.

Your treatment will work out logically if you keep the following principles in mind:

- If in doubt refer or admit.
- Screen for diabetes (RBS) and immunosuppresion (WCC).
- **Never underestimate** a fascial space infection. In fact, never call it a 'dental abscess' as this terminology will put you, the anaesthetist, and theatre staff in the wrong state of mind and a lower gear of alertness. It is a 'fascial or cervical space infection'.
- Do not underestimate the rapidity with which these infections can come to threaten the airway. If you suspect the airway may potentially be threatened, do not 'wait and see' by treating with antibiotics. Electively secure the airway with endotracheal intubation and drain the abscess.
- Never treat a fascial space infection of an identifiable cause with antibiotics alone, try to remove the cause.
- If a collection has formed, it will never resolve with antibiotics alone, but requires incision and drainage. The space containing it must be incised and drained, with appropriate drains left *in situ*.

Indicators of advanced infection and admission include:
- **trismus**
- **difficulty swallowing**
- **difficulty talking**
- **inability to protrude the tongue**
- **swollen eyelids**
- **gross swelling**
- **systemic upset**.

Trismus
This is an important sign and should always be taken seriously, especially in infections. Trismus is limitation in mouth opening due to muscle spasm. Most commonly, the spasm is in the masseter muscle, but it can occur in the medial pterygoid or temporalis muscles instead. It is a marker indicating that the infection is aggressive and is often taken as a sign that the patient needs admission. Untreated it will progress, eventually resulting in dysphagia and potential airway problems. Anaethetists need to be aware of this if the patient is going to theatre, as often skilled **fibre optic intubation** is required.

Trismus in the absence of an infection may be the presenting sign of an underlying tumour—take it seriously.

☼ The acutely swollen neck

Ludwig's angina

This is a rapidly spreading, tense cellulitis of the submandibular, sublingual, and submental spaces bilaterally. When advanced it is an obvious diagnosis with gross swelling both in the neck and the mouth. Earlier infections still need to be treated seriously and often need admission. **Ludwig's angina is a potential airway emergency, which if not diagnosed and treated quickly has a mortality rate of around 75% within the first 12–24 h**. With aggressive surgical intervention, good airway control, and antibiotics, this has now dropped to 5%.

Usually the cause is a submandibular space infection secondary to an infected wisdom tooth. Other causes are infected mandibular fractures and submandibular sialadenitis. From the submandibular space, the infection spreads to the ipsilateral sublingual space around the deep lobe of the submandibular gland. It then passes to the contralateral sublingual space and thence to the adjacent submandibular space. The submental space is affected by lymphatic spread. Infection can also originate in the sublingual space. Left untreated, oedema and cellulitis spread backwards in the space between the hypoglossus and genioglossus to the epiglottis and larynx, resulting in **respiratory obstruction**.

Clinical features
- Systemic upset.
- Massive firm swelling bilaterally in the neck.
- Swelling in the floor of the mouth, forcing of the tongue up onto the palate.
- Difficulty in swallowing, talking and eventually breathing.
- Inability to protrude the tongue.

Management
The first consideration is the airway, which can rapidly obstruct. **Difficulty in swallowing and talking, and gross swelling are all indications to call an anaethetist urgently**. Refer to maxillofacial team urgently. Further management includes IV fluids (patients often present after a few days and have not been able to drink), IV antibiotics (e.g. penicillin and metronidazole), together with surgical drainage of the submandibular and sublingual spaces and removal of the underlying cause.

Peritonsillar abscesses (Quinsy)

These are common infections arising when infection of the tonsil spreads to the surrounding tissue. Initially there is tonsillitis (sore throat, fever, and malaise), which progresses to a **unilateral, asymmetric bulge in the palate, with displacement of the uvula to the opposite side**. Often they can be drained in casualty but if they threaten the airway GA is required. Tonsillectomy is generally not indicated for a single peritonsillar abscess, but recommended if it recurs.

Necrotizing fasciitis

This is a rare but potentially life-threatening mixed infection, characterized by necrosis of the fascia and subcutaneous tissues Untreated the condition can spread rapidly with a mortality approaching 40%. Although it is more commonly seen in the groin, it can occur in the neck where it is nearly always due to an underlying dental infection. Patients often have an underlying predisposition such as diabetes, alcoholism, or chronic malnutrition.

Clinically, the overlying skin is often pale and mottled or may appear dusky due to thrombosis of underlying vessels. Blisters and ulceration may develop. Complications include:

- systemic toxicity
- lung abscess
- carotid artery erosion
- jugular vein thrombosis and mediastinitis.

Treatment involves intravenous antibiotics, wide surgical debridement, and hyperbaric oxygen. Any underlying predisposition must be managed as well.

☼ Deep-neck infections

These usually arise following penetrating injuries, untreated tonsillitis, or wisdom tooth infections. Once established the infection can rapidly spread throughout the neck, into the chest, and become life-threatening. When this occurs, mortality is high. In the early stages diagnosis can be difficult.

Signs and symptoms

Fever, malaise, and lethargy are common and patients rapidly become very ill. A **very high WCC (>20)** is an ominous sign and often indicates tissue necrosis and likely mortality. **Pain on swallowing** should be taken seriously, which can be so severe that the patient sits, drooling, and unable to swallow their own saliva. There may be **cellulitis**, but because of the overlying fascial planes, *deep* abscesses do *not* fluctuate. Instead **swelling** presents with a 'dough-like' consistency. Initially the fascia may direct swelling medially, compromising the airway. Other signs of symptoms of deep-neck infections include **dysphagia and trismus**.

Untreated, if **airway obstruction** or sepsis does not kill the patient, erosion into the carotid vessels can result in **septic emboli** and CVA.

Indicators of severe infection include:
- difficulty breathing
- shock
- pyrexia
- malaise
- dyspahagia/drooling
- trismus
- dysphonia
- inability to protrude the tongue
- high WCC.

Management

Assess for airway obstruction and where necessary consider intubation or a surgical airway. Once secure assess the patient's hemodynamic status and give fluids. Often they have sat at home for a few days unable to eat and drink, so will probably be **at least mildly dehydrated**. These patients need to be admitted. **Consider immunosupression** (diabetes, alcoholics, long term steroids, HIV, etc.).

CT or MRI of the neck and chest is usually required to determine the extent of infection, notably into the mediastinum. **Aggressive surgical drainage** and removal of dead tissue is usually required, even if there is only cellulitis. By opening tissue planes not only is pus released but tissue perfusion is improved by reducing tension. The surgical approach depends on the location of the abscess. Some can be drained intra-orally, eliminating a scar. However, drainage via a neck incision is more common, allowing identification of the great vessels and placement of large drains.

There is some evidence that **hyperbaric oxygen** may be beneficial, but this is a controversial issue. Only in very mild cases can patients be managed conservatively, if so they must be watched very closely. In selected cases ultrasound guided aspiration may avoid aggressive surgery.

Antibiotics

Since many infections originate as dental, pharyngeal, or tonsillar infections, coverage should include organisms known to affect these areas. Most infections will be mixed and will include Gram-positive cocci and anaerobes.

⊙ Infections of the parotid glands

Acute parotid sialadenitis

Mumps is the commonest cause of parotid swelling, even unilaterally. It has a peak incidence in childhood, but can occur in adults. In teenagers, coxsackie and echoviruses can cause acute sialadenitis. Clinically there is pyrexia and malaise. Pain is the most striking symptom. There is diffuse swelling of the gland and often trismus. Treatment is supportive.

Acute suppurative parotid sialadenitis

This is the result of salivary stasis either form duct obstruction (calculus or stenosis), glandular disease (sjogrens, chronic sialadenitis), or a decrease in saliva production. Major predisposing factors are dehydration, the infirm or elderly, and poor oral hygiene. It was more prevalent in the past in old, debilitated, and dehydrated hospitalized patients. The chief agent is *Staphylococcus aureus*. Treatment is rehydration of the patient, encourage salivary flow (lemon drops), gland massage, and antibiotics (e.g. rifampicin or clindamycin). If an abscess occurs, it will need surgical draining.

Chronic recurrent sialadenitis

This is an incompletely understood entity. It is characterized by recurrent unilateral or bilateral diffuse swelling of the parotids in children and adults. Some go on to develop sjogrens.
- The sialogram is useful, showing sialectasis.
- Treatment is conservative monitoring, troublesome glands may be removed.

HIV salivary gland disease

This clinically resembles Sjogrens in that it is bilateral diffuse enlargement of both glands. It has characteristic multi-centric cystic appearances. Positive HIV serology will confirm the diagnosis.

ⓘ **Infections of the submandibular glands**

Acute submandibular sialadenitis

The majority of infections are secondary to a calculus in the duct. Other causes include surgical scarring or strictures secondary to radiation. The whole gland swells up and there is malaise, pyrexia, and pain. Submandibular calculi are opaque in 80% of cases, so a radiograph may aid in the diagnosis. Antibiotics are required. If the stone is easily felt in the mouth it can be removed intra-orally. If the infection leads to a collection, then incision and drainage of the submandibular space must be carried out, and the gland removed electively later.

Chronic submandibular sialadenitis (Kuttner's tumour)

This results from repeated episodes of acute sialadenitis. The structure, parenchyma, and function of the gland are gradually destroyed. The gland ends up feeling very hard to palpation. Treatment is by surgical excision.

ⓘ Mastoiditis

Mastoiditis is an extra-cranial complication of aggressive or untreated acute otitis media, where the infection passes to the mastoid air cells causing further suppuration and bone necrosis. It should be remembered that an infection that can track to the mastoids might also travel elsewhere—always consider other possible complications of acute otitis media with your diagnosis.

- Intra-cranial (meningitis, brain abscess, extra and subdural abscess, lateral sinus thrombosis).
- Extra-cranial (labyrinthitis, facial nerve paralysis, mastoiditis).

Presentation

Patients complain of a **persistent and throbbing pain with increasing deafness**. A discharge (otorrhoea) is present, which is usually creamy and may be profuse. Clinical signs include:

- systemic upset: unwell/pyrexia/tachycardia;
- tenderness over the mastoid prominence often with a post auricular swelling that pushes the pinna forwards.

Investigation

- **Otoscopy:** may show bulging of the roof or posterior wall of the external auditory canal. The tympanic membrane is usually red, perforated and discharging.
- **Full blood count:** will show a raised white cell count (neutrophils).
- **Mastoid XRs:** will show opacity of the air cells.
- **CT scans** will give far more information but are not always indicated.

Treatment

First line of treatment is admission to hospital for intra-venous antibiotics, fluid resuscitation, control of pyrexia, and analgesia. If the causative organism is unknown, then broad-spectrum antibiotics are given, e.g. amoxicillin and metronidazole. In the absence of a rapid or complete response to antibiotics, or if a subperiosteal abscess develops, surgery is indicated. Cortical mastoidectomy is performed, the objective being to drain the mastoid air cells and remove any necrotic debris, while leaving the middle ear intact.

⊙ Otitis media

Inflammation of the middle ear (otitis media) is a common condition, usually occurring bilaterally, which may be acute or chronic. Acute otitis media is commonly seen in children, often following an upper respiratory tract infection. It may be viral or bacterial in origin. *Streptococcus pneumoniae* and *Haemophilus influenzae* are common bacterial pathogens.

Acute otitis media (AOM)

AOM begins with mucosal inflammation and oedema, resulting in exudates in the middle ear. Oedema prevents drainage of the Eustachian tube and, as pus accumulates, pressure builds up. This causes the eardrum to bulge. Untreated, necrosis occurs, and the tympanic membrane eventually perforates. As the middle ear can now drain, the infection will slowly resolve.

Presentation

Patients complain of a throbbing earache (otalgia), which progresses in intensity until perforation of the drum relieves some of the pressure. A conductive deafness is present, possibly with tinnitus. Patients are often systemically unwell. The tympanic membrane ranges in appearance from the loss of the light reflex, to red and bulging, culminating in perforation with discharge (otorrhoea). **Deafness in children is a treatable cause of developmental delay—early detection and appropriate investigation and treatment is therefore imperative**.

Management

- **Antibiotics**—penicillins are often the first line of treatment, but culture and sensitivities of known pathogens may alter this.
- **Analgesics/antipyretics**—paracetamol, NSAIDs.
- If a bulging tympanic membrane persists, despite adequate antibiotic therapy, **myringotomy** under general anaesthetic enables the ear to drain.
- Patients who present with a discharging ear (perforation) should be started on broad-spectrum antibiotics after microbiology swabs have been sent for culture and sensitivities.
- If signs and symptoms do not resolve, consider altering the choice of antibiotic and consider infection elsewhere (mastoid, nasopharynx, sinuses).

Otitis media with effusion (OME): 'glue ear'

This condition is said to affect 30–40 % of children at some stage in their development, and presents with deafness and a mild otalgia, occasionally associated with tinnitus. OME is due to a build-up of fluid in the middle ear and, although many cases will spontaneously resolve, a short course of antibiotics may prove useful if there is suspicion of underlying infection.

If pain or hearing loss persists for over 10 weeks, surgery should be considered:

- **Myringotomy and grommet insertion**. Under GA, a small incision is made in the tympanic membrane and a plastic grommet (drainage tube) is inserted. These often self-extrude after an average period of 6 months—repeated insertions may be necessary if the effusion persists.
- **Adenoidectomy** may be beneficial in the long-term treatment of 'glue ear'.

☼ Intra-cranial infections

Meningitis

Patients with meningitis can deteriorate extremely rapidly, so immediate attention is necessary. Consider it in any irritable child with a rash.

Meningitis is inflammation of the linings of the brain and spinal cord (the meninges) with infection of the cerebrospinal fluid (CSF). Most frequently the pathogen is viral and may vary with age and social environment. Bacterial pathogens include:

- Neonatal:
  - *Streptococcus* (group B)
  - *Escheria coli*
  - *Listeria monocytogenes*.
- Children (<14):
  - *Neisseria meningitidis*
  - *Strep. Pneumoniae*
  - *Haemophillus influenzae*.
- Adults:
  - *Neisseria meningitidis*
  - *Strep. Pneumoniae*.

Bacterial meningitis may arise in a variety of clinical settings:

- spontaneous;
- post traumatic especially skull fractures;
- post-surgical;
- device associated, e.g. CSF shunts for hydrocephalus.

Spontaneous meningitis may be difficult to diagnose, as initially the prodrome state is indistinguishable from many viral infections—malaise, lethargy, fever, anorexia. Usually within 24 h (or often more rapidly) sinister signs develop.

Clinical features

- Pyrexia.
- Tachycardia/tachypnoea/shock.
- Headache.
- Photophobia.
- Irritability.
- Fits.
- Vomiting.
- Neck stiffness.
- +ve Kernig's sign (a strong sign of meningeal irritation)—pain occurs with attempts at passive knee extension with the hips fully flexed.
- Maculo-papular rash (meningococcal meningitis).
- Deteriorating conscious level in late cases.

Focal neurology and epileptic fits are usually absent. The diagnosis might be difficult in young children, where irritability and lethargy might be the initial presenting features.

Management

- Resuscitation, IV fluids.
- Antibiotics should be given as soon as the diagnosis is suspected and continued until the CSF white cell count is normal. Discuss choice with microbiologist/neurologist.

- Blood cultures.
- CT scan to determine safety of LP and rule out other pathology.
- LP for CSF analysis.
- Contact Tracing (Public Health Department)—for single cases treat close contacts only ('kissing contacts'). Usual regimes: rifampicin 600 mg twice daily for 2 days (adult dose), ciprofloxacin 500 mg single dose.

Subdural empyema

Most cases of subdural empyema are secondary to sinusitis or middle ear infection. Patients initially present with an illness similar to meningitis, but usually develop a hemiparesis due to cortical venous thrombosis. Fitting is also common and might be refractory to treatment.

Management

This should follow the same pathway as for meningitis, but an **LP should never be performed** due to the risk of coning.

A **CT scan** will usually show a thin subdural collection, and pus often accumulates along the falx. The size of the collections is much less than with chronic subdural haematomas.

Patients should be resuscitated and referred for prompt neurosurgical drainage of the pus, usually via a craniotomy.

Brain abscess

Sinusitis and middle ear infections are common causes of brain abscesses, by direct spread. Haematogenous infection can also occur. Well-recognized causes include infective endocarditis and dental caries. In some cases the cause is never determined.

Clinical features

- Headache.
- Vomiting.
- Focal neurology.
- Epileptic fits.
- Deteriorating conscious level in late cases.
- Pyrexia is often absent. If present it is more likely to be due to the causative infection.

Investigations

The **white cell count is often normal** as the brain is outside the lymphatic system.

CT scans show an enhancing ring lesion with surrounding oedema. In contrast to gliomas, abscesses are usually perfectly circular with a wall of uniform thickness. Abscesses may be multiple. An **LP should never be performed** due to the risk of coning.

The diagnosis is usually suspected on the basis of an enhancing circular lesion on a CT scan of a patient with an infection known the cause brain abscesses.

Patients should be referred for prompt neurosurgical drainage. If their consciousness is deteriorating, patients should be fully resuscitated and given steroids and mannitol prior to transfer.

⑦ Oral infections presenting as white and red lesions

This largely refers to candidiasis, a fungal infection. The most common species is *Candida albicans*. It is an oral commensual, present in around 90% of the population, which becomes pathogenic during prolonged use of antibiotics. Immonosupression, diabetes mellitus, pregnancy, steroid use, denture use, xerostomia, and radiotherapy, also predispose to infection. **HIV** presents in a form, that has the characteristics of both acute and chronic candidiasis.

Oral manifestations are divided as follows.

Acute candidiasis
- **Pseudomembranous:** also known as thrush. Painless creamy soft plaques can be wiped away leaving behind an erythematous, ulcerated surface.
- **Atrophic:** dekeratinization of the mucosa, also known as antibiotic glossitis.

Chronic candidiasis
- **Atrophic:** this is seen in patients wearing poorly fitting dentures. There is a prediliction for the underlying palatal mucosa, which appears bright red.
- **Angular cheilitis** is often seen with the atrophic group. This is a mixed infection of candida and skin commensal, which leads to painful cracking at the corners of the mouth. It can be associated with iron deficiency, diabetes and worn dentures.
- **Hyperplastic** often involves the dorsum of the tongue, known as median rhomboid glossitis.

Mucocutaneous candidiasis
- **Localized**. This is a persistant form also affecting the nails and skin. It is often resistant to treatment.
- **Familial** is transmitted as an autosomal dominant and is associated with an endocrinopathy such as Addison's, diabetes mellitus, and hypothyroidism.
- **Syndrome-associated** is very rare, consisting of a triad of candidiasis, myositis, and thymoma. Diagnosis is usually clinical, but a smear or biopsy with PAS will demonstrate the fungus.

Treatment includes removal of the underlying cause and topical antifungals. Persistent chronic and systemic infections require antifungals such as amphoterecin b and ketoconazole, all of which are hepatotxic. **Consider underlying disease in anyone presenting with *Candida*, especially if resistant to infection.**

⊘ Infections presenting as verrucal lesions

- **Condylomata lata** are one of the many expressions of secondary syphilis. It presents as an exophitic papillary lesion in the mouth.
- **Oral warts** are caused by human papilloma virus (HPV). They are found on the lips and any mucosal surface. They consist of cauliflower-like surfaces. Treatment is surgical removal or laser ablation.
- **Condylomata acuminata** are also caused by an HPV subtype, but are normally found in the ano-genital region. Presence in the mouth is increased in HIV infected patients.
- **Focal epithelial hyperplasia** (Heck's disease) is also caused by an HPV subtype. More common in native populations in the Americas. The lesions consist of numerous soft small nodules, are asymptomatic. Affects people of all age groups. No treatment is necessary.

⑦ Sinuses and fistulas

A sinus is an abnormal, blind-ending tract, opening onto an epithelial surface. This does not mean skin only, but includes any epithelial surface, including mucosa (mouth, pharynx, anus, rectum, vagina, etc.), intestinal epithelium, bronchial epithelium, bladder epithelium, and so on. Contrast this to a fistula, which is an abnormal communication between two epithelial surfaces.

When an abscess is left long enough, it enlarges throughout the path of least resistance, usually the connective tissue fascial planes. Eventually it will erode through mucosa to drain intra-orally, or outwards to form a sinus through the skin. Any untreated abscess may result in a discharging sinus.

Therefore a sinus tract may be the result of:
- a dental abscess;
- a chronically infected dental root;
- chronic osteomyelitis;
- a foreign body in the skin such as a wood splinter;
- an infected osteosynthesis plate;
- a necrotic lymph node;
- an underlying **tumour;**
- a carbuncle;
- congenital cysts.

Clinically a sinus on the skin appears as a small opening, often with adjacent scarring. When the underlying cause is quiescent, it often heals over, but later recurs. There is often a discharge of pus from the sinus, or debris within it, such as sequestrum. A fistula may occur if the abscess drains both intra-orally and onto the skin.

A microbiological swab should be taken from any discharge. If there is no obvious dental or jaw pathology, a sample should be taken to exclude actinomycosis. This is a chronic granulomatous, suppurative and fibrosing disease caused by anaerobic, Gram-positive, filamentous bacteria, the commonest being *Actinomyces israeli*. Clinically, this is classically described as 'sulphur granules' discharging onto the skin, but they are not always present.

The treatment of a sinus is primarily the elimination of the underlying condition, very much like the treatment of an abscess. Incision and drainage without removal of the underlying cause will result in recurrence. The sinus is excised and the tract is dissected out and followed to its point of origin. The underlying pathology is simultaneously removed. If the excision results in a oro-cutaneous communication, this is closed in layers (mucosa, deep tissues, then skin). A specimen for histopathology should always be sent.

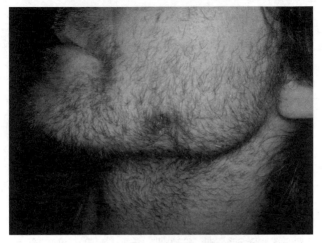

Fig. 3.2 A discharging sinus. Consider infections (especially teeth, skin, and bone) and malignancy.

⑦ 'At risk' patients

This is a group of patients with underlying systemic disease that predisposes them to infections, either opportunistically or following a surgical intervention.

Cardiovascular disease

Infective endocarditis affects principally the heart valves, but any part of the endocardium can be affected. It is normally preceded by damage to the valves.

Patients at risk from infective endocarditis, requiring antibiotic prophylaxis:
- **previous infective endocarditis;**
- **previous rheumatic fever;**
- **damaged heart valves from any other cause;**
- **mitral valve prolapse;**
- **prosthetic heart valves;**
- **congenital heart disease.**

Any pathology that damages the endocardium can potentially predispose to endocarditis. Examples include rheumatoid conditions (systemic lupus erythematosus, ankylosing spondilitis, etc.), Marfan's syndrome, and syphilis.

Procedures requiring antibiotic prophylaxis in 'at risk of endocarditis' patients:
- **tooth extraction and any oral surgery;**
- **periodontal surgery;**
- **scaling;**
- **re-implantation of teeth;**
- **surgical placement of titanium implants;**
- **intra-ligamentary injections.**

Patients NOT requiring antibiotic prophylaxis:
- following coronary artery bypass grafts;
- following myocardial infarction;
- secundum atrial septal defect repaired more than six months previously;
- patent ductus arteriosus that has been repaired more than six months previously;
- if more than six months have passed following heart transplant;
- cardiac pacemakers or defibrillators.

Antimicrobial prophylaxis regime for 'at risk' patients: consult the BNF as the regime sometimes changes from year to year.

Endocrine disease

Diabetes mellitus predisposes to an increased risk of spreading infection. Abscess will more readily spread into adjacent fascial spaces than in a non-diabetic. The pathophysiology behind this is complex, but the core problem is that neutrophil chemotaxis is markedly reduced.

In the elective surgical patient healing is compromised and the possibility of secondary wound infection significantly increased. Glucose

Table 3.1 Antibiotic prophylaxis in cardiovascular disease. (Always check with current guidelines in the BNF.)

Local anaesthesia		General anaesthesia		
No allergy to penicillin	Allergy to penicillin	No special risk	At increased risk*	*
		Not allergic to penicillin	No allergy to penicillin	Penicillin allergy
Amoxycillin orally 3 g	Clindamycin orally 600 mg or teicoplanin 400 mg	Amoxycillin 1 g IM followed by 0.5 g oral 6 h later	Amoxycillin 1 g IM with gentamycin 120 mg IM followed by amoxycillin 0.5 g oral 5 h later	Vancomycin IV 1 g with gentamycin 120 g

* Refers to cases which have had previous infective endocarditis or prosthetic heart valves.

control in these in-patients must be closely monitored, and insulin carefully titrated with a sliding scale. These are now provided on a proforma in most hospitals, but you must understand their basic mechanism, and be especially aware of the effect of insulin and glucose on potassium levels.

Diabetic patients presenting with serious infections tend to loose control of their blood glucose, serum glucose levels shoot up beyond the control of their daily insulin regime. They must immediately be placed on a sliding scale. If left alone, the natural progression will be to a ketoacidotic coma and death.

Suspect diabetes and check the random serum glucose level in all patients presenting with oro-facial infections, especially fascial space infections or carbuncles and furuncles.

Renal disease
Chronic renal failure patients are very susceptible to infections. Any sign of an infection should be treated without delay.

Renal transplantations are very susceptible to opportunistic infections due to immunosuppressive drug regimes.

The immunosuppressed patient
These patients are conveniently divided into:
- **Primary**, whereby a genetic or developmental pathology leads to an immunodeficient state. These are rare, and are not discussed.
- **Secondary** to an acquired pathology or from immunosupressant drugs. This is common.

⑦ The acquired immunodeficiencies

Immunosupressive therapy

Patients on a range of drugs, such as corticosteroids, cyclosporin, and anti-cancer drugs or anti-rejection drugs, are at risk. These affect predominantly cell-mediated immune responses. Patients are not only at risk of infections but also tumours, the commonest being lymphoma and Kaposis sarcoma.

The commonest opportunistic infections in immunocompromised patients are

- **Viral:**
  - herpes simplex
  - varicella zoster
  - cytomegalovirus
  - Epstein–Barr virus
  - papilloma virus
  - hepatitis viruses.
- **Bacterial:**
  - *Mycobacteria*, e.g. TB
  - *Pseudomonas*
  - *Klebsiella*
  - *Staphylococci*.
- **Fungal:**
  - *Candida*
  - *Cryptococcus*
  - *Aspergillus*
  - Histoplasma.
- **Parasitic:**
  - *Pneumocystis*
  - *Toxoplasma*.
- **Asplenic patients**. Sepsis is usually from pneumococcal organisms and rarely from oral flora.
- **Leucopenias** secondary to immunosupressants or from leukaemias/lymphomas predispose to opportunistic infections.
- **Chronic debilitating conditions**, such as uraemia (chronic renal failure), diabetes mellitus, malnutrition, underlying cancer, and so on.

HIV and AIDS

Compromise the immune system by infecting the CD4 T-lymphocytes, thereby crippling cell-mediated immunity. This predisposes to the viral, mycobacterial, fungal, and parasitic infections listed above, as well as to neoplasms such as Kaposis sarcoma, lymphomas, and squamous cell carcinomas.

Diagnosis of HIV can often be made clinically from the history and oral examination. The following infections or infective processes are seen in and around the mouth in HIV and AIDS:

- acute and chronic candidiasis;
- cervical lymphadenopathy;
- primary herpes simplex, varicella zoster, cytomegalovirus;

- hairy leucoplakia on the lateral borders of the tongue associated with Epstein–Barr virus (hairy leucoplakia is also seen in other immunosupressed states such as in renal transplants);
- warts from papilloma viruses;
- periodontal disease, such as necrotizing ulcerative gingivostomatitis;
- aphthous-like ulcers;
- salivary gland disease with xerostomia, or salivary gland enlargement (on MRI or CT these appear as multicentric cystic areas in the glands);
- molluscum contagiosum;
- lymphoma;
- Kaposi's sarcoma.

ⓘ Skin and soft tissue infections

Cellulitis

This is a spreading infection in the subcutaneous tissues and skin. The most common cause is *Streptococcus pyogens*. Streptoccocal infection of the skin of the face is called **erysipelas**. Hyaluronidase produced by the organism allows rapid spread. Treatment is with penicillin. Cellulitis of the face is commonly caused by trauma to the skin or from an infected skin appendage (hair follicle, etc.). However, remember that it may also be caused by a fascial space infection of dental origin that tracks to the sub-cutaneous tissues of the face.

Boils or furuncles

These are infections of hair follicles, commonly with *Staphylococcus aureus*. They are mostly found in the face, neck, buttock, and axilla, but can occur in any hair-bearing area of the body. Boils are recurrent and although it is tempting to try flucloxacillin for resistant, recurrent cases, systemic antibiotics do not help and are therefore not indicated.

Treatment is by eradication of the *Staphylococcus aureus* by using antiseptic soaps and naseptin (mupirocin and neomycin) cream to the skin and nose (as in the treatment of methycillin-resistant *Staphylococcus aureus*—MRSA). Those that are large and painful should be incised.

Carbuncles

This is an extensive infection of the hair follicles caused by *Staphylococcus aureus*, involving several adjacent follicles and the subcutaneous tissue. Look for an underlying cause such as diabetes. Flucloxacillin and surgical incision is necessary.

☼ Necrotizing fasciitis (see The acutely swollen neck)

Although this is immediately apparent in the skin (usually of the neck) it arises from a deep focus of infection—the wisdom teeth or tonsils. This is a severe infection that can rapidly spread into the face, undermining the skin itself and resulting in considerable loss of tissue. This is a devastating condition, but fortunately very rare in the head and neck.

Clinically the overlying skin is often pale and mottled or may appear dusky due to thrombosis of underlying vessels. Blisters and ulceration may develop. Complications include:

- systemic toxicity;
- lung abscess;
- carotid artery erosion;
- jugular vein thrombosis and mediastinitis.

Treatment involves intravenous antibiotics, wide surgical debridement, and hyperbaric oxygen. Any underlying predisposition must be managed as well.

Cold sores

These are due to recurrent infections from the herpes simplex virus, usually type 1. The herpes viruses are a large family of viruses. Seven types affect humans and six of the seven affect the head and neck.

- Herpes simplex virus type I causes oral, perioral, and occasionally genital infections.
- Varicella zoster virus causes chickenpox and herpes zoster.
- Epstein–Barr virus has been linked to infectious mononucleosis, burkitt's lymphoma, nasopharangeal carcinoma, and oral 'hairy' leukoplakia.
- Cytomegalovirus is associated with salivary gland pathology and systemic infections in immunocompromised patients.

Herpes simplex virus (HSV) infections

This is a common cause of vesicular eruptions on skin. In healthy individuals it is self-limiting. Two forms occur, the primary (systemic) herpes and secondary (localized) herpes. Spread is by physical contact.

Primary HSV

This is a vesicular eruption of perioral skin, vermillion border, or oral mucosa.

Secondary or recurrent HSV (cold sores)

Prodromal symptoms of pain, burning, and tingling precede multiple small vesicles within hours of eruption. These may develop after a period of 'stress' such as a recent illness. Generally they heal without scarring, but can get secondarily infected. The lesions are infective.

Immunodeficient patients may present with repeated attacks of secondary herpes with a predisposition to bacterial and fungal infections of the vesicles.

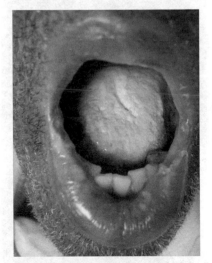

Fig. 3.3 Primary HSV. When severe patients may not be able to swallow and occasionally need admission.

Herpetic whitlow refers to secondary HSV infection of the fingers and was seen classically on clinicians hands, especially dentists, prior to the advent of rubber gloves.

Treatment is usually unnecessary other than analgesia, fluids, and rest. Prompt topical application of 5% acyclovir ointment reduces slightly the duration of infection. Transplant patients benefit from prophylactic systemic acyclovir in reducing secondary HSV infections.

Varicella zoster (VZ) infections

Varicella (chickenpox)

This is the primary infection with the VZ virus. Usually its occurs in childhood. A rash involving the head, neck, and most of the body erupts with fever and general malaise. The rash develops into a general vesicular eruption, which turns into pustules and ulcerates. It is self-limiting. Rarely, and mostly among the very young or the immunosupressed, varicella can be severe progressing to encephalitis, pneumonitis, and death. **Infection during pregnancy leads to fetal abnormalities**.

Herpes zoster (shingles)

This is an acute herpetic infection often in the Vth cranial nerve. It is the secondary manifestation of VZ. This usually affects older age groups.

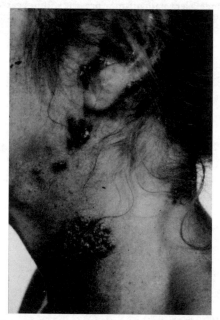

Fig. 3.4 Shingles involving the cervical plexus.

It specifically affects a particular sensory dermatome. Thus on the face it can erupt in the distribution of any of the branches of the trigeminal nerve, or cervical plexus. It is very painful and debilitating with severe complications if it affects the ophthalmic branch. **It has a very high incidence in the immunosupressed**.

Clinical features

Burning, tingling pain with occasional lancinating components felt in the skin. Pain may precede or follow herpetic eruptions and last from one to several weeks.

Ramsay Hunt syndrome

This is VZ involvement of the facial and auditory nerves, in which facial paralysis is accompanied by vesicles in the ipsilateral external ear, tinnitus, deafness, and vertigo. **This can sometimes be confused with Bells palsy** (which may require steroids). To differentiate between the two consider the history and carefully examine for vesicles in the external meatus.

   Treatment is supportive. If immunocompromised, **acyclovir or vidarabine** can be given systemically.

Chapter 4

The head

⑦ The head—basic anatomy and physiology

The scalp

Anatomists describe the SCALP as having five layers: Skin, Subcutaneous tissue, Aponeurosis, Loose areolar tissue and Pericranium. Functionally, it can be considered as two layers:

- a superficial layer from the skin to the galea apponeurotica; and
- a deep layer consisting of the areolar tissue and pericranium.

It is between these layers that the scalp moves. Most scalp lacerations extend the full thickness of the upper layer. The vessels and nerves lie in the subcutaneous tissue (anteriorly—supra-orbital and supratrochlear; laterally—superficial temporal artery and auriculotemporal nerve; posteriorly—posterior auricular artery and occipital artery). The scalp has a rich blood supply and can bleed profusely. In children blood loss can result in shock.

The skull

The skull consists of the calvarium, which contains the brain, and the facial skeleton. The calvarium consists principally of eight bones:

- frontal
- sphenoid (2)
- temporal (2)
- parietal (2)
- occipital bones.

A small part of the ethmoid bone completing the skull base anteriorly.

The skull is thickest over the vertex. It is **thinnest in the temporal region and where it forms the roof of the orbits and nose**. (See for yourself. Get a real skull and hold it up to daylight. This graphically demonstrates how fragile some areas are.) Skull thickness and sinus volume can vary from person to person.

Internally the skull is divided into the anterior, middle, and posterior cranial fossae.

The **anterior cranial fossa** contains the anterior part of the frontal lobe of the brain. It extends back to the lesser wing of the sphenoid bone, and lies above the orbits and nose. The anterior fossa is perforated by the olfactory nerves only (cranial nerve I).

The **middle cranial fossa** is the largest. It is continuous with the anterior fossa above the lesser wing of the sphenoid. It is separated from the posterior fossa by the tentorium cerebelli. The middle fossa is filled by the temporal lobes of the brain and above them contains the remainder of the frontal lobes, the parietal and occiptal lobes. The carotid arteries enter the skull and the cranial nerves II to VI leave the skull via the middle fossa floor.

The **posterior cranial fossa** lies below the tentorium cerebelli. It contains the midbrain, pons, medulla, and cerebellum. The major venous outflow of the brain is through the posterior fossa, where the sigmoid sinus continues as the internal jugular vein. Cranial nerves VII to XII also exit through the posterior fossa. The medulla continues with the spinal cord through the foramen magnum, which is also where the vertebral arteries and spinal root of the accessory nerve enter the skull.

The meninges

The inner surface of the skull is lined by the **dura mater**, which is a tough fibrous membrane ('pachy' or thick meninges). It becomes more firmly attached to the skull with age. The dura is reflected internally to form:
(1) the falx cerebrum, which separates the two cerebral hemispheres;
(2) the tentorium cerebelli, which separates the middle and posterior cranial fossae; and
(3) the falx cerebelli, which separates the two cerebellar hemispheres.

The extradural space, external to the dura, is a potential space only: normally it does not exist.

Large **venous sinuses**, which provide the major venous outflow of the brain, lie within the dura. The superior sagittal sinus and inferior sagittal sinus lie along the upper and lower margins of the falx, respectively. The inferior sagittal sinus continues as the straight sinus, which lies where the falx joins the tentorium. The straight and superior sagittal sinuses join at the confluence of the sinuses, or torcula, which lies internal to the external occipital protruberence. The sinuses continue laterally as the transverse sinuses, which lie in the lateral margin of the tentorium. The anatomical arrangement of the confluence results in most of the blood from the superior sagittal sinus passing to the right transverse sinus and from the straight sinus to the left. The transverse sinuses continue as the sigmoid sinuses, which curve through the posterior fossa to the jugular foramen.

The cavernous sinuses lie alongside the sella tursica (pituitary fossa) and communicate with the sigmoid sinuses via the superior and inferior petrosal sinuses, which lie along the upper and lower borders of the petrous temporal bone. **The cavernous sinuses receive some venous drainage from the face and are thus a route whereby extra-cranial infection can gain access intra-cranially**. The importance of the venous sinuses is that they can bleed profusely if damaged. Particular care need to be taken if they have been potentially damaged, e.g. by depressed fractures.

The **arachnoid mater** lies deep to the dura. It is a flimsy membrane and consists of the parietal layer of the 'lepto' (or thin) meninges. The sub-dural space lies between the dura and arachnoid and is usually empty, although the two membranes are not adherent. The subarachnoid space lies deep to the arachnoid and contains the cerebrospinal fluid (CSF). This helps to support and cushion the brain. At various places, mostly around the base of the brain, the subarachnoid space is very wide and forms the 'basal cisterns'.

The **pia mater** is the visceral layer of the leptomeninges. It is firmly attached to the brain.

Cerebral blood supply

The internal carotid and vertebral arteries supply the brain. The **internal carotid** arteries divide into the anterior and middle cerebral arteries. The anterior cerebral artery supplies the inferior surface of the frontal lobe and the anterior part of the medial surface of the hemisphere, extending a short distance onto the lateral surface. This includes the leg area of the motor cortex. The middle cerebral artery supplies most of the lateral surface of the hemisphere. This includes the trunk, arm and face areas of the motor cortex, speech area (on the dominant side) and auditory cortex.

The two **vertebral arteries** unite to form the basilar artery, which divides into the two posterior cerebral arteries. The latter supplies the inferior surface of the temporal and occipital lobes and the posterior part of the medial surface of the hemisphere, also extending a short distance onto the lateral surface. This includes the visual cortex. The vertebro-basilar system also supplies the cerebellum, and brainstem.

The brain

Each of the cerebral hemispheres is divided into four lobes. The central sulcus separates the frontal lobe from the parietal lobe, the parieto-occipital fissure separates the parietal and occipital lobes, and the Sylvian fissure separates the temporal lobe from the frontal and parietal lobes. The cortical surface is highly convoluted into gyri (the folds) and sulci (the clefts). This increases the area of the cortex, which is where the higher functions are organized.

Cortical functions are crossed, with one hemisphere dealing with the function of the other side of the body. The left hemisphere is dominant for speech in 99% of right-handed individuals (as the right hemisphere is dominant in 1%, dysphasia can occasionally be caused by a right cerebral lesion). There is a 50:50 likelihood of either hemisphere being dominant for speech in left-handed individuals, but right hemisphere dominance is more likely if there is a strong family history of left-handedness.

Localization of cortical functions:

- **Primary motor area**. Pre-central gyrus of frontal lobe (body image inverted with leg area on the medial hemisphere surface). The basal ganglia are also highly important.
- **Primary sensory area**. Post-central gyrus of parietal lobe (body image inverted with leg area on the medial hemisphere surface).
- **Speech motor area**.* (Broca's area) infero-lateral frontal lobe (just above tip of temporal lobe).
- **Speech interpretation area**.* (Wernicke's area) inferior parietal lobe and upper temporal lobe (behind primary sensory area).
- **Visual cortex**. Tip of occipital lobe, especially medial surface.
- **Auditory cortex**. Superior temporal gyrus.
- **Higher intellectual functions**. Tip of frontal lobe (unilateral lesion causes minor deficit only).
- **Emotions**. Inferior frontal lobe, tip of temporal lobe and cingulated gyrus (on medial surface above corpus callosum). Other deep parts of the limbic system are also involved (a series of structures that surround the lateral ventricle, including the hippocampus, amygdala and fornix).
- **Olfactory function**. Infero-medial temporal lobe.

- **Other parietal lobe functions**: (dominant) numeration, calculation; (non-dominant) body image and awareness of external environment.

* Dominant hemisphere only.

The two hemispheres are connected by the commisures, the largest and most important of which is the corpus callosum. Descending white matter tracts from the cortex converge to form the internal capsule en route to the brainstem. The motor fibres are condensed into the posterior limb. **A small lesion here can produce a major deficit**. Ascending sensory fibres (except olfaction) relay in the thalamus, which is lateral to the internal capsule. The other basal ganglia are concerned with motor function, and have complex interconnections.

The hypothalamus is concerned with autonomic function and endocrine control through the pituitary gland.

Cerebellum

The cerebellum is concerned with **balance and coordination**. It consists of two hemispheres and the midline vermis. It is divided into three lobes (anterior, posterior, and flocculonodular lobe), but these divisions are not usually obvious on external inspection.

- Damage to the vermis causes ataxia and unsteadiness on sitting (truncal ataxia).
- Damage to the cerebellar hemispheres causes incoordination on the same side of the lesion.

Brainstem

The midbrain, pons, and medulla contain nuclei for the third to twelfth cranial nerves, together with descending and ascending fibre tracts. The midbrain contains a gaze-control centre. The brainstem **reticular formation** contains centres for the vital functions (wakefulness, pulse and blood pressure control, breathing).

Ventricular system

The two lateral ventricles are C-shaped cavities within the cerebral hemispheres. They connect via the foramen of Monro with the midline, slit-like third ventricle. This, in turn, connects via the cerebral aqueduct with the pyramidal fourth ventricle, between the brainstem and cerebellum. The exit from the fourth ventricle is via the median foramen of Magendie and the lateral foramina of Luschka.

Each of the ventricles contains the frond-like choroid plexus, which produces **CSF**. The total volume of CSF in a normal adult is 150 ml, but only 22 ml are in the ventricles, the rest being in the sub-arachnoid space. CSF production is **450 ml per day** so CSF is replaced three times per day. CSF is absorbed through the arachnoid villi over the cortical surface by a passive, pressure-dependent process. Blood in the CSF can block this process resulting in **raised intra-cranial pressure (ICP).**

⊘ The head—neurological examination

Neurological examination cannot be considered in isolation from the rest of the body. For instance, poor respiratory or cardiac function can impair neurological function by causing cerebral ischaemia (hence you **cannot accurately assess 'D' until 'A, B & C' have been optimized**.) Remember focal neurological dysfunction might be related to lesions elsewhere; e. g. metastases, brain abscesses.

Neurological examination should be carried out as appropriate. The following should be considered:

- **Glasgow coma scale**: orientation, eye opening and verbal response;
- **cranial nerve examination**;
- **limb function**:
  - appearance (deformity, wasting, abnormal movement);
  - muscle tone;
  - power in each muscle group;
  - limb reflexes;
  - sensation (touch, pain, vibration, temperature) in each dermatome;
- **co-ordination:**
  - Rhomberg's test for equilibrium;
  - gait;
- **Higher cerebral functions:**
- language ability: expressive, receptive and nominal **dysphasia**;
- reading ability: **dyslexia**;
- writing ability: **dysgraphia**;
- calculation ability: **dyscalculia**;
- object recognition: **agnosia**;
- ability to perform specific tasks: dressing, geographical (follow route) and constructional (copy drawing) **apraxia**;
- **memory** test: immediate, short-term, long-term, verbal, and visual memory (cannot be tested if confused or dysphasic);
- **reasoning and problem solving ability**;
- **mental state**: degree of anxiety, mood, emotional behaviour, inhibition, speed of thought and response.

Examination of the unconscious patient

Neurological examination is limited in unconscious patients, but the following should be assessed:

- resuscitation status;
- Glasgow coma scale;
- pupil responses;
- eye movements and fundoscopy;
- signs of injury;
- abnormal skin colour (cyanosis, jaundice, rubor in carbon monoxide poisoning);
- needle-stick marks (drug overdose);
- smell of breath (alcohol, ketosis, uraemia, cyanide);
- brainstem reflexes;
- limb tone;
- limb movements (spontaneous, localizing, flexion, extension, or absent);
- limb reflexes and plantar response.

Glasgow coma scale (GCS)

The importance of the GCS, like many investigations, is that it is a 'snapshot' of the patient's condition at the time it was taken. To be of use it must be repeated again and again at suitable intervals. Only this way will it be possible to quickly pick up any improvements or deterioration in the patient's condition.

The GCS was devised as a means of consistently describing the depth of unconsciousness and monitoring any change. It involves assessing three responses:

- eye opening
- motor
- verbal.

Patients should be described according to the three responses, as this gives a clearer indication of their status (e.g. eye opening to speech, disorientated, and localizing pain and not just 'GCS 12').

Progression down the scale indicates a worsening condition and a worsening prognosis. Following trauma, a person who has no eye opening, no motor, and no verbal response (GCS 3) is unlikely to survive (see Table 4.1).

Glasgow coma scale in young children

In young children the modifications shown in Table 4.2 can be used.

Table 4.1 Glasgow coma scale

Eye-opening response	Motor response	Verbal response	Score
	Obeys commands		6
	Localizes pain*	Orientated‡	5
spontaneous	normal flexion	confused	4
To speech	Abnormal flexion	Words only	3
To pain	Extension	Sounds only	2
Nil	Nil	Nil	1

* Must bring hand higher than chin to supra-orbital pain.

‡ Orientated to time, place and person.

Table 4.2 Glasgow coma scale in young children

Eye-opening Response	Motor response	Verbal response	Score
	Spontaneous movement		6
	Localizes pain	Usual vocalization	5
Spontaneous	Normal flexion	Reduced vocalization	4
To speech	Abnormal flexion	Cries only	3
To pain	Extension	Moans only	2
Nil	Nil	Nil	1

When discussing the GCS make it clear which score you are using. The original GCS had a maximum score of 14 not 15. Some units may still use this score, so be clear, especially if you are transferring or receiving a patient elsewhere.

The cranial nerves
See Table 4. 3. Note the following:
- CNIII—gaze deviation and ptosis are only seen in a conscious patient.
- Pupillary inequality can occur in 20% of normal people; both pupils will react to light in this case.
- CNVII—taste is via the nervus intermedius, which joins the trigeminal (CNV3) for distribution to the tongue.
- Weber's test: place tuning fork in centre of forehead. If sound is heard best in deaf ear, deafness is conductive.
- Rinne's test: hold tuning fork by ear until sound inaudible, then move fork to mastoid process. If sound is heard deafness is conductive.

Cranial nerve (brainstem) reflexes
Pupillary reflexes
Afferent II, efferent III parasympathetic: shine a torch into each eye in turn and watch for pupillary constriction. If one eye is blind there will be no response in that pupil (direct reflex) or the opposite pupil (consensual reflex), but the affected pupil will constrict to light in the opposite eye. If there is a III palsy, that pupil will not react to light in either eye, but the opposite pupil reacts to light in both eyes.

Corneal reflex
Afferent V, efferent VII: stroke the cornea with cotton wool and watch for blinking.

Grimace reflex
Afferent V, efferent VII: press on the supra-orbital nerve at the orbital margin and watch for facial grimacing. Any limb or autonomic (pulse rate and blood pressure elevation) responses should also be recorded.

Gag reflex
Afferent IX, efferent X: stimulate the posterior pharynx and watch for gagging.

Oculocephalic and oculovestibular reflexes
Afferent VIII, efferent III, IV, and VI: these are the same reflex pathway stimulated by different methods.

In the **occulocephalic (dolls eyes) reflex** the head is turned briskly to one side; if the reflex is preserved the eyes will turn to the opposite side as if maintaining gaze on the same point. This cannot be tested on conscious patients as voluntary control over gaze predominates.

In the **oculovestibular reflex** ice cold water is irrigated into the external auditory canal, after ensuring it is not blocked by wax or that the ear drum is perforated; if the reflex is preserved nystagmus will develop due to stimulation of the semicircular canals by convection currents. This should not be tested on conscious patients as severe vertigo and vomiting will result.

Table 4.3 The cranial nerves

No	Nerve	Function	Test	Palsy
I	Olfactory	Smell	Various smell bottles (test each nostril separately)	Loss of smell (anosmia)
II	Optic	Vision	Visual activity, visual fields, pupillary responses, fundoscopy	Blind eye, visual field defect or loss of acuity, papilloedema
III	Occulo-motor	Eye movements	Eye movement in all directions, pupillary responses	Ptosis, eye deviated down and outwards, unreactive dilated pupil
IV	Trochlear	Eye movements	Eye movement down when looking medially	Inability to look down when looking medially
V	Trigeminal	Facial sensation Muscles of mastication	Sensation in three trigeminal divisions, corneal reflex, jaw movement	Loss of facial sensation, loss of corneal reflex Jaw weak and deviates to side of lesion of opening, wasting of mastication muscles (chronic)
VI	Abducent	Eye movements	Eye movement laterally	Inability to look laterally
VII	Facial	Facial movements Taste to anterior tongue	Facial movements Sweet, bitter, salt taste	Loss of facial movement UMN: forehead spared substances LMN: forehead affected Loss of taste
VIII	Vestibulo-cochlear	Hearing Equilibrium	Hearing, Weber's and Rinne's tests balance and equilibrium	Deafness nystagmus, loss of equilibrium
IX	Glosso-pharyngeal	Pharyngeal posterior tongue sensation and taste motor to upper pharynx	Pharyngeal sensation, gag reflex	Loss of gag reflex and pharyngeal sensation
X	Vagus	Visceral parasympathetic supply (extensive) Larynx and pharynx motor function	Pharyngeal movement, gag reflex Laryngoscopy	Loss of gag reflex and pharyngeal movement Hoarse voice, vocal cord paralysis
XI	Accessory	Trapezius and sternomastoid motor function	Trapezius and sternomastoid power	Weakness of trapezius and sternomastoid
XII	Hypo-glossal	Tongue movements	Tongue movements	Tongue deviates to side of lesion

UMN = upper motorneurone, LMN = lower motorneurone.

⑦ Head injuries—pathophysiology

The brain is the most sensitive organ in the body to hypoxia and ischaemia. Therefore it is essential to maintain an adequate supply of well oxygenated blood to the injured brain.

Autoregulation maintains a constant supply of blood to the brain between a mean blood pressure (BP) of 50 and 160 mmHg. However, this mechanism is usually **impaired following head injury**. The **cerebral perfusion pressure** (CPP) is the force driving blood through the brain and is normally over 70 mmHg. It is related to the BP and intra-cranial pressure (ICP) by:

$$CPP = BP - ICP.$$

A developing **intra-cranial mass lesion** will initially be compensated for by displacement of venous blood and CSF, so the ICP will not rise. When this compensatory mechanism has been exhausted the ICP will rise and the CPP fall. The **Cushing reflex** then comes into play, increasing the BP to maintain cerebral blood flow. The pulse rate also falls due to a vagal reflex. When this compensatory reflex fails progressive cerebral ischaemia will occur leading to cerebral infarction and brain death. A vicious circle becomes established with hypoxia, hypotension and cell breakdown products, which worsen cerebral oedema, contributing to the deterioration.

Brain herniation

Three types of herniation can occur when a mass lesion develops intra-cranially.

- **Sub-falcine herniation**. One hemisphere is displaced beneath the falx, which is seen as midline shift on a CT scan. This can obstruct the foramen of Monro anteriorly, causing unilateral ventricular dilatation and compress the posterior cerebral artery against the falx posteriorly, causing a posterior cerebral infarct.
- **Trans-tentorial herniation**. The uncus of the medial temporal lobe herniates through the tentorial notch. This compresses the occulomotor nerve (dilatated pupil), and the midbrain.
- **Tonsilar herniation**. The cerebellar tonsils herniate through the foreman magnum causing brainstem compression (coning). This is the ultimate cause of brain death.

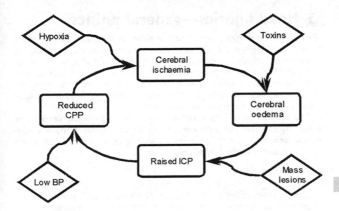

Fig. 4.1 Complex interplay of factors regulating ICP.

☠ Head injuries—general points

'Primary' brain injury occurs **at the time** of the trauma. As clinicians there is nothing we can do about this. Prevention is the only way to reduce this. However, **'secondary' brain injury** occurs after the initial event and is due to complications such as hypoxia, hypercarbia, hypotension, raised intra-cranial pressure (haematomas or cerebral oedema), cerebral herniation of infection. One way or another these all result in either hypoxia or inadequate cerebral perfusion.

The aim of head-injury management is to prevent secondary injury by regular observation and rapid correction if any deterioration occurs. This helps promote a physiological milieu that encourages natural recovery of the primary injury.

Primary brain injury

Primary brain injury can take the form of:

- **Cortical lacerations (burst lobe)** usually results also in an acute subdural haematoma together with a cerebral haematoma and surrounding contusions. The affected brain usually swells markedly. A craniotomy is necessary for evacuation of the subdural and debridement of the damaged brain. The prognosis is usually poor due to the extent of the primary brain damage.
- **Cerebral contusions**. This is discussed under Intra-cranial haematomas
- **Diffuse axonal injury** consists of widespread disruption of axon sheaths due to a high-energy impact. It is particularly associated with a rotational element to the force. **Concussion**, a transient impairment of consciousness following a minor or moderate head injury is probably a mild diffuse axonal injury. The CT scan in diffuse axonal injuries can be normal, but more often shows a tight swollen brain with or without petaechial haemorrhages. The degree of brain swelling usually increases over the 48 h post-injury. The prognosis for diffuse axonal injury is poor.

The commonest causes of head injuries are:

- motor vehicle collisions;
- assaults;
- falls from a height;
- sporting accidents.
  Alcohol is involved in about 30% of head injuries.

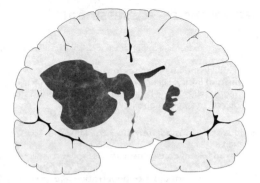

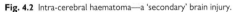

Fig. 4.2 Intra-cerebral haematoma—a 'secondary' brain injury.

① Head injuries—assessment

History
The following are extremely important and should be determined in all cases:
- **Time of injury and any changes in condition.**
- **Mechanism of injury:** suddenly stopping (a deceleration injury) will transfer more energy to the brain than a stationary person struck by a moving object (an acceleration injury):

    $E = \frac{1}{2}mv^2$.

- **Conscious state immediately after the injury**: for baseline observation.
- **Any delayed loss of consciousness**: this implies complications are developing.
- Any suggestion of **compound or penetrating injury:** bleeding from the ears, CSF loss from the nose or ears. Penetrating injuries through the orbit can be easily overlooked.
- Period of **post-traumatic amnesia:** for prognostic reasons.
- **Any ongoing symptoms.**

Examination
- **Resuscitation status**: any deficiency needs immediate correction—before taking a history if necessary.
- **Conscious state**: Glasgow coma scale.
- **Focal neurology**: cranial nerve and limb neurology. Unequal but reactive pupils occur in 20% of normal individuals. A dilated unreactive pupil is usually on the side of a mass lesion (a true localizing sign). The usual sequence is initial pupillary constriction as the III nerve is irritated followed by dilatation as a palsy occurs. A hemiparesis can be caused by a mass lesion pressing on the opposite motor cortex, or a mass on the same side compressing the opposite cerebral peduncle against the edge of the tentorium. **Thus, a hemiparesis does not help in determining the side of a mass lesion and is considered a false localizing sign**.
- Local signs of injury.
- CSF rhinorrhoea or otorrhoea, bleeding from the ear: a compound skull base fracture.
- Battle's sign (bruising over the mastoid process): a fractured petrous bone.
- Panda eyes (well circumscribed peri-orbital bruising): an anterior fossa skull base fracture.
- Scalp lacerations, abrasions, swelling; etc. Consider whether a laceration overlies a fracture.
- Examination for other injuries: this should be repeated when the patient has been stabilized.

Investigations
Plain skull X-rays need not be performed if the patient is to have a CT scan.
Skull X-ray indications:
At the time of writing these are undergoing major review in the UK by the National Institute of Clinical Excellence (NICE).

- any loss of consciousness or amnesia;
- suspected penetrating injury;
- CSF or blood loss from nose or ear;
- significant scalp laceration, bruise, or swelling;
- violent mechanism of injury, including >60 cm fall in a young child;
- persisting headache and/or vomiting.

CT scan indications:
- reduced GCS or neurological signs persisting after resuscitation;
- neurological deterioration in resuscitated patient;
- skull fracture or suture diastasis;
- epileptic fits;
- diagnosis uncertain;
- tense fontanelle in a child.

Head injury classification

Head injuries are classified for management, epidemiological, and research purposes as minor, moderate, and severe, based upon the total GCS score. **When discussing the GCS, make it clear which score you are using. The original GCS had a maximum score of 14 not 15. Some units may still use this score, so be clear, especially if you are transferring or receiving a patient elsewhere.**
- Minor: GCS 13–15.
- Moderate: GCS 9–12 (or 7–8 with eye opening).
- Severe: GCS 8 or less.

:❂: Skull fractures

The main worry in interpreting skull X-rays lies in distinguishing fractures from vascular marks and sutures.

- **Vascular marks** usually run upwards and posteriorly from the skull base and their margins are usually less well-defined (they are due to a cylindrical vessel indenting the bone and so the thickness of the skull overlying them varies across their diameter).
- **Sutures** lie in well-defined locations, but sometimes additional sutural bones might be present. Their margins are highly tortuous.
  Sometimes following a head injury, a suture might become separated (diastasis of a suture) and this should be managed as a fracture.

Linear fractures

These are usually relatively straight with well-defined margins and are usually several centimetres long. The margins of long fractures might be separated by several millimetres. Skull fractures heal slowly and it might not be possible, from its appearance, to determine how old a fracture is, particularly if an individual is prone to multiple head injuries. However, a new fracture will be painful and tender and there will often be a degree of scalp swelling. Fractures of the skull base are difficult to see on plain skull X-rays and should be suspected on the basis of clinical features.

The main significance of linear skull fractures is that they signify an increased risk of developing an intra-cranial haematoma. They are managed the same as a minor head injury without a fracture—observation and basic care. They should be scanned and can be discharged when asymptomatic.

Basal skull fractures

A greater degree of force is required to produce a basal fracture than a vault fracture. They are difficult to see on plain skull X-ray and are usually diagnosed on clinical grounds. They are usually visible on a fine cut CT scan with bone windows.

Basal fractures without a CSF leak are managed similar to vault fractures. CSF otorrhoea usually settles conservatively. CSF rhinorrhoea also frequently settles, but the fistula might re-open with a risk of late meningitis, sometimes years later. Surgical repair should therefore be discussed with the patient, especially if a large defect is seen on a coronal CT scan. Prophylactic antibiotics are not indicated as they have not been shown to prevent meningitis (antibiotics penetrate poorly into CSF in the absence of infection) and they lead to colonisation by resistant organisms.

Depressed fractures

These are usually round with linear fracture lines radiating from the centre, resulting in several fragments. All fractures should be evaluated further by CT scanning. They are usually compound in adults, but can be closed in young children ('ping-pong ball' fracture). Compound fractures should be elevated if they are depressed by an amount greater than the skull thickness. The principal aim of surgery is wound toilet and removal of any foreign bodies to reduce the risk of infection, and so surgery should be performed within 24 h. There is a risk of long-term epilepsy, which increases if there was a dural tear, an intra-cranial haematoma, over 24 h of post-traumatic amnesia and whether there were any early fits. Closed depressed fractures can be left alone unless they are in a cosmetic area or a significant depression is associated with a neurological deficit, although abnormal neurology is very rare in depressed fractures.

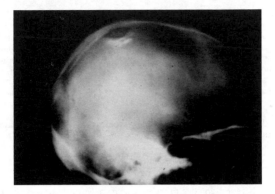

Fig. 4.3 Depressed skull fracture.

☠ Intra-cranial haematomas

The risk of developing an intra-cranial haematoma had been determined with relationship to the orientation of the patient and the presence of a skull fracture (see Table 4. 4). One of several different types of haematoma might develop.

① Concussion

This is a temporary disturbance in brain function following relatively minor head injuries. Structurally the brain remains undamaged. Typically the patient is 'knocked out' for several minutes. Prolonged episodes of unconsciousness are rare. In any event the **patient rapidly wakes up and makes a full recovery**. So long as there are no other complicating medical or social factors such patients can go home providing they can be carefully observed. **If the patient does not fully recover do not treat this as concussion**.

☠ Extradural haematomas

Extradural haematomas are **usually associated with a skull fracture or suture diastasis**. The commonest site is temporal, due to a tear of the middle meningeal artery, but they can also occur in the frontal and occipital regions. They are rare in young children, as their skull fractures are not sharp enough to damage the artery, and in the elderly, as their dura is usually firmly adherent to the skull. They classically present with delayed deterioration due to the dura being only slowly stripped from the skull. However, only a minority of patients are completely asymptomatic during this '**lucid interval**'.

Extradural haematomas are lentiform (lens) shaped on CT scans and are mostly high density. Low-density areas within them are said to be due to unclotted blood.

Very small extradurals with minimal symptoms can often be left alone (although they should all be transferred to neurosurgical units for observation), but most need a craniotomy for evacuation. The prognosis is very good if they are treated early enough.

☠ Acute subdural haematomas

Acute subdural haematomas are due to:
- a tear of a bridging vein between the brain and skull, in which case the prognosis is good with prompt treatment; or
- a laceration of the brain surface (burst lobe), which has a worse prognosis.

There **need not be a skull fracture** with subdural haematomas. They are commoner than extradurals and can extend over a wide area of the lateral cortical surface. They are crescent-shaped on CT scans.

All patients with acute subdurals should de transferred to neurosurgical units for management. Thin subdurals can be treated conservatively with close observation, but significant ones need a craniotomy as the clotted blood is too thick to drain via burr holes.

Cerebral contusions and haematomas

In cerebral contusions blood is interspersed between the neurones and glia, whereas with cerebral haematomas the bleeding forms a cavity within the brain. However, cerebral contusions can enlarge and result in a haematoma. Contusions often occur at the poles of the brain due to a contra-coup injury; i. e. the brain striking the inner surface of the skull after it has come to an abrupt stop.

They can be associated with marked oedema and a greatly raised intracranial pressure (ICP). They are usually treated conservatively, but a lobectomy (or evacuation of an intra-cerebral haematoma) can be performed if the ICP cannot be controlled and only one lobe is involved.

The affected brain usually resorbs to form a porencephalic cyst. The prognosis is usually poor, with survivors often having some degree of cognitive, personality or memory change.

① Chronic subdural haematomas

Chronic subdural haematomas are thought to be due to repeated minor bleeding following a minor head injury several weeks previously. The **head injury can be so trivial that it cannot be remembered in 50% of cases**. They usually occur in the elderly, but can also occur in babies due to non-accidental injuries. They are often associated with coagulopathies and alcoholism.

They can cause a wide variety of symptoms, including headaches, reduced consciousness, and focal neurology. **Therefore, consider this in all elderly patients with intermittent confusion** Chronic subdural haematomas are usually treated by burr hole drainage and have a good prognosis but might recur, especially with a persistent coagulation disorder.

Criteria for SXR

At the time of writing these are undergoing major review in the UK by the National Institute of Clinical Excellence (NICE).
May vary with different units—check local policy:
- mechanism of injury;
- LOC;
- vomiting;
- severe headache;
- visual disturbance;
- fits, faints, neurological deficit;
- GCS < 15;
- difficulty in assessment (child, C_2H_5OH);
- amnesia (retrograde vs anterograde);
- penetrating injury;
- ?FB;
- battles sign;
- CSF oto/rhinorrhea;
- 'panda' or 'racoon' eyes.

Table 4.4 Risks of intracranial haematoma following head trauma

	Orientated	Confused or worse
No skull fracture	1:6000	1:120
Skull fracture	1:32	1:4

One of several different types of Haematoma might develop.

Criteria for admission

May vary with different units—check local policy:
- skull fracture (proven or suspected);
- GCS less than 15;
- FND;
- epilepsy;
- unable to assess;
- elderly;
- infants;
- ?NAI;
- ethanol;
- mechanism of injury;
- social;
- risk factors, e. g. warfarin.

Criteria for neurosurgical consultation/CT scan

May vary with different units—check local policy:
- skull fracture + GCS < 15;
- penetrating injury;
- depressed fracture;
- deterioration;
- pupillary asymmetry;
- FND;
- Cushings;
- compound fracture;
- FB;
- coma;
- GCS > 15 after 8 h;
- anaesthetised + any head injury.
- coma after resuscitation.

Possible outcomes

- Death.
- PVS/FND/post-concussion syndrome.
- Epilepsy.
- Irritability/personality change.
- Pyrexia.
- Diabetes insipidus.
- Hydrocephalus.
- Meningitis.
- ARDS/stress ulcer.

① Head injuries—definitive care

Scalp lacerations

Scalp lacerations should be thoroughly cleansed and closed, in two layers if possible. The use of tissue glue is acceptable for small lacerations. The possibility of foreign bodies or an underlying fracture should be considered if the patient has not been X-rayed. Also remember anti-tetanus prophylaxis. Scalp sutures can usually be removed after 7 days.

Observations should be performed hourly, and half-hourly in higher risk patients. Most patients can be discharged the following day if asymptomatic. Stable patients who need longer admission can have their observation frequency reduced to 2-hourly. Patients not admitted should receive written guidelines of when to return and should only be discharged with a responsible adult who can call for assistance when required.

Transfer arrangements

- **Fully resuscitate ABCs in all patients before transfer**—this may include a laparotomy or pelvic fixation to stop bleeding.
- Intubate and ventilate comatose patients.
- If patients are being transferred for observation only, avoid intubation and sedation (discuss with neurosurgeons), if safe to do so.
- Intravenous mannitol can be given to gain time by reducing intra-cranial pressure.
- Transfer with experienced anaesthetist.
- Transfer promptly!

Advanced head injury management

On intensive care (ICU) patients will have at least the following inserted:
- endotracheal tube;
- ICP monitor;
- arterial catheter—BP monitoring;
- CVP line;
- urinary catheter;
- Naso-gastric catheter.

If the ICP is difficult to control, a jugular venous oximeter (JVO_2) may also be inserted. This is passed up to the jugular bulb at the skull base and measures the amount of blood being extracted from the brain. If the patient is being vigorously hyperventilated to reduce the ICP, cerebral vasoconstriction can occur, worsening cerebral ischaemia. This can be detected on JVO_2 by an increase in the amount of oxygen being extracted by the brain and the amount of hyperventilation reduced.

ICP management

The following measures can be used to lower ICP in severe head injuries. The first four are commonly used; the other measures are increasingly less successful and less frequently used:
- ventilation- to maintain a normal pO_2 and normal pCO_2;
- removal of mass lesions;
- diuretics;
- mannitol;
- frusemide;

- inotropes- maintain CPP by BP elevation;
- hyperventilation—reduce pCO_2 to 3.5 kPa;
- barbiturates—lowers cerebral metabolism;
- hypothermia—lowers cerebral metabolism;
- CSF drainage (the ventricles are usually small and difficult to cannulate so this is not often used);
- decompressive craniotomy—allows additional space for the brain to expand into.

CSF leaks

Facial fractures that extend into the base of the skull (e.g. Le Fort II, Le Fort III, naso-ethmoidal and occasionally fractures involving the mandibular condyle) can tear the dural lining and allow cerebral spinal fluid (CSF) to leak from the nose (rhinorrhoea) or from the ear (otorrhoea). Clear CSF tends to mix with blood and presents as a heavily blood-stained, watery discharge. This trickles down the side of the face, where peripherally the blood tends to clot while the non-clotted blood in the centre is washed away by CSF. This creates two parallel lines referred to as **'tramlining'**. One test for CSF is the 'ring test' (allow drops to fall on blotting paper, blood clots centrally, the CSF diffusing outwards to form a target sign). Other tests include examining for eosinophils and sugar. This is helpful in distinguishing between CSF and mucous. More sensitive indicators include B2 transferrin and tau protein, although practically it is easier to simply assume that a leak is present. **Tell the patient not to blow their nose for three weeks. If they do the increased pressure can force air intra-cranially through the tear, which then cannot escape. This is the neurosurgical equivalent of a tension pneumothorax!**

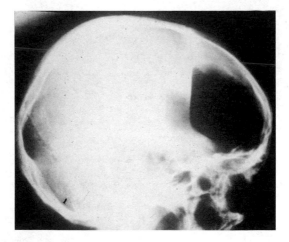

Fig. 4.4 A 'tension' pneumocephalocele.

Head injuries in children

These can be difficult to assess. Many of the features, which would lead to concern in adults are often present even with minor injuries (vomiting, drowsy, headaches, etc.). Carefully consider the mechanism of injury, other injuries present and whether the parents are capable of taking the child home for close observations. Interpretation of skull X-rays can be difficult as large fractures may be confused with wide sutures or vascular markings. CT scans are difficult to get and nearly always require general anaesthesia in an uncooperative child. If in doubt either refer or admit. **Remember NAI.**

Headaches

① Headaches

'Facial pain' conditions may also present as a headache. This can be a clinical entity in its own right or the manifestation of extra-cranial disease. **Take headaches seriously. Although the majority have a benign cause, if not assessed thoroughly, serious pathology may be missed.**

Headache is a common presenting symptom and may be attributable to an obvious diagnosis (e.g. meningitis, subarachnoid haemorrhage), or described as a feature of a less obvious local cause (e.g. TMJ dysfunction).

Most headaches are benign and self-limiting, but a few headaches are due to serious pathology, which may prove fatal or result in significant disability without prompt treatment.

Headaches persisting for longer than 6 weeks with abnormal physical signs should be thoroughly investigated, including:
- FBC with ESR (to exclude temporal arteritis);
- chest X-ray for bronchial carcinoma;
- CT scan to exclude space occupying lesion.

In all cases consider:
- **intra-cranial infections:**
  - meningitis
  - brain abscess
  - subdural empyema
- **mastioditis**
- **intra-cranial haemorrhage:**
  - subarachnoid haemorrhage
  - intra-cerebral haemorrhage
- **brain tumours**
- **hydrocephalus**
- **headache due to raised intra-cranial pressure**
- **dural venous thrombosis:**
  - cavernous sinus thrombosis
  - saggital sinus thrombosis
- **post-traumatic haematomas:**
  - extradural haematomas (small)
  - subdural haematomas (acute and chronic)
- **cerebral contusions**
- **migraine**
- **cluster headaches (migrainous neuralgia)**
- **tension headache**
- **post-concussion headache**
- **temporal (giant cell) arteritis**
- **glaucoma.**

① Temporal arteritis

Temporal arteritis (giant cell arteritis) is a vasculitic disease predominantly affecting the over-sixties. It is an important diagnosis in the elderly patient who presents with severe headache because of the potential for blindness if left untreated.

Aetiology and pathology

The aetiology of temporal arteritis is unknown; however, many patients report a prodromal flu-like illness. It may be that the systemic manifestations of the disease have a viral infection as their cause, although no distinct virus has been implicated.

Histologically there is a panarteritis with giant cell granuloma formation in a disrupted internal elastic lamina. The intimal thickening causes reduced vessel calibre or obliteration, and the vessels are enlarged and nodular. Involvement of the arteries is often patchy, with the description of 'skip lesions' often been made—this is an important feature when undertaking temporal artery biopsy for diagnostic purposes.

Clinical features

Patients present with a headache that may be a generalized 'tension' type or severe and well-localized over the region of the temporal arteries, often with burning or tenderness of the scalp. Jaw claudication with pain on chewing is another common feature and is thought to be due to involvement of the facial artery. Patients may also complain of an altered sensation of the oro-pharynx and a loss of taste. Systemic problems are also common and often made manifest with weight loss, arthralgia and fever.

Of great importance is the particular danger of the **sudden irreversible loss of sight** and optic complications may occur within weeks of the onset of systemic features of the disease. Often the presenting feature is of a visual field disturbance, which becomes progressively worse. Blindness is thought to occur as a result of ischaemic optic neuritis caused by arteritis of the ophthalmic arteries.

Temporal arteritis generally affects medium- and large-sized arteries with an internal elastic component. Branches of the carotid arteries are the commonest sites of involvement, but the vertebral, meningeal, and intra-cerebral vessels can be involved leading to hemiplegia, epilepsy, or local lobe lesions.

Investigations

The clinician has to be astute to the possible diagnosis of temporal arteritis, particularly in the patients with impending visual problems.

ESR—erythrocyte sedimentation rate, is usually markedly raised in excess of 90 mm/h in these patients.

Temporal artery biopsy—will help to confirm the diagnosis on the basis of the pathological findings. However, it must be remembered that the disease generally shows 'skip lesions' and therefore a negative biopsy does not exclude a diagnosis, particularly in the presence of a raised ESR.

Management

The aims of management are to reduce the pain and distressing symptoms of the condition and the prevention of complications, particularly blindness.

Steroids—usually high dose (40–60 mg daily) given urgently to suppress symptoms. Dosage can be titrated against the ESR, and affect on symptoms, but it is often necessary to continue treatment for 2–3 years with a gradually reducing dose until there is no evidence of the disease.

① Polymyalgia rheumatica (PMR)

Is a clinical condition of middle-aged and elderly patients which has a recognized association with temporal/giant cell arteritis and is characterized by:

• systemic upset—weight loss, fever, fatigue;
• severe arthralgia—pain and stiffness, usually bilateral and symmetrical;
• ESR—elevated;
• clinically, a rapid response to small doses of corticosteroids.

Around 50% of patients with temporal arteritis have symptoms of PMR, whereas a range of 15–50% of patients with PMR has giant cell arteritis. The clinical entities are more common in the elderly, particularly women, with a reported incidence in the region of 1 in 10 000.

Glaucoma

Patients may complain of facial pain in and around the eyes and it is important to consider ophthalmic conditions as a possible cause especially glaucoma.

Migraine

Migraine is a severe headache that may present as a facial pain affecting the cheek, orbit, or forehead. However, classical migraine with preceding visual disturbances and an aura rarely affects the face. 'Common' migraine is ten times more frequent and is described as a severe pulsatile headache invariably associated with nausea.

Migraine is episodic in nature and is thought to affect approximately 10% of the population. It is more common in females (3:1), usually begins around puberty, and continues into middle-age, and there may also be a family history.

Classic migraine is described as starting with an impending sense of ill health and a visual aura (e.g. flashing lights). The throbbing, severe, sharp, unilateral headache is associated with anorexia, nausea and vomiting, photophobia, and withdrawal—the patient often wants to just go into a darkened room and sleep.

Associations have been made with such trigger factors as stress, diet (chocolate, cheese, red wine), hormonal state (pre-menstrual, OCP), emotions (anger, excitement), and barometric changes.

Management

Recognizing and removing precipitating causes, with simple analgesics in the first instance. Anti-emetics may also be used to reduce nausea. If attacks are frequent and affect routine daily activities, then prophylactic treatment can be considered with, for example, oral pizotifen at night, or daily beta blockers. In severe cases, patients may be prescribed sumatriptan to use in the prodrome state.

① Cluster headaches (migrainous neuralgia)

So called because attacks generally occur in clusters, usually at night for 1–3 weeks, every 12–18 months. More common in men between 20 and 40 years, it may be precipitated by alcohol. Typically the patient is woken at night by a severe unilateral stabbing or burning pain, which may be frontal temporal, around the eye, or over the cheek. Nausea is not a common feature but there is frequently rhinorrhoea, unilateral nasal obstruction, and the eye may be red (conjunctival injection) with lacrimation.

Cluster headaches often respond to ergotamine.

① Tension headache

Tension headaches are described as a feeling of pressure, or a 'band-like' tightness that varies in intensity, frequency, and duration. It is often felt bilaterally over the forehead or temples but may affect the vertex, occiput, or eyes. Commonest in middle-aged women with associated stress or depression, it may be chronic or episodic and is only occasionally helped with simple analgesics (NSAIDs). Definite reassurance and a thorough normal physical examination are often therapeutic.

① Post-concussion headache

May have features of a tension type headache but is often associated with dizziness and loss of concentration.

☼ Headache due to raised intra-cranial pressure

Usually due to tumour, haematoma, or abscess, the headache is often associated with vomiting, is worse on waking, and improves a few hours after rising. Straining, coughing, or sneezing may exacerbate the headache, although simple analgesics are often useful.

☼ Hydrocephalus

Hydrocephalus is classified as:
- **Communicating hydrocephalus:** there is free flow of CSF from the ventricular system to the subarachnoid space. The hydrocephalus is usually due to failure of CSF absorption. It is safe to perform a lumbar puncture. A shunt is the only treatment option available.
- **Non-communicating hydrocephalus:** there is an obstruction within the ventricular system so that the CSF cannot reach the subarachnoid space. It is **not safe to do a lumbar puncture in this group**. Treatment options include a third ventriculostomy to bypass the obstruction internally.

Clinical features
- Headache.
- Vomiting.
- Visual disturbance.
- Deterioration in consciousness.

Investigations
- A **CT scan** will show ventricular dilatation. The forth ventricle is usually dilated in communicating hydrocephalus, but is small in non-communicating hydrocephalus. The cause of the obstruction might also be visible.
- An **MRI scan** might be necessary, particularly if a third ventriculostomy is being considered, to visualise the anatomy of the basal cisterns.

Management
- **Shunts:** divert CSF into the peritoneum, or less commonly the right atrium.
- **Third ventriculostomy:** creates an internal bypass by forming a stoma between the floor of the third ventricle and the basal cisterns through the lamina terminalis.
- **External ventricular drainage:** the CSF drains via a manometer to an external collecting system. This is usually only performed if there is infection or bloodstained CSF preventing shunt insertion, or in an emergency when there is insufficient time to insert a shunt (it can be done at the bedside with the appropriate equipment).

☼ Shunts and shunt complications

Shunts consist of:
• ventricular catheter;
• subcutaneous reservoir—for sampling CSF;
• valve—this might have a pumping chamber, depending upon the type;
• distal catheter—most commonly to the peritoneum (VP shunt),
  but occasionally to the right atrium via the internal jugular vein, etc
  (VA shunt).

Shunt assessment

• **CT scan:** to look at the ventricular size. It is most useful to compare
  the scan with a previous scan taken when the shunt was known to be
  functioning. However, in patients who have had multiple-shunt revisions,
  the ventricular wall can become stiff and might not dilate.
• **Shunt series:** plain X-rays of the whole of the shunt to look for
  breakages, disconnections, or migration of the shunt from its usual
  location.
• **Shunt palpation:** if the pumping chamber can be emptied, but does
  not refill, it suggests the ventricular catheter is blocked. If the pumping
  chamber cannot easily be emptied, the distal catheter is blocked.
  However, if the shunt is old and the materials have lost their
  compliance this is unreliable.
• **Shunt tap:** a needle is inserted into the subcutaneous reservoir
  (not the valve pumping chamber) to:
  • measure CSF pressure using an LP manometer. If there is no flow
    the ventricular catheter is blocked;
  • sample CSF for microbiology.

☼ Shunt obstruction

The commonest site of a blocked shunt is the ventricular catheter (due to
choroid plexus), followed by the valve (due to CSF debris) and the distal
catheter (due to omentum in VP shunts and clot in VA shunts). A blocked
shunt usually presents with similar symptoms to the patients original
hydrocephalus, but the **symptoms often progress more rapidly**. CT
scan usually confirms the diagnosis, but a shunt tap might be necessary in
symptomatic patients with small ventricles. **All symptomatic patients
should be admitted** for observation until their symptoms have settled.
The obstructed component, or preferably the whole shunt, will need to
be replaced. Attempts to clear the obstruction usually fail.

☼ Shunt infection

Shunt infections usually develop within a few weeks of the last shunt operation and are due to contamination from skin bacteria. An infected VP
shunt will usually become obstructed by omentum localizing the infection.
Patients therefore present with **symptoms of a blocked shunt accompanied by a fever**. They usually do *not* have meningism. An infected VA
shunt will usually not block and so the infection may continue undetected
for a long period. The symptoms of an infected VA shunt usually consist of
vague ill health and a low-grade temperature. Diagnosis is by a shunt
tap, with CSF microscopy and culture. The CSF white cell count might be

normal, as CSF flow flushes the bacteria away from the ventricles. Antibiotics alone are insufficient to clear a shunt infection. Removal of the shunt and external ventricular drainage are also necessary, with a new shunt being inserted when the CSF is sterile.

Prophylactic antibiotics have not been shown to prevent shunt infections.

① **Shunt overdrainage**

Occasionally a shunt will drain excessive CSF, so that the patient develops low-pressure headaches, which are **worse when upright and are eased by lying down**. If the ventricles are very large, the low pressure can cause them to collapse, tearing cortical bridging veins and causing subdural haematomas. These patients usually have symptoms of raised intra-cranial pressure with a hemiparesis.

Low-pressure headaches are treated with reassurance and advising a high fluid intake. The shunt can be revised if the symptoms persist.

☼ Subarachnoid haemorrhage

Aetiology

- 70% intra-cranial saccular (Berry) aneurysm (often remain asymptomatic—2% finding in routine post-mortems)
- 15% no identifiable cause;
- 5–15% arteriovenous malformation;
- Rare causes, for example:
  - inflammatory vascular disease;
  - cerebral amyloid angiopathy;
  - drug abuse;
  - scorpion bite!

One-third of aneurysmal subarachnoid haemorrhage (SAH) patients die from the initial bleed. Another third (half of the survivors) will have another bleed within 6 weeks, and 50% of the re-bleeds will be fatal. The likelihood of further bleeds in the remaining patients gradually falls over a year to a baseline level of 1% per year. It is therefore vital not to miss the diagnosis, as these patients remain at risk of sudden death.

The risk of re-bleeding in AVMs is much less at 6% in the first year and 3% for each subsequent year, so treatment can be delayed until the patient has settled.

Clinical features

- 'Thunder clap' headache—a sudden severe occipital headache radiating over the head and down the neck.
- Impaired conscious level—ranging from transient loss of consciousness to comatose, dependent on site and size of bleed.
- Meningism and neck stiffness.
- Photophobia.
- Vomiting.
- Fitting.
- Hemiparesis and/or dysphasia (in poor grade cases)—focal neurology will only occur if bleeding has also occurred into the brain substance.

Some patients report a sudden onset headache, that eased within a few hours, several weeks before a major SAH—a 'herald bleed'. **All patients with a sudden-onset headache should therefore be investigated for SAH, even if the headache eased within a few hours.**

Management

- **Resuscitation**, IV fluids, clotting studies.
- **Analgesics, anti-emetics**.
- **CT scan**. This should be performed as soon as possible after the bleed, when it will be diagnostic in 90% of cases. A delay in performing the scan reduces its diagnostic rate as the blood lyses. **A normal CT scan does not rule out a SAH**.
- **Lumber puncture (LP)**. This is required in all suspected cases if the CT scan is normal, but if performed too soon, the CSF can be normal, as the blood has not reached the lumbar region. The LP should not therefore be performed within 6 h from the bleed. The diagnostic

finding is xanthochromia, but all cases with bloodstained of equivocal CSF should be discussed with the neurosurgical unit.

- **Oral nimodipine**. Improves outcome by reducing the risk of ischaemic complications.
- In the neurosurgical unit, **cerebral angiography** will be performed to determine the cause.
- Aneurysms are secured by either **surgical clipping or endovascular embolization**. AVMs can be excised, embolized, or treated with extremely high-dose, finely localized radiation (**stereotactic radiosurgery**), which leads to gradual obliteration over a 2-year period. If no structural cause is found, the patient can be reassured that they are not at risk of further bleeds.

☼ Intra-cerebral haemorrhage

Intra-cerebral haemorrhage, a form of stroke, is most commonly due to **hypertension**. Bleeding disorders, AVMs, aneurysms, tumours, and venous hypertension due to central venous thrombosis can also be responsible.

Clinical features

These include the following, but not all need be present:
- headache
- loss of consciousness
- focal neurological deficit.

Management

- **Resuscitation**, IV fluids, clotting studies.
- **CT scan**. This should be performed as soon as possible after the bleed, especially if the patient is unconscious or an aneurysmal SAH is a possibility. MRI scans are best avoided, as the appearance of a haematoma on them is variable. An LP is unnecessary and potentially dangerous.
- **Angiograms** might be performed, especially if the clot is close to the Circle of Willis or Sylvian Fissure (possible aneurysmal cause) in younger non-hypertensive patients (possible AVM), or if surgical evacuation is being considered.
- **Surgical evacuation**. The role of surgery is controversial, as evacuating a cerebral haematoma has not been proven to improve the outcome. Most neurosurgeons would evacuate the haematoma in a semi-conscious patient, or a patient who starts in good condition but deteriorates later due to cerebral oedema.
- **Stroke rehabilitation**. This will be necessary in the majority of patients.

:Ö: Cavernous sinus thrombosis

Often fatal in the pre-antibiotic era, cavernous sinus thrombosis is essentially a septic thrombosis within the cavernous sinus. **It usually arises from an infection in the face**, most commonly the peri-orbital region, but can also arise from paranasal sinus infection. Propagation of an infected thrombus to the cavernous sinus occurs against venous flow, because of the absence of valves in the facial, angular, ophthalmic, and pterygoid plexus of veins. Thrombosis might spread to other venous sinuses and the infection may spread to cause subdural empyema or meningitis. Infective endocarditis and thrombosis of the internal carotid artery can also occur.

Clinical features
- Systemic upset: swinging pyrexia/tachycardia/rigors/sweats.
- Facial or peri-orbital pain.
- Venous obstruction—eyelid oedema/dilated facial veins.
- 'Pulsating exophthalmus' a transmitted carotid pulse with periorbital oedema.
- Blindness with papilloedema and retinal haemorrhages.
- Ophthalmoplegia: classically abducens (VIth) first followed by IIIrd and IVth.
- Obvious site of infection: usually unilateral initially; most commonly a peri-orbital cellulitis.
- Central signs—developing evidence of meningeal irritation.
- Bilateral signs develop with contra lateral extension of thrombus.

Investigations
- CT or MRI scans: usually show brain swelling and possible local infection. An occluded sinus might be visible on MRI scans.
- Coagulation studies.
- Cerebral angiogram, with venous phase (if diagnosis uncertain).
- Investigations into the cause of the infection.

Management
- Antibiotics and drainage of any collection of pus.
- Neurosurgical opinion.
- Anticoagulation.
- Thrombolytic therapy might be given if the patient is deteriorating.

✪ Saggital sinus thrombosis

Saggital sinus thrombosis can affect any age and either sex, but most commonly affects young and middle-aged females. It can be caused by trauma with depressed fractures overlying the sinus, tumours invading the sinus, and post-neurosurgery.

Clinical features
- Headaches, especially of a morning.
- Visual disturbance.
- Papilloedema.

Investigations
CT or MRI scans might show brain swelling. The 'delta' sign is a triangular filling defect in the sinus on a contrasted CT scan. An occluded sinus is usually visible on MRI scans. Infarction or haemorrhage due to venous hypertension might also be visible.

Management
- Anticoagulation.
- Thrombolytic therapy might be given if the patient is deteriorating.
- CSF diversion: might be necessary later if benign intra-cranial hypertension results.

:⚙: Cerebral tumours

There are a large number of brain tumours and cysts, both benign and malignant. However, they all present with one of three syndromes (or a combination of them):

- **raised intra-cranial pressure:**
  - worsening headaches, especially in the morning;
  - vomiting;
  - visual disturbance;
- **falling consciousness—in late cases**
- **progressive neurological deficit:** usually a hemiparesis ± dysphasia; patients do not usually notice cortical blindness or deafness;
- **epileptic fits:** especially late onset or focal fits.

Investigations

MRI scan is now the investigation of choice and will invariably be required before surgery, but a CT scan, without and with contrast, is usually easier to obtain. Tumours are seen as irregular enhancing lesions that might be cystic or solid, with mass effect and surrounding oedema. The three commonest tumours are:

- **metastases**, which are small round 'canon ball' lesions, usually multiple;
- **gliomas**, which are usually large irregular lesions; and
- **meningiomas**, which have a large dural attachment.

Chest X-rays should be obtained in all cases in view of the possibility of metastases.

Management

- Dexamethasone 4 mg four times daily.
- Anticonvulsants should be given if the patient has had fits. Not all neurosurgeons use prophylactic anticonvulsants in other cases.
- Neurosurgical referral. Excision of the tumour is the preferred treatment, but might not be possible due the site of the tumour or frailty of the patient, in which case a biopsy will be performed. Post-operative radiotherapy is given for high grade malignant tumours.
- If the patient has symptoms of raised intra-cranial pressure, but the scan looks normal, they might have benign intra-cranial hypertension and so should be referred for an opinion.

Emergency treatment

It the patient is deteriorating rapidly, intravenous mannitol and a massive dose of dexamethasone should be given pending neurosurgical transfer and emergency surgery.

Chapter 6

The neck

☼ Penetrating injuries of the neck

Penetrating neck trauma can be a life-threatening injury. **Never explore a neck wound under local anaesthetic if it is deep to the platysma.** Many important underlying structures are at risk, especially when the injury is at the root of the neck. The neck is divided into zones:

- zone I is located below the cricoid cartilage;
- zone II is between the cricoid cartilage and the angle of mandible;
- zone III is located above the angle of the mandible.

Depending on the clinical picture and patient's condition, management varies. Prior to exploration, zones I and III injuries may be evaluated with CT or angiography as surgery is difficult and risky. Zone II injuries may require CT angiography, MRI angiography, esophagoscopy, bronchoscopy, barium swallow, USS, or angiography depending on the injuries suspected.

Consider:

- **site and depth:**
  - anterior triangle;
  - posterior triangle;
  - zone (root of neck can also involve the chest and arm);
- **vascular structures:**
  - active bleeding;
  - hypovolemia;
  - haematoma (?expanding, or pulsatile);
- **peripheral pulses (compare with other side):**
  - distal carotid;
  - superficial temporal;
  - brachial or radial;
  - bruit;
- **larynx/trachea, esophagus:**
  - haemoptysis (ask patient to cough and spit on paper);
  - air bubbling through wound (ask patient to cough)/subcutaneous emphysema;
  - hoarseness;
  - pain on swallowing;
  - haematemesis;
- **nervous system:**
  - GCS;
  - localizing signs: (pupils, limbs);
  - spinal cord;
- **assess cranial nerves:**
  - facial;
  - glossopharyngeal (check mid-line position of soft palate);
  - recurrent laryngeal (hoarseness, effective cough);
  - accessory (shrug the shoulder);
  - hypoglossal;
- **spinal cord and brachial plexus;**
- **Horner's syndrome (myosis, ptosis, anhydrosis, enophthalmos).**

Indications for exploration include:
- expanding haematoma;
- pulse deficit;
- active bleeding;
- haemoptysis;
- haematemesis;
- hoarseness;
- surgical emphysema
- cause of injury: (bullet, knife, other);
- suspected foreign body.

:⚙: **The larynx—injuries**

The larynx is a semi-rigid structure consisting of a horse shoe-shaped hyoid bone and collection of small cartilages connected by fibrous tissue. It contains the vocal cords, 'supraglotic', and 'subglotic' spaces. The 'paraglotic' space lies between the lining mucosa and cartilages. **This space is potentially very distensible from bleeding and oedema**. The cricoid cartilage lies below the larynx and is the only complete ring in the respiratory tract.

Airflow through a tube varies according to Pouiselle's law:

$$flow = p\pi r^4/8ln,$$

where p is the pressure, r is the radius of the tube, l is its length, and n is the coefficient of viscosity. This formula strictly applies to fluids, but the principle also applies to air. **Small changes in the radius (e.g. from swelling/oedema) can therefore have profound effects on the flow of air through the larynx.** This is important at the vocal cords, the narrowest part of the upper airway, where the mucosa can swell considerably.

The **hyoid bone** is most commonly fractured following attempted strangulation. A fracture separating the cricoid from the trachea is referred to as laryngo-tracheal separation and is most commonly due to a clothesline type injury.

Common causes of injury include:

- road traffic accidents;
- sports (eg martial arts and racket sports);
- assaults;
- knife wounds;
- attempted suicide;
- inhalation of smoke, hot air or steam.

Types of injury

- **Oedema or haemorrhage**. This occurs particularly after thermal inhalation with rapid reductions in airflow. Early intubation is often necessary.
- **Fractured larynx**. In young patients, the larynx is elastic and flexes rather than fractures. Blunt injuries tend to bend and displace the larynx, which springs back to its normal position. However the epiglottis may become avulsed. In older patients the cartilages become calcified and fractures may occur.
- The **trachea can be avulsed** from the cricoid cartilage. Displacement is usually rapidly fatal, however if it springs back, the airway may be maintained but may displace later.
- **Surgical emphysema** of the neck and face may be seen after penetrating or blast injuries.

Clinical features

- Dyspnoea/stridor.
- Pain/tenderness.
- Hoarse voice.
- Dysphagia.
- Surgical emphysema.
- Palpable displacement of the larynx.

Management

First control the airway. Where there is airway distress a tracheotomy (not ostomy) may be necessary. Endotracheal intubation (ETT) is worth a try, but may cause further damage. ETT and cricothyroidotomy may not provide an airway in a patient with laryngo-tracheal separation.

In minor laryngeal injuries, humidified oxygen enriched air and steroids may be required. Severe injuries need the airway securing by either intubation or tracheostomy (after intubation).

Indications for surgery include:

- tracheal injuries;
- laryngeal displacement;
- swelling of laryngeal soft tissues;
- most cases of surgical emphysema.

Beware the patient who presents with surgical emphysema. If this is not allowed to drain, air can accumulate in the chest and result in tension pneumothorax or cardiac tamponade. Tracheostomy is required.

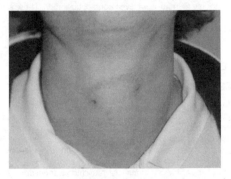

Fig. 6.1 Dog bite to the neck. Patient had a sore throat, tenderness, and palpable crepitus.

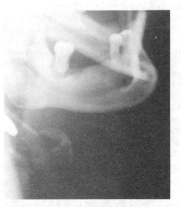

Fig. 6.2 Fracture of the hyoid—remember the potential for associated soft tissue swelling.

⑦ The larynx—loss of voice

Laryngeal disorders can present with a 'hoarse voice' (dysphonia), which untreated can progress to stridor. **A change in voice lasting over 4 weeks should be investigated**. Causes of dysphonia include:

- **Acute laryngitis**—usually associated with a respiratory tract infection or overuse. Usually painful, with a cough. Resolution is often spontaneous.
- **Carcinoma.**
- **Juvenile respiratory papillomata.**
- **Myasthenia gravis.**
- **Rheumatoid arthritis.**
- **Recurrent laryngeal nerve palsy (iatrogenic).**
- **Habitual dysphonia**—overuse of vocal cords can result in inflammation, oedema, nodule formation, or even contact ulceration. These are initially reversible but may become permanent if the overuse continues.
- **Psychogenic dysphonia.**

⑦ Deep neck infections—general points and clinical anatomy

Terminology can be confusing. Variation exists in the literature.

The neck may be regarded as containing superficial and deep fascial planes. These divide it into several specific compartments.

The **superficial cervical fascia** does not play a major role in deep neck infections. It encircles the neck blending with the fascia overlying the platysma muscle. Superiorly it blends with the muscles of the face comprising part of the 'SMAS' (superficial musculo aponeurotic system). This layer is important in certain types of 'face lift' procedures.

The **deep cervical fascia** is subdivided into three additional layers:

- The most superficial layer of the deep cervical fascia is also known as the **investing cervical fascia**. This encircles the neck, attaching and enclosing the sternocleidomastoid, trapezius, and omohyoid muscles, and parotid and submandibular glands. Posteriorly it attaches to the superior nuchal line. It can only distend a small amount.
- The middle layer of the deep cervical fascia is also known as the **visceral layer**. It encircles the strap muscles and the viscera of the neck, i.e. the larynx, pharynx, trachea, and thyroid gland. Part of this layer covers the pharyngeal constrictors and the buccinator muscle—the buccopharyngeal fascia.
- The deep layer of the deep cervical fascia is also called the **pre-vertebral fascia**. It lies just anterior to the pre-vertebral muscles of the spine allowing the pharynx to glide over them during neck movements and swallowing.

Both the middle and deep layers pass into the chest. Notably, the space between the buccopharyngeal and the pre-vertebral fascia (retropharyngeal) **extends into the mediastinum**.

The deep fascial planes divide the neck into several compartments. In the early stages, these limit the spread of infection to the defined compartment. However, untreated infection will eventually perforate the fascia and spread more rapidly.

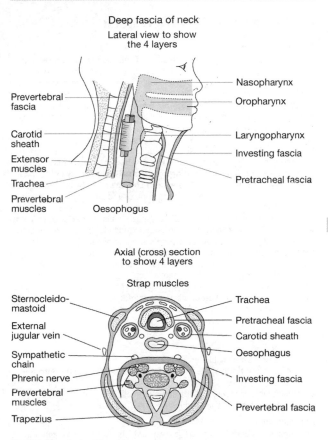

Fig. 6.3 Deep fascia of the neck.

☼ The acutely swollen neck

Ludwig's angina

This is a rapidly spreading, tense cellulitis of the submandibular, sublingual, and submental spaces bilaterally. Usually there is no abscess formation, but instead firm induration of the floor of the mouth with surrounding perioral oedema. It is clinically important because the muscular sling (mylohyoid muscle) attached to the mandible prevents tissue oedema from spreading downward. Instead swelling pushes the base of the tongue backwards, resulting in airway obstruction.

When advanced, this is an obvious diagnosis with gross swelling, both in the neck and the mouth. Earlier infections need to be treated seriously and often need admission. **Ludwig's angina is a potential airway emergency, which if not diagnosed and treated quickly has a mortality rate of around 75% within the first 12–24 h**. With aggressive surgical intervention, good airway control and antibiotics this has now dropped to 5%.

Usually the cause is a submandibular space infection **secondary to an infected wisdom tooth**. From the submandibular space, the infection spreads to the sublingual space on the same side around the deep lobe of the submandibular gland. It then passes to the contralateral sublingual space and thence to the adjacent submandibular space. The submental space is affected by lymphatic spread. Infection can also originate from the sublingual space. Other known causes are infected fractures and submandibular sialadenitis. Left untreated, the infection, oedema, and cellulitis spread backwards in the space between the hypoglossus and genioglossus to the epiglottis and larynx, resulting in respiratory obstruction.

Clinical features
- Systemic upset.
- Massive firm swelling bilaterally in the neck.
- Swelling in the floor of the mouth, forcing of the tongue up onto the palate.
- Difficulty in swallowing, talking and eventually breathing.
- Inability to protrude the tongue.

Management

The first consideration is the airway, which as in burns can rapidly obstruct. **Difficulty in swallowing and talking, and gross swelling are all indications to call an anaethetist urgently**. Refer to maxillo-facial team urgently. Further management includes IV fluids (patients often present after a few days and have not been able to drink), IV antibiotics (eg penicillin and metronidazole), together with surgical decompression of the submandibular and sublingual spaces and removal of the underlying cause.

Peritonsillar abscess (quinsy)

These are common infections arising when infection of the tonsil spreads to the surrounding tissue. Initially there is tonsillitis (sore throat, fever, and malaise), which progresses to a **unilateral, asymmetric bulge in the palate with displacement of the uvula to the opposite side**. Often they can be drained in casualty but if they threaten the airway GA is required. Tonsillectomy is generally not indicated for a single peritonsillar abscess, but recommended if it recurs.

Necrotizing fasciitis

This is a rare but potentially life-threatening mixed infection, characterized by **necrosis of the fascia and subcutaneous tissues.** Untreated the condition can spread rapidly with a **mortality approaching 40%.** Although it is more commonly seen in the groin, it can occur in the neck where it is usually due to an **underlying dental infection**. Patients often have an underlying predisposition such as diabetes, alcoholism or chronic malnutrition.

Clinically the overlying skin is often pale and mottled or may appear dusky due to thrombosis of underlying vessels. Blisters and ulceration may develop. Complications include:
- systemic toxicity and multi-organ failure;
- lung abscess;
- carotid artery erosion;
- jugular vein thrombosis and mediastinitis.

Treatment involves intravenous antibiotics, wide surgical debridement and hyperbaric oxygen. Any underlying predisposition must also be managed.

Fascial tissue spaces

Fascial spaces related to the mandible

The mylohyoid muscle has been described as the 'diaphragm' of the mouth. It divides the floor into two large (and two of the most commonly involved) spaces. These are the sublingual space above the muscle—(see The acutely swollen mouth), and the submental and submandibular spaces below it.

Submandibular space

This is triangular in shape, bounded by the mylohyoid muscle medially, and laterally by the mandible above and the deep cervical fascia below. It contains lymph nodes, the superficial lobe of the submandibular glands and blood vessels. It communicates with the sublingual space above, the superficial facial space laterally and the deep pterygoid space posteriorly.

Surgical access can be made 2–3 cm below the lower border of the mandible (to avoid injury to the mandibular branch of the facial nerve). Skin and subcutaneous tissues are incised and sinus forceps are used to penetrate the deep cervical fascia towards the lingual side of the mandible.

Submental space

This is contained by the two anterior bellies of the digastric muscles. Above is the mylohyoid muscle and below the deep cervical fascia covered by platysma and skin. It contains submental lymph nodes and communicates posteriorly with the submandibular space.

Surgical access is obtained behind the chin prominence in the neck.

Deep neck infections

These usually arise following penetrating injuries, untreated tonsillitis, or wisdom tooth infections. Once established the infection can rapidly spread throughout the neck, into the chest, and become life-threatening. When this occurs mortality is high. In the early stages diagnosis can be difficult.

Signs and symptoms

Fever, malaise, and lethargy are common and patients rapidly become very ill. A **very high WCC (>20)** is an ominous sign and often indicates tissue necrosis and likely mortality. **Pain on swallowing** should be taken seriously, which can be so severe that the patient sits drooling and unable to swallow their own saliva. There may be **cellulitis**, but because of the overlying fascial planes, *deep* abscesses do *not* fluctuate. Instead **swelling** presents with a 'dough-like' consistency. Initially the fascia may direct swelling medially, compromising the airway. Other signs of symptoms of deep neck infections include **dysphagia and trismus**.

Untreated, if **airway obstruction, sepsis** or **mediastinitis** does not kill the patient erosion into the carotid vessels can result in **septic emboli and CVA.**

Indicators of severe infection include:
• difficulty breathing
• shock
• pyrexia
• malaise
• dyspahagia/drooling
• trismus
• dysphonia
• inability to protrude the tongue
• high WCC.

Management

Assess for airway obstruction and where necessary consider intubation or a surgical airway. Once secure, assess the patient's haemodynamic status and give fluids. Often they have sat at home for a few days unable to eat and drink, so will probably be **at least mildly dehydrated**. These patients need to be admitted. **Consider immunosupression** (diabetes, alcoholics, long-term steroids, HIV, etc.).

CT or MRI of the neck and chest is usually required to determine the extent of infection, notably into the mediastinum. **Aggressive surgical drainage** and removal of dead tissue is usually required, even if there is only cellulitis. By opening tissue planes, not only is pus released but tissue perfusion is improved by reducing pressure. The surgical approach depends on the location of the abscess. Some can be drained intra-orally, eliminating a scar. However, drainage via a neck incision is more common, allowing identification of the great vessels and placement of large drains.

There is some evidence that **hyperbaric oxygen** may be beneficial, but this is a controversial issue. Only in very mild cases can patients be managed conservatively, if so they must be watched very closely. In selected cases ultrasound guided aspiration may avoid aggressive surgery.

Antibiotics—since many infections originate as dental, pharyngeal, or tonsillar infections, coverage should include organisms known to affect these areas. Most infections will be mixed and will include gram positive cocci and anaerobes.

☼ The cervical spine in the trauma patient

Initial considerations

Thorough assessment of the cervical spine is essential following trauma. In all patients with injuries *above the collar bones* there should be a high index of suspicion of an associated spinal injury. Always assume there is one, until proven otherwise.

Injuries to the spine occur when the force applied is greater than that which can be resisted by the vertebral bones *or* supporting structures. **Serious injuries can therefore be *either* bony or ligamentous in origin. The latter is especially important since the patient may have a normal looking X-ray.** Forces may be applied in any one or a combination of directions:

- compression flexion;
- vertical compression;
- distraction flexion;
- compression extension;
- distraction extension;
- lateral flexion.

When considering cervical spine trauma the *mechanism of injury* provides important clues. For instance following a road traffic accident (RTA) consider:

- the speed,
- the vehicle (motorcycle, pedal bike, lorry, 4×4, open top sports car, etc.);
- nature of the impact (head-on, side blow or glancing);
- ejection from the vehicle;
- seat belt use;
- bulls-eye breakage of the windscreen;
- air bag deployment;
- head restraint;
- how long trapped in the vehicle;
- if walked about after the accident;
- alteration in movement and sensation of the limbs since or worsening neck pain.

Remember the possibility of other injuries. So long as the spine is correctly immobilized, imaging can wait until more pressing injuries are dealt with (this may include laparotomy, craniotomy, or rarely thoracotomy).

Full c-spine immobilization includes not just the neck but *immobilization of the entire spine*. Movement lower down the spine will result in a degree of movement in the neck. Furthermore, injuries of the c-spine may be associated with spinal injuries elsewhere, which also need to be protected.

See Fig. 6.4. Following significant injuries most patients arrive supine with

- **spinal board**—solid inflexible plastic board the length and width of the patient with straps that hold the patient rigid across the chest, pelvis and legs;

- **blocks**—usually foam filled rubber coated blocks about the size of a shoe box, on both sides of their head, preventing the neck from rotating, radiolucent to allow radiographic examination of the spine;
- **tape**—often simple elastoplast tape but more commonly two purpose-made straps, one across the mandible, the other across the forehead, holding the head down on to the spinal board;
- **hard collar**—stiff plastic neck collar that holds the cervical spine more stable by reducing flexion, extension, and lateral flexion of the neck.

Go to your A&E department, and ask to see these items, be familiar with how they are applied and taken off. Better to learn now than have to learn during the real thing!

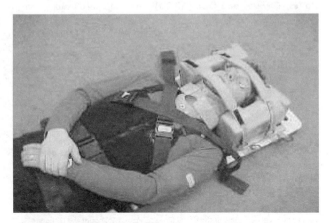

Fig. 6.4 Correct spinal immobilization.

Cervical spine film interpretation

Unlike almost any other clinical examination for a fracture where we Look, Feel, Move, then X-ray, in the examination of the suspect *trauma* cervical spine **X-ray first.** The key view is the lateral, and this should be obtained first as part of the initial assessment according to the Advanced Trauma Life Support protocol. However, before a cervical spine can be cleared *radiologically* you need adequate anterioposterior and odontoid peg views. Do not interfere with the immobilization until you have seen a film, unless other life threatening conditions demand.

Adequacy

First determine whether the film is adequate. Do not feel embarrassed in rejecting a film and asking for improved views. All radiographers involved in trauma know how difficult it is to obtain good films. You are about to make a vital decision.

An adequate film demonstrates all seven of the cervical vertebrae, skull base, and the superior aspect of T1.

There are various ways of getting better views of the C7-T1 level. The experienced radiographer will know them. Different protocols exist between units but they include:

- coned view with greater penetration of the film;
- swimmers view—one arm raised forward as if the patient is doing the crawl;
- pull-down view—gentle firm traction on both arms allowing the shoulders to be removed from the lateral view;
- trauma obliques—sometimes known as 'scottie dog views', these consist of two films taken at 90 degrees to each other but each one an oblique of the spine rather than a true lateral;
- computed axial scan (CT scan).

Consider things in a logical order. A useful approach is **Alignment, Bones, Cavities and Disc (ABCD).** This is a difficult radiograph to interpret, and deserves time.

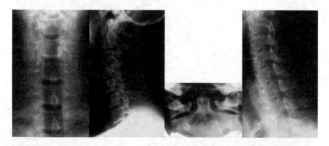

Fig. 6.5 (a)–(b) Anterioposterior (A–P), lateral, odontoid peg and trauma oblique views of the cervical spine. Is the lateral film adequate? No, count the number of vertebral bodies visible.

Alignment

There are four curves to follow. Let your eyes follow your index finger as you trace each one out. This allows you to concentrate on specific areas in turn, rather than be flooded with information all at once.

- Anterior line of the vertebral bodies (greater than 3 mm mal-alignment indicates a possible dislocation).
- Posterior line of the vertebral bodies.
- Posterior spinal canal (width of canal at least 13 mm, but age and sex dependent).
- Tips of the spinous processes.

Bones

Examine in turn:

- Vertebral body—any cortical discontinuity, normal height, wedged >3 mm between anterior and posterior height, retropulsion into spinal canal.
- Atlas and Axis (C1 and C2)—posterior aspect of C1 on lateral should not be greater than 3 mm from the anterior aspect of the odontoid peg on the lateral film.
- Posterior elements—facet joint dislocation, laminal fracture, pedicles splayed or clay shoveler fracture of spinous process tip.

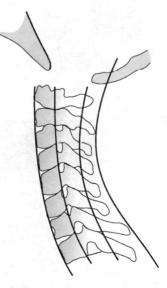

Fig. 6.6 Diagram of the lateral view of the cervical spine showing the four curves needed to check alignment.

Cavities

These include:

- a pre-vertebral space of more than 3 mm in the proximal spine, 5 mm in the mid segment and 10 mm in the distal segment is highly suspicious of free blood implying an underlying fracture;
- normal fat stripe should be present. loss may indicate oedema or haemorrhage at that level;
- an increased angle between the spinous processes could imply a ruptured interspinous ligament—look for the potentially associated anterior disruption.

Disc

Intervertebral disc (height, even width, an angle between the end plates of more than 11 degrees is suspicious, calcification).

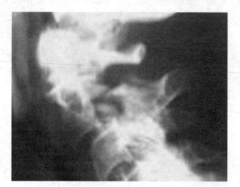

Fig. 6.7 Anterior subluxation of C2 due to lamina fracture (Hangman's fracture).

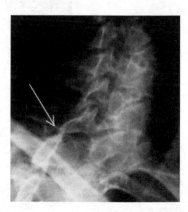

Fig. 6.8 'Clay shovellers' fracture of the tip of C 7. This is not a normal lateral film but a trauma oblique.

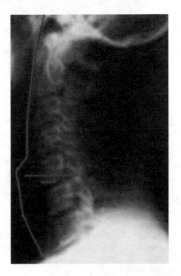

Fig. 6.9 Lateral view of cervical spine, the red line demonstrates the soft tissue swelling.

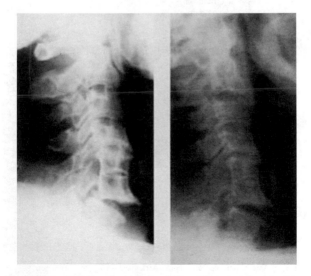

Fig. 6.10 (a) and (b) Note the angulation of C6 on C7 is greater than 11 degrees.

Examination

Unlike almost any other clinical examination for a fracture where we Look, Feel, Move, then X-ray, in the examination of the suspect *trauma* cervical spine *X-ray first*. The key view is the lateral, and this should be obtained first as part of the initial assessment according to the Advanced Trauma Life Support protocol. However, before a cervical spine can be cleared *radiologically* you need adequate anterioposterior and odontoid peg views. Do not interfere with the immobilization until you have seen a film, unless other life threatening conditions demand.

Following the primary survey if radiologically clear reassess the patient.

- **Talk** to the them. This will tell you whether the airway is patent, part of the Glasgow Coma Scale, improves patient cooperation, and tells them what you are going to do.
- **Look**—remove tapes, head blocks and undo collar **but** keep the head and neck stationary by in line manual immobilization. Do **not** allow movement at this stage. Are there any wounds, swellings, bruising, or unusual posture?
- **Feel**—start by standing above the patient and feel the trachea and hyoid bone. Progress along the line of the mandible posteriorly, then inferiorly to the clavicles. Palpate along the posterior aspect of the neck from occiput to thoracic spine. At this stage you may detect:
  - deviated trachea;
  - fractured larynx/hyoid bone;
  - surgical emphysema;
  - strap muscle haemorrhage;
  - great vessel haematoma;
  - soft tissue or bone pain.

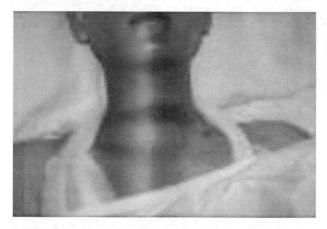

Fig. 6.11 Anterior abrasion on patient's neck may be a sign of more serious cervical or vascular injury.

Finally place a gloved finger in the mouth of the patient (this depends on their level of co-operation and GCS) and feel for a 'boggy swelling' or pain at the back of the throat. This is highly suggestive of an underlying fracture and haematoma.

- **Move**—if all of the above fail to demonstrate any significant problems, it is reasonable to attempt to 'clear' the c spine **(see 'Clearing' the c spine).** Ascertain whether the patient has head control; are they able to comfortably move their neck or is there muscle spasm, fear or instability preventing this? Do not force the patient to move. Allow them time to truly assess what they can do. Assess flexion, extension, lateral flexion and rotation.
- **Listen**—over the carotids for bruits, especially if there has been a direct blow to the front of the neck. Blunt carotid injury is seldom thought of and therefore frequently missed.

'Clearing' the c.spine

Always follow local protocol. Assess the neurological state of the limbs:

- **tone**—lower motor neurone lesion, i.e. cut peripheral nerve = flaccid, upper motor neurone lesion, i.e. cerebrovascular accident = increased;
- **strength**—medical research council grading;
- **sensation**—soft touch and pinprick (spinothalamic tract);
- **reflexes**—look for qualitative reduction or quantitative absence, compare and contrast sides;
- **proprioception** (posterior columns) and **coordination** are included in the perfect neurological examination, but seldom practically needed here.

In addition:
- **Examine relevant X-rays.**
- **Are there any other injuries? (Distraction from neck pain.).**
- **Has analgesia (especially opiates) been given? (May mask cervical pain.).**
- **Is there any spinal tenderness?**
- **Is the patient mentally alert? (HI/alcohol/drugs, etc.).**
- **If all the above are normal/excluded, take the collar off.**
- **Assess active movement first** (i.e. get the *patient* to move their neck—not you). Lateral flexion first, then rotation, then lift head off bed. Take your time, the neck will be a bit stiff at first if they have been laying on a trolley with collars, blocks, etc., for some time.
- **Any neurological Sx or pain**—not cleared—replace immobilization and refer. Consider the mechanism of injury and possible need to X-ray the whole spine.

Neurological injuries

These can be considered as:
- complete
- incomplete.

Or anatomically as:
- anterior cord syndrome (motor function lost but sensation preserved);
- posterior cord syndrome (seldom seen);
- central cord syndrome (upper limbs affected more than lower);
- Brown–Sequard syndrome (ipsilateral loss of motor and propioception, with contralateral loss of pain and temperature sensation).

Frankel classification of spinal cord injury
- Complete loss (no motor or sensory function).
- Incomplete loss (no motor but useful sensory function).
- Incomplete loss (some motor function but not useful below injury level).
- Incomplete loss (reduced but useful motor function below injury level).
- Normal.

Specific fractures

Atlas (C1)
- Posterior arch.
- Anterior arch.
- Jefferson fracture (blow-out fracture through anterior and posterior arches).
- Transverse process fracture.
- Lateral mass fracture.

Odontoid peg (C2) Anderson and D'Alonzo classification
- Tip of the odontoid process.
- Through the base of the odontoid
- Through the odontoid and extends into the body of the vertebra.

C2 Posterior elements hangman's fracture produced by extension and distraction (Levine classification)
- Minimally displaced.
- Displaced greater than 3 mm.
- Fracture associated with unilateral or bilateral facet dislocation of C2 on C3.

Vertebral body
- Wedge compression.
- Burst.
- Tear-drop.

Facet joints
- Occipital–cervical dislocation.
- Atlanto-axial subluxation (normal atlanto anterior arch, and odontoid distance is less than 3 mm).
- Unilateral facet dislocation (25% displacement of the superior vertebra on the inferior or malalignment of the spinous processes on the anterior-posterior film).
- Bilateral facet dislocation (50% displacement of the superior vertebra on the inferior).

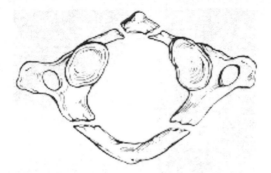

Fig. 6.12 Blow out fracture of C1 Jefferson type.

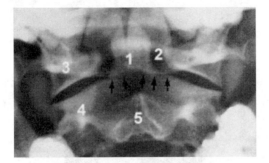

Fig. 6.13 Type II odontoid fracture.

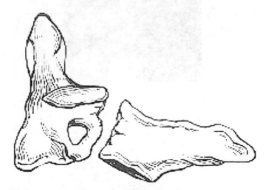

Fig. 6.14 Lateral diagram of Hangman's fracture.

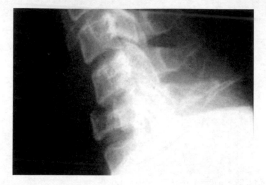

Fig. 6.15 Burst fracture of C7.

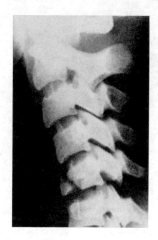

Fig. 6.16 Tear-drop fracture of C6.

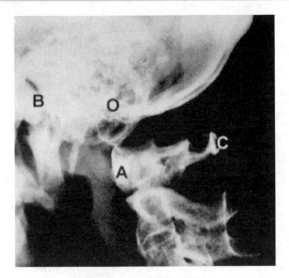

Fig. 6.17 Occipital-cervical dislocation.

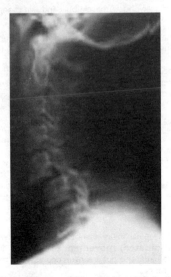

Fig. 6.18 Bilateral facet dislocation of C5 on C6. Note 50% overlap.

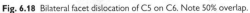

① Examination of minor injuries

Initial considerations

Although the ATLS dictates complete immobilization of the spine, this is clearly not necessary (or practical) in *every* patient complaining of neck pain. 'Clinical common sense', together with a high index of suspicion based on the mechanism of injury will allow most cases to be managed appropriately. If in doubt, err on the side of caution and seek advice. Useful clues include:

- **age**—young patients are more commonly associated with trauma and congenital malformation, older ages with degenerative causes;
- **position**—are they standing, sitting or lying down;
- **posture**—do they turn their head to see you or does their whole body turn?
- **clothing**—velcro fastening on a blouse vs tiny intricate buttons (pre-existing neurological problems);
- does the patient use any **prostheses**?—walking aids, standing frame, soft collar, etc.. these also give clues about pre existing pathology and psychology of the patient;
- **the hands**—are these the hands of a rheumatoid patient?

Look

- Can they look you in the eye or is there a cervical spondilosis?
- Is this a case of congenital unifacet dislocation and sternocliedomastoid spasticity resulting in a torticollis?
- Can you see the incision from an anterior approach to cervical spine?
- How flexed is the cervical spine?
- Note any thoracic kyphosis, muscle bulk and skin changes.

Feel

Most palpation in the cervical examination can be done from behind. It is often less tiring for the patient, and easier for you, if they are sitting down.

Start at the occiput working your way down over the erector spinea and spinus processes. The highest bone you will feel will be C2. Work down to T1, the most prominent bone in the neck. This is sometimes over shadowed by C7. To work out if you are on T1 or C7 ask the patient to extend the neck slightly—C7 glides back, T1 does not.

Palpate laterally, around and over trapizeius into the supraclavicular fossae. Continue advancing till your fingers meet in the mid-line anteriorly. Be gentle, do not throttle the patient!

Feel the top of the manubrium sterni and advance upwards towards the thyroid gland. Continue upwards, remember the hyoid bone is a landmark for C3–4 level. Assess the tension in sternoclideomastoid continue under the angle of the mandible proceed forwards feeling for nodes till you reach the point of the chin.

Move

Only possible if a spinal injury is not suspected. **Always start with active (patient initiated) movement** to avoid hurting the patient. If necessary, ask the patient to put a tongue depressor in their mouth to act as a guide to the range.

Ask the patient to hold their head in a comfortable position, does this differ from neutral? Ask the patient to put their 'chin on chest' for forward flexion—usually about 75 degrees (but varies with age). Then 'look up at the ceiling' for extension usually about 50 degrees.

Assess lateral flexion, 'put your right ear on your right shoulder' and the opposite for the left. Look at the rise of the shoulder and compare sides. The range of motion is usually about 90 degrees. Assess rotation—'put your right chin on your right shoulder'. This is just short of 90 degrees.

Passive movement is very useful but this is not a chance to move the head a little further and demonstrate that full range of motion does exist. Consider it in two ways:

- **physiological motion**—assessing the static elements of the neck (i.e. are the ligaments, joint capsule, roots, etc.. the cause of pain and limitation?);
- **mobility motion**—assessment of not only the flexibility of the cervical spine but the rhythm and cadence of the motion.

Power
You have assessed the control of the neck, now assess the power in all the planes of movement, 'push against my hand'.

Neurology
Comprehensive neurological examination of upper and lower limbs is required. Remember tone, power, sensation, coordination proprioception and reflexes. Are the limbs held flaccid or is there a spastic posture? Coordination and proprioception expose central pathology, chronic alcohol abuse, infarct, metastasis, cord compression, and so on.

⑦ Special cases
Cervical rib
This may present with unilateral vascular changes in the hand. Such changes include cold, white, mottled, or blue skin discolouration, trophic ulcers, or tapering of the pulp, and so on (cf. Raynaud's which is more often bilateral). Feel the radial pulse, and apply gentle traction to the arm to see if it is altered. Compare sides. Hold the arm across the body, feel the radial pulse and ask the patient to look towards you and take a deep breath, again assess both sides and compare any alteration. Finally listen for a bruit with a stethoscope in the supraclavicular fossa.

Cord compression
Look for the following:
- **Hoffmann's test**—flick the terminal phalanx of the middle finger into extension suddenly and watch and see if index and thumb flex;
- **dynamic Hoffmann's test**—the same flick as above but get the patient to flex/extend the neck at the same time; these tests demonstrate cortico-thalamic tract dysfunction;
- **Lhermitte's** test is positive if flexion–extension of the neck produces neurological feelings in the legs of burning, electric shock, etc.;
- **clonus** occurs when the foot is rapidly brought up into dorsiflexion from a planter position—it is counted as normal if there two or three beats; more than this indicates an abnormality.

Whiplash

This is a very difficult diagnosis to prove or disprove, and is a potential minefield when it comes to litigation. Consider it as a sprain of the surrounding neck muscles, notably trapezius and the deep extensors. Anyone who has had whiplash will appreciate how painful it is. During the injury, muscle fibres are torn resulting in intense painful spasm. The neck is held still by this spasm and the muscles feel hard. Sometimes the head is rotated to one side due to the pull of the sternomastoid.

Radiographs can be difficult to interpret if the neck is twisted, which of course should be immobilized. One clue is the loss of the cervical lordosis, with staightening of the vertebra on the film. This does not confirm a whiplash injury and should be regarded as a marker that the neck has potentially sustained a serious injury. There should be no bony tenderness or neurological features.

Management of whiplash involves NSAIDs and a soft collar. It should settle after a few days.

Vertebrobasilar insufficiency

Osteophyte formation with increasing age can gradually compress the vertebral vessels. This can result in positional dependent vertigo or blackouts in which movement of the neck results in the symptoms. This is a useful clinical sign but be careful when eliciting it!

⑦ Lumps in the neck

Applied anatomy

The neck is divided into anterior and posterior triangles by the obliquely running sterno-cleido-mastoid (SCM) muscle. This muscle has two heads of origin inferiorly, one from the manubrium sterni and the other from the medial clavicle. These pass supero-posteriorly, fuse to form a fleshy belly, which inserts into the mastoid process and the superior nuchal line of the occipital bone. The sterno-cleido-mastoid is supplied by the spinal part of the accessory nerve (mostly C2 and C3), and receives its blood supply from the superior thyroid and occipital arteries.

Tips

- The triangular gap between the two heads of origin of SCM overlays the internal jugular vein—this site may be used for central venous access.
- The strip of anatomy deep to SCM should not be forgotten. Essentially the lower half covers the carotid sheath containing the common carotid artery, the internal jugular vein, and the Vagus, and the upper half lies over the emerging cervical plexus.

The deep cervical lymph nodes

These are classified into five groups or 'levels' denoted by Roman numerals:
- **level I**—nodes in the anterior submandibular or submental triangle;
- **level II**—jugulodigastric node(s);
- **level III**—nodes immediately above the intermediate tendon of omohyoid;
- **level IV**—nodes below the intermediate tendon of omohyoid;
- **level V**—nodes in the posterior triangle.

Levels II to IV simplistically divide the SCM into upper, middle and lower thirds.

Overview of the anterior triangle

Boundaries:
- upper—lower border of the mandible;
- back—anterior border of the SCM muscle;
- front—the mid-line.

This may be further sub-divided into submental, digastric, carotid, and muscular triangles by the digastric muscle and the hyoid bone. However, from a practical point of view this is not necessary. More useful is the simple sub-division into the submandibular triangle lying between the lower border of the mandible and the digastric muscles. Below the digastrics lies a more elongated inferior triangle with its apex inferiorly.

Contents of importance—these are all deep to platysma

- **Suprahyoid muscles**—digastric, stylohyoid, geniohyoid, mylohyoid (forming the diaphragm of the floor of the mouth).
- **Infrahyoid muscles** (the 'strap muscles')—sternohyoid, omohyoid, thyrohyoid, sternohyoid.
- **Carotid sheath**—runs from the level of the sterno-clavicular joint to the bifurcation of the common carotid artery (at the level of the upper border of the thyroid cartilage—C3 vertebra).

- **Common carotid artery** divides to give the
  - **internal carotid** (no extra-cranial branches);
  - **external carotid artery**: gives the following branches thyroid, lingual, facial, occipital, posterior auricular, ascending pharyngeal artery.
- **Internal jugular vein**—surface markings run from the ear lobe to the sternal end of the clavicle. Deep cervical lymph nodes are adjacent to the vein throughout its course. On the left-hand side the Thoracic duct crosses behind the vein at the level of C7 vertebra.
- **Anterior jugular veins**—commencing beneath the chin, running inferiorly to the suprasternal region.
- **Vagus nerve**, runs in the groove between the common carotid artery and the internal jugular vein.
- **Phrenic nerve** 'C3, 4 and 5 keeps the diaphragm alive'.
- **Hypoglossal nerve**—emerges between the ICA and the IJV in the upper part of the neck. It lays on the carotid sheath deep to the posterior digastric and passes forwards beneath the tendon of digastric to provide motor innervation to the tongue.
- **Cervical lymph nodes**: levels I to IV (see above).
- **Submandibular salivary gland**—this comprises a large superficial part and smaller deep part that wraps around the posterior border of mylohyoid. Its duct runs forwards in the floor of the mouth, crossing the lingual nerve, to open in the anterior floor of mouth.
- **Parotid**—the lower pole, or tail, can pass into the neck, just below the earlobe. The lower branches of the facial nerve pass through and both can be injured by penetrating injuries in this region.
- **Thyroid**—a bi-lobed endocrine gland united in the mid-line by its isthmus, overlying the 2nd to 4th tracheal rings. Pathological enlargement of the gland may displace other structures in the neck.
- **Parathyroids**—small glandular tissue lying on the posterior aspects of the lateral thyroid lobes—normally four (90% of population).

Mid-line structures
- **Trachea**—continues from larynx at the level of C6. A vital site for urgent and elective surgical airways.
- **Oesophagus**—behind the trachea, a continuity of the pharynx at the level of C6. The recurrent laryngeal nerves run on each side in the groove between the oesophagus and trachea.

Overview of the posterior triangle
Boundaries:
- front—posterior border of SCM;
- back—anterior border of trapezius muscle;
- below—the lateral part of the clavicle.

The posterior triangle is a spiral that passes from its apex at the back of the skull to its base in the front at the root of the neck. Its roof is formed by the investing layer of deep cervical fascia, and its floor by the pre-vertebral fascia.

Contents of importance
- **Third part of the subclavian artery**—runs very low in the posterior triangle at the level of the clavicle; just above the clavicle the suprascapular and transverse cervical vessels pass.

- **External jugular vein**—runs through the anterior/inferior part of the triangle to drain into the subclavian vein which lies more inferiorly and is not included in the posterior triangle.
- **Occipital, transverse cervical, suprascapular and subclavian arteries.**
- **Accessory nerve** emerges from the posterior border of SCM at the junction of its upper and middle thirds. It runs vertically down (over levator scapulae) to enter the anterior border of trapezius usually 5–6 cm above the clavicle.
- **Cervical plexus branches:**
  - muscular branches;
  - a loop from C1 to hypoglossal;
  - C2/3 branches to S–C–M and C3/4 to trapezius;
  - inferior root of ansa cervicalis.
- **Phrenic nerve** (C3, 4, and 5)—runs from lateral to medial over scalenus anterior:
  - cutaneous branches;
  - lesser occipital nerve (C2)—posterior part of the neck to the superior nuchal line, and behind the auricle;
  - great auricular nerve (C2 and 3)—skin over the angle of the mandible and parotid gland, and the auricle;
  - transverse cervical (C2 and 3)—skin in the mid-line of the neck;
  - supraclavicular nerve (C3 and 4)—root of neck/upper chest.
- **Brachial plexus** trunks—the three trunks of the brachial plexus along with the cervical plexus are held down to the pre-vertebral muscles by the covering of pre-vertebral fascia that forms the floor of the posterior triangle. Strictly speaking they are *not contents* of this triangle, but are mentioned, however, because of their anatomical importance in penetrating injuries.
- **Omohyoid muscle**—posterior belly. From its origin at the hyoid bone it passes deep to SCM, coming to lie over the carotid sheath. As it overlies the IJV the fibres form a flat tendon (the 'intermediate tendon') that are a useful maker during neck dissections to the vein's position. The muscle is held down to the clavicle at the intermediate tendon by a fascial sling.
- **Cervical lymph nodes:** level V

Lymphatic drainage

When lymph nodes are enlarged secondarily to disease elsewhere, which node is involved depends on the site of the primary pathology. For this reason, it is important to know the lymphatic drainage patterns of the various anatomical sites in the head and neck:

- **pre-auricular**—eyelids, orbit, temple and vertex of scalp;
- **occipital**—posterior pinna, back of scalp;
- **bucco-facial**—cheek, lower eyelids;
- **submental**—anterior lower lip, tip of tongue, floor of mouth, lower anterior teeth (bilateral drainage);
- **submandibular**—anterior 2/3 tongue, lips, anterior neck, centre of forehead, nose, teeth, paranasal sinuses;
- **supraclavicular**—occipital nodes, axillary nodes, breast, upper anterior body wall;
- **infraclavicular**—lower neck, breast, body wall.

Deep nodes
- **Jugulo-digastric**—subcutaneous nodes, tonsillar area/pharyngeal wall.
- **Jugulo-omohyoid**—submental and submandibular groups, all of tongue.
- **Lymphadenopathy in the neck (especially supraclavicular) can arise from disease both above and below the collar bones.**

General considerations

One of the most important considerations in an adult presenting with a lump in the neck is, it may represent a metastatic lymph node. In such cases the primary cancer is often in the upper respiratory or alimentary tract. The risk is increased in smokers and heavy drinkers. The primary tumour must then be found quickly but open biopsy of the node should not be done. Fine needle aspiration cytology may be useful.
- In patients over 40, 75% of lateral neck masses are caused by malignant tumours.
- In the absence of obvious infection, a lateral neck mass is malignant until proven otherwise (metastatic squamous cell carcinoma or lymphoma).
- The primary tumour can usually be found in half of patients by clinical examination alone. Endoscopy of the upper aerodigestive tract will find it in another 10–15%.
- Fine needle aspiration biopsy is a useful investigation.
- Biopsy of cervical metastases results in a 2–3 times increased incidence of recurrence. Most studies suggest that open biopsy of a metastatic node have an adverse effect on survival. It also makes subsequent examination of the neck more difficult and encourages fungation.
- Biopsy of parotid tumours risks damage to the facial nerve and recurrence may develop up to 20 years later.

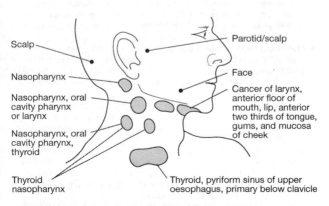

Fig. 6.19 Lymphatic drainage is generally predictable. This helps determine the possible source of lymph node swelling (especially infection of malignancy).

Causes of lumps in the neck
- **Developmental**—branchial cyst, haemangioma, laryngocoele.
- **Skin and subcutaneous tissues**: sebaceous cyst, lipoma.
- **Infected lymph nodes**—viral: Epstein–Barr virus, HIV, bacterial (Staphylococcus, tuberculosis, cat scratch, brucella), protozoa (toxoplasma, leishmaniasis), fungal (histoplasmosis, blastomycosis, coccidiomycosis).
- **Neoplastic lymph nodes**—lymphoma, metastasis.
- **Granulomatous lymph nodes** sarcoid, foreign body reaction.
- **Carotid sheath: aneurysm, carotid body tumour, vagal or sympathetic neuroma.**
- **Salivary gland (parotid or submandibular)**—infective (sialadenitis, sialolithiasis), autoimmune (Sjögren's syndrome), neoplastic, miscellaneous (AIDS related disease).

History

Even with obvious lumps, take a full medical history. This will ensure that other pathologies are not missed and may pick up important details relevant to the patient's further management. Tuberculosis, for example, has relevance in terms of previous lung disease and the safe administration of general anaesthesia, and may also be relevant as an infective cause of cervical lymphadenopathy. Smoking and alcohol are important in head and neck malignancy. Some animals (cats) can pass on infections (toxoplasmosis)

Useful information in diagnosing neck lumps
- **Age.** This may be a useful guide:
  - **<16 years**: cervical lymphadenopathy secondary to infection is the commonest cause of neck swellings at this age group followed by congenital and developmental lesions (more so in the younger age groups). Neoplastic disease can still occur (especially leukaemia/lymphoma) but is less common.
  - **16 to 40 years**: inflammatory lesions are still the most common followed by developmental lesions. Neoplasia is next most common with benign disease seen slightly more than malignant disease.
  - **>40 years**: neoplasia is the most common cause of neck swellings with malignant disease predominating.
- **How long has the lump been present?** Was it acute in onset or a gradual increase over many months or years. Developmental lesions tend to gradually increase in size becoming increasingly troublesome. Inflammatory causes tend to develop rapidly and are often associated with pain.
- **Is it painful?** Cervical lymphadenopathy secondary to infection and inflammatory salivary gland disease often present with painful swellings. Metastatic lesions in the neck are rarely painful unless associated with secondary infection or malignant invasion of local nerves.
- **Does it vary in size?** Has the lump gradually increased in size or does it increase and then decrease in size at different times of the day? Ask particularly about mealtimes as obstructive sialadenitis secondary to sialolithiasis (salivary stones) is quite common and often presents as submandibular swelling around mealtimes.
- Does the patient have **foul breath (halitosis) or a foul taste** in their mouth? Submandibular gland infection may discharge pus in the mouth,

resulting in a foul tasting discharge. Similarly, a pharyngeal pouch can become secondarily infected as a result of food stagnation; the patient (usually elderly) will present with halitosis, dysphagia and a painful neck swelling just anterior to SCM.

- Ask about **sore throat, unilateral hearing loss, earache, and hoarseness**. These may indicate underlying malignancy.
- **Other symptoms of systemic upset.** Are there other infective symptoms present: malaise, fever, and lethargy? Cervical lymphadenopathy may represent a generalised viral infection, e.g. glandular fever (late teens).
- **Has the patient travelled overseas recently?**
- **Are there other features of malignant disease?** Weight loss/cachexia, lethargy, malaise. Generalized lymphadenopathy, sweating, skin itching associated with lymphoma.
- **Are there features of thyroid disease?** Thyrotoxic (tremor, tachycardia/AF, perspiration, lid lag, thyroid eye disease, bruit.), hypothyroid (dry hair/skin, xanthelasma, puffy face, croaky voice).

Examination

Examine the entire head and neck including the mouth (infections and malignancy). You may also need to examine other body sites and systems (lymphadenopathy, abdominal masses, liver, spleen, etc.).

The patient must be:

- comfortable—as relaxed as possible and in a warm room;
- sitting upright;
- uncovered—so that you can see the clavicles;
- well illuminated.

Look

- Start by standing back and simply observing the patient from the front and then the lateral views.
- Is there an obvious lesion/lump? Note its site, size, and shape—think of underlying anatomical structures.
- Does the ear lobe stick out? (Parotid swelling.).
- Get the patient to drink some water (if not an emergency!)—does the lump move up on swallowing? If so it must be attached to the tongue or upper airway.
- Get the patient to stick out their tongue. If the lump moves up it will be attached to it somewhere (classically seen in thyroglossal cysts).
- Is the overlying skin normal or changed? Is the skin tethered or is there a discharging sinus?
- Look at the scalp, the skin of the face and in the mouth—are there any lesions that could cause inflammatory or metastatic neck swellings (lymphadenopathy)?
- Is there evidence of systemic disease? Is the patient anaemic, cachexic, or are there signs of thyroid disease?
- Look at the nursing charts—what is the temperature?

Feel

Examine as many necks as possible until you are familiar with the 'normal'. All necks have irregularities, palpable lumps, depressions, etc., which are normal findings. For instance, you can often feel ptotic submandibular glands in the elderly. Only when you are familiar with the normal are you likely to pick up abnormal findings.

There are different ways to examine the neck. Some clinicians feel both sides simultaneously for asymmetry, others feel each in turn—that way you can laterally flex the neck and feel deep into the submandibular triangle. Try both and decide for yourself but don't throttle the patient!

Standing behind the patient, gently but firmly rest your fingertips under the lower border of the mandible under the chin. Palpate the submental area moving posteriorly to the submandibular areas feeling for abnormal or painful masses. Feel *along the side* mandible as well as below, lymph nodes are commonly found in the lower face, but should be considered as part of the neck. Palpate the depression behind the ramus, below the ear lobe—an important site for parotid swellings. Follow on by feeling down the anterior border of sterno-mastoid to the sternal notch, and then staying in the mid-line move back superiorly to the submental area where you started. Palpate the posterior triangle behind the SCM, the supraclvicular areas, and the occipital scalp for lymphadenopathy/masses. By laterally flexing the neck *gently* grab the SCM and try to feel deep to it—this is an important and often missed area of examination. It is where many lymph nodes lay.

If there is an unusual mass, note:
- site, size, shape, including nature of surface;
- fixed or mobile;
- consistencey, e.g. cystic or solid, soft or hard, fluctuance;
- tender;
- pulsatile;
- transillumination.

Other useful examination techniques
- Fibre optic nasendoscopy—to assess the nasopharynx for occult primary tumours to complete the head and neck examination.
- Auscultation—listen over the mass with a stethoscope. Is there a thyroid bruit present?
- Illumination—cystic hygromas (congenital cavernous lymphangioma) transilluminate brilliantly.

Investigations

Fine needle aspiration (FNA)

A fine-bore needle ('green' gauge) attached to a 20 ml syringe is passed into the mass while it is immobilized between the fingers of the other hand. Negative pressure is applied by withdrawing the plunger of the syringe, thus collecting cells from the lesion into the needle/syringe. A sample is then placed on a microscope slide and a thin film made by passing a second slide over it—this may then be air dried or fixed, depending on local protocols. The slide is then viewed by an experienced histopathologist to give a report on the nature of the cells of the lesion. Comment can be made as to whether the cells show malignant features or not, although a definitive diagnosis cannot be made as the architecture of the lesion cannot be seen. This is quite an 'operator sensitive' technique and on occasion a non-diagnostic sample is made.

Caution should be applied to the use of FNA in assessing salivary gland tumours, especially when there is some doubt as to whether the presenting lesion is benign or malignant.

Ultrasound

Ultrasound is useful for distinguishing between solid and cystic lesions and may be used to guide biopsy needles to sample masses or aspirate collections. It proves particularly useful for the investigation of salivary gland lesions as it has particular value in assessing suspected inflammation and tumours. Ultrasound may also be able to distinguish whether a suspected tumour is benign or malignant: benign masses, such as adenomas, are generally echo-poor with well-defined margins, whereas malignant conditions are generally ill defined, and are often lobulated with a heterogeneous echo texture.

Sialogram

Sialography involves the injection of a radiopaque medium into salivary ducts and the use of plain radiographs. It is a useful process in the investigation of neck swellings when salivary gland aetiology is suspected. It may be used to demonstrate salivary calculi or duct strictures when there is an obstructive history. It may also show pathological processes within the gland, or sometimes outside, compressing it. A plain film should be taken prior to the procedure (a 'control' film). This may show obvious calculi and so negate the need to proceed to formal sialography.

Acute infection and iodine sensitivity are contra-indications to sialography.

Computerized tomographic scanning (CTS)

CT scanning is exceptionally useful in assessing the extent of neck swellings particularly invasion into deeper tissues. However, artefact produced by metal in dental restorations often cause problems when investigating lesions in the floor of the mouth and upper neck.

Magnetic resonance imaging (MRI)

MRI is useful in the head and neck as it produces images with excellent soft tissue definition and so is particularly useful for the assessment of salivary glands and other neck masses. It has the advantage of not using radiation. Its use is contra-indicated in patients with metal implants such as aneurysm clips or cardiac pacemakers.

Radio-isotope imaging

In the assessment of neck swellings this technique is useful in the assessment of salivary and thyroid function. The images however do give relatively poor spatial resolution and the radiation dose can be relatively high so its use is limited.

Lymphadenopathy

Enlarged cervical lymph nodes—cervical lymphadenopathy, represent the most common cause of swellings in the neck. Lymphadenopathy in the neck (especially supraclavicular) can arise from disease both above *and* below the collar bones (eg Bronchial/gastric malignancy).

Possible causes of enlarged, palpable lymph nodes include:
- **local causes:**
  - infection—dental infections, tonsillitis, skin sepsis, TB neck nodes;
  - neoplastic—lymphoma or metastatic (anywhere in the head and neck);
  - parotid nodes;
  - developmental;
- **generalized causes:**
  - infection—URTI, infective mononucleosis, toxoplasma, cat-scatch fever, HIV;
  - sarcoidosis;
  - **Hodgkin's disease, non-Hodgkin's lymphoma, lymphatic leukaemia.**

Infection

Acute infections are the commonest cause of lymph node enlargement in patients under 40. They are generally viral (colds, glandular fever, etc.) or bacteriological (dental infections, tonsillitis, scalp infections such as impetigo). Tuberculosis is a chronic inflammatory cause that has seen an increase in incidence in recent years. TB lymph nodes tend to be firm and indurated and often give rise to sinuses.

Neoplastic

Primary: Hodgkin's disease and non-Hodgkin's lymphomas
Lymphomas are malignant neoplasms of lymphoid tissue. They are broadly divided into Hodgkin's and non-Hodgkin's type with further subdivisions made on histological and immunological criteria. Hodgkin's disease is a neoplastic process affecting the lymphatics—in 80% of case the cervical lymph nodes are involved. Some patients present with systemic symptoms such as weight loss, fever, and night sweats (type B symptoms). Diagnosis is confirmed by biopsy.

Secondary: metastatic disease
Enlarged cervical lymph nodes, secondary to head and neck malignancy are a common cause of neck swellings. It has been shown that in approximately 90% of cases spread to the cervical lymph nodes occurs in an ordered fashion (superior nodes being involved before inferior nodes). The pattern of cervical lymph node involvement not only dictates the nature of treatment, but is also the single most important prognostic factor in determining patients' survival. Of particular importance is the level and frequency of node involvement and the presence (or absence) of extra-capsular spread.

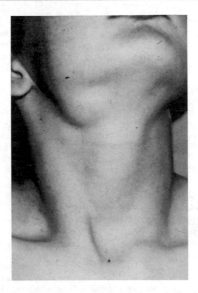

Fig. 6.20 Submandibular swelling. Is it an enlarged salivary gland or lymphnode?

Congenital
Cystic hygroma—also termed a cavernous lymphangioma is said to be a congenital lesion arising from an embryonic remnant of the jugular lymph sac. Approximately 65% are present at birth and the remainder become apparent before the child's second birthday. On clinical examination these lesions are classically described as being able to transilliminate. Haemangioma can also present in the neck. If deep, discolouration may not be that obvious.

Thyroid/thyroglossal cyst
The thyroid gland lies in the mid-line of the lower third of the neck behind the pre-tracheal fascia; it is a bi-lobed gland with a central isthmus. Assessment of a thyroid lesion essentially involves two questions:

- **Is it a generalized enlargement of the gland or a solitary nodule?**
  - Enlargement of the whole gland is called a 'goitre'.
  - A solitary nodule may be benign or malignant (primary or secondary).
- **What is the patient's thyroid status?**
  - Euthyroid, i.e. normal.
  - Thyrotoxic, i.e. over-active—tiredness, weight loss, anxiety, palpitations and tremor.
  - Myxoedematous, i.e. under active: such patients tend to be overweight, have thick skin and thinning hair, and be slow in thought and speech.

Goitres
- **Physiological**—seen during pregnancy, at puberty and in conditions of iodine deficiency (less commonly seen in present day).
- **Inflammatory**—De Quervain's Thyroiditis, Hashimoto's Thyroiditis, Riedel's Thyroiditis.
- **Nodular**—this is a simple benign enlargement of the thyroid gland and only necessitates treatment if the patient becomes thyrotoxic, concerned with its appearance, or presents with symptoms of compression of adjacent structures, e.g. dysphagia or dyspnoea. Malignant change is possible and may present with a local increase in size or hoarseness of the voice due to recurrent laryngeal nerve involvement.
- **Toxic**—Graves' disease.

Solitary thyroid nodule
- **Cyst**—usually a degenerative part of a nodular goitre although true cysts are seen. Haemorrhage into the cyst is a common complication and will present with pain and rapid enlargement that may compress adjacent structures.
- **Adenoma**—may produce thyrotoxicosis if functioning. Subdivided into histological type: papillary, follicular, embryonal, and hurtle cell.
- **Papillary adenocarcinoma**—seen in younger age groups; low grade and rarely fatal.
- **Follicular adenocarcinoma**—a malignancy of middle age; bony metastases are common.
- **Anaplastic carcinoma**—an aggressive malignancy of the elderly; metastatic disease at presentation is common.
- **Medullary carcinoma**—seen in all age groups with equal sex incidence; moderate malignant potential spreading to lymph nodes.
- **Malignant lymphoma**—may occur in lymphatic tissue within the thyroid gland or as secondaries.
- **Secondary**—direct spread from adjacent malignancies or metastatic spread, most commonly from breast, renal, colon, lung.

Thyroglossal cyst

During embryological development the thyroid gland reaches its final anatomical position in front of the 2nd and 3rd tracheal rings having descended through the neck from its origin at the foramen caecum. Epithelial remnants along this embryological pathway may persist and form thyroglossal cysts. Clinically the vast majority of patients present with a mobile, painless neck swelling that transilluminates and fluctuates. **Because of its links with the thyroid gland the lesion will move in the vertical plane with swallowing. If it remains attached to the tongue it will also move up on tongue protrusion.** Other features include:

- commonest age of presentation is 5–10 years;
- 90% are mid-line lesions, although 10% lie laterally (frequently left);
- 75% are pre-hyoid;
- 25% are at the level of the thyroid or cricoid cartilage;

Management involves the surgical removal of the cyst and its tract that may incorporate the central portion of the hyoid bone (sistrunk procedure).

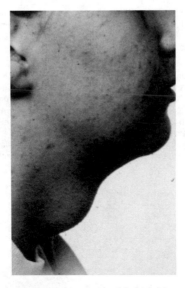

Fig. 6.21 Thyroglossal cyst. Ask the patient to stick out their tongue.

Carotid body tumour

Tumours of the carotid body (chemodectomas) are rare, slow-growing ovoid lesions arising in the carotid bifurcation, distorting and encasing the carotid vessels. They occur over a wide age range although are most commonly seen in patients in their fifties. Chronic hypoxia has been reported as a causal factor and the tumours are said to have a high incidence in high altitude areas, such as Mexico City and Peru. A familial tendency has also been reported, around 30% of familial tumours are said to be bilateral. Of the non-familial tumours 10% are bilateral.

Carotid body tumours are slow growing, although they may eventually become locally invasive or even metastasise via the lymphatics or the blood. The incidence of metastases has been reported between 2.5 and 50% and indeed some surgeons consider all these tumours as malignant. Left untreated about 5–10% will develop metastases within 10 years.

Clinical features

Patients are usually aged over 50 years and present with solitary or bilateral lumps in the neck at the level of the carotid bifurcation. The tumours are just in front of and deep to the anterior border of the sternocleidomastoid muscle, usually at the level of the hyoid bone. The lesion will transmit the carotid pulse rather than being pulsatile itself. It can be moved laterally (displacing the carotid pulse) but not vertically. Occasionally pressure on the carotid sinus by the tumour may cause fainting attacks.

Investigations

Carotid arteriography is the investigation of choice and will show a splayed carotid bifurcation containing a highly vascular tumour; it is useful in defining the extent of the tumour and also in establishing the adequacy of collateral blood flow through the other carotid artery.

Management

Surgical excision is the management of choice in the young patient as left untreated carotid vessel obstruction may ensue; there is also a greater risk of malignancy as their size increases, and the larger the tumour the more difficult the surgery. It is often possible to dissect the tumour away from the carotid vessels; if it is necessary to sacrifice the vessels graft replacement of the artery is performed.

In the elderly, frail patient, these slow growing tumours are often simply watched as the surgery to remove them is certainly not without risk.

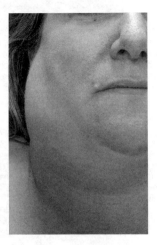

Fig. 6.22 Branchial cyst.

Branchial cyst

After the thyroglossal cyst, the branchial (lateral cervical) cyst is the second most common congenital swelling in the neck. It is thought that branchial cysts develop from remnants of the second branchial cleft in the neck, and in some cases tracts are found running from the deep surface of these cysts to the pharyngeal wall. However, it has also been postulated that branchial cysts are simply cystic degeneration in cervical lymphatic tissue, as almost all branchial cysts are found to have lymphoid tissue in their walls; hence the alternative name of lateral cervical cyst.

Clinical features

Most lesions present in the third decade of life and show equal sex distribution. Patients complain of an enlarging mass arising from behind the anterior border of the junction of the upper and middle thirds of the sternomastoid muscle. Frequently the cyst may appear as a swelling during an upper respiratory tract infection, which may be painful and persist after the infection has been treated. Recurrent infections can result in a firm, fixed mass which are adherent to surrounding structures such as the jugular vein, proving difficult to excise surgically.

Investigations

Diagnosis is usually made on the basis of the history and the site of the swelling. However, fine needle aspiration biopsy can prove useful by producing an opalescent fluid containing cholesterol crystals or frank pus.

Management

Surgical excision of the lesion is the treatment of choice following management of infections with appropriate antibiotics. All of the cyst lining should be removed as any remaining remnants may result in recurrence or a chronic discharging sinus from the wound.

Branchial sinus/branchial fistula

A branchial sinus is a small opening found over the anterior border of sternomastoid, which may discharge a mucous secretion. They are generally present at birth but may present in later life as a consequence of a ruptured, chronically infected branchial cyst (a secondary branchial cyst). The sinus can extend supero-medially between the internal and external carotid arteries to open onto the lateral wall of the pharynx forming a branchial fistula.

Pharyngeal pouch

This is a mucosal protrusion (diverticulum) of the pharyngeal wall through part of the inferior pharyngeal constrictor muscle (thyropharyngeus and cricopharyngeus). Patients often give a history of a hiatus hernia (with heartburn and acid reflux). It is thought that the pouch arises as a result of a relative obstruction or spasm at the level of cricopharyngeus caused by hypertrophy of the muscle attempting to prevent overflow of reflux contents into the larynx.

A weak area between thyropharyngeus and cricopharyngeus known as Killian's dehiscence, is situated posteriorly. It is here the pouch originates, above the spasm of cricopharyngeus.

Clinical features

More commonly seen in males and the elderly where they often have a long, symptom-free development. Patients complain of dysphagia (difficulty swallowing), associated with regurgitation of undigested food and consequent weight loss. Often the first mouthful is easily swallowed, but as the pouch becomes full it obstructs the oesophagus and hence dysphagia develops with regurgitation. A palpable neck swelling low down in the anterior triangle may be felt which produces a characteriztic squelch on pressure and gurgling on auscultation due to free fluid in the pouch. Recurrent respiratory infections are a common feature along with coughing fits, especially at night, due to inhalation of regurgitated contents of the pouch. Neoplasia has been reported in less than 1% of pouches.

Investigation

Diagnosis of a pharyngeal pouch is easily confirmed by a barium swallow of the upper neck.

Management

Surgical management is by excision of the pouch along with release of the cricopharyngeal spasm by myotomy. Nasogastric feeding should be continued for five days to reduce the chance of fistula formation.

In high-risk patients, excision of the pouch (diverticulectomy) may be replaced by simple inversion and oversewing. However, this procedure does not allow for the histological assessment of the pouch and a carcinoma may be missed.

Cervical rib

In approximately 0.5–1% of the population, the costal element of the lowest (7th) cervical vertebra overdevelops to form a cervical rib. This may range from a fibrous strand to a fully formed bone attaching to the first rib. In 50% of cases the cervical rib is seen to be unilateral, usually on the right, and anteriorly can be palpated as a fixed, hard swelling in the supraclavicular fossa where it can mimic neoplastic disease.

The cervical rib itself rarely cause symptoms, but its presence may cause disturbance of the function of the adjacent subclavian vessels and the brachial plexus resulting in symptoms of **thoracic outlet syndrome**.

Clinical features

The condition occurs equally in both sexes and is usually first noticed in the late teens when the neck extends and the shoulders droop. The patient may be aware of tenderness or swelling in the neck along with pain on the affected side due to vascular insufficiency. Exercise will exacerbate these symptoms, especially if the arm is pulled down, and the hand may be cold and pale as a result of distal ischaemia. Rarely the patient may present with a neurological deficit, including paraesthesia in the forearm and weakness of the hand. Close examination may reveal signs of ischaemia or emboli in the hand and the radial pulse may disappear if the arm is elevated. Auscultation may elicit a bruit over the subclavian artery.

Investigation

A cervical spine radiograph (X-ray) will show a bony cervical rib. In the absence of a bony rib close examination of the film may show a prominence of the anterior tubercle of the 7th cervical vertebra which could be associated with a fibrous band.

Post stenotic dilatation of the subclavian artery caused by the cervical rib may be demonstrated by angiography, particularly if the arm is elevated.

Management

Physiotherapy may improve muscles that elevate the arm and support the upper limb girdle in case where cervical rib causes mild neurological symptoms. Surgical excision should be considered if a cervical rib is causing vascular or marked neurological symptoms.

Subclavian aneurysm

Aneurysms of the subclavian artery were originally described in dock labourers and coal heavers where the strain of lifting heavy loads produced raised thoracic pressure causing the subclavian artery to be constantly occluded against the clavicle. Mechanization has now almost abolished this particular occupational hazard. Aneurysyms at this site are now generally found in association with a cervical rib as a post stenotic dilatation: a 'false' aneurysm.

Clinical features

The patient may present with the features of a cervical rib and thoracic outlet syndrome. They may have noticed a mass or pulsation in the neck and clinically a bruit may be heard over the artery in the supraclavicular fossa. The bruit may vary in differing degrees of abduction of the arm. Emboli from a subclavian aneurysm have the potential to cause patchy necrosis and gangrene of the hand and digits.

Investigation

Arteriography to show the extent of the aneurysm.

Management

Treatment of the cause, i.e. excision of the cervical rib if present. Following this the limits of the aneurysm are defined and the vessel is isolated before it is cross-clamped and the aneurysm resected. Often it is necessary to replace the aneurysm by a segment of long saphenous vein or a prosthetic graft.

Salivary glands

Any swelling of the glands may present as a swelling in the neck. It is unusual for the sublingual gland to produce a true neck swelling except in the case of a plunging ranula which is essentially a huge mucous extravasation pseudo-cyst of the sublingual gland.

The causes of salivary gland swelling are in essence threefold: obstructive, infective, and neoplastic. These may occur in isolation although more frequently may co-exist: for example, a neoplasia may produce obstructive symptoms.

Obstructive

Obstruction of any part of the salivary gland duct system may result in a build up of salivary secretions and hence a swelling. The degree of the swelling depends on the site of obstruction and to what degree the obstruction blocks drainage. With recurrent bouts of obstruction infection may supersede due to stagnation of secretions.

The classic history is of swelling associated with meal times as gustatory secretion is stimulated—the patient may report that the swelling settles a few hours after the end of eating.

Salivary calculi

Form as a result of calcium deposition around a nidus of organic material. Of salivary stones, 80% form in the submandibular gland and 10% in the parotid; they are usually unilateral and males are affected twice as often as females. Of submandibular gland stones, 20% are radiolucent, in which case sialography is indicated to locate them. Those in the floor of the mouth may be removed through a local incision under local anaesthetic. However, recurrent damage to the gland may necessitate its removal.

Duct strictures

Usually formed as a result of chronic trauma or iatrogenic injury (poor surgical technique), but may also be caused by ulceration around a salivary calculus. As a result fibrosis ensues and leads to duct stenosis which produces obstructive symptoms.

Neoplasia

May present with obstructive symptoms.

Infective

Infective causes of salivary gland swelling usually present with painful, red, warm, tender swellings at the site of the main gland. The regional lymph nodes may be enlarged and tender and a pustulous discharge may exude from the duct orifice. Patients generally present with progressive malaise and systemic upset.

Mumps

Bilateral painful parotid swelling due to a paramyxovirus; highly infectious generally affecting children, with an incubation period of 21 days. Immunity is long lasting after an attack.

Suppurative parotitis

Seen in debilitated patients, particularly post-operatively, as a result of xerostomia secondary to dehydration. Management includes rehydration and appropriate antibiotic therapy.

Chronic sialadenitis

Usually a complication of duct obstruction.

Neoplastic

Salivary gland tumours are the second most common neoplasms of the head and neck after oro-pharyngeal squamous cell carcinomas. The current incidence in Europe of salivary gland cancer is reported at 1.2 per 100 000 population. Of all salivary gland tumours 70–80% arise in the parotid—of these 75% are pleomorphic adenomas and 10–15% are malignant.

⑦ Difficulty in swallowing (dysphagia) and aspiration

Normal swallowing

In order to better understand dysphagia, it is helpful to first understand the mechanism and stages of a normal swallow. On average, people swallow once or twice every minute, to clear saliva and mucous from the oro- and naso-pharynx. It takes approximately one second. Dysphagia, even when only mild or intermittent, affects the ability to enjoy almost all other aspects of life. Aspiration is the intrusion of food or liquid into the unprotected airway below the level of the vocal folds. This can lead to infections of the respiratory system, pnemonitis and pneumonia.

1 The pre-oral stage

Normal requirements

Sight, smell, taste, co-ordination.

Problems

- Loss of smell and taste following surgery and/or radiotherapy.
- Xerostomia following irradiation of salivary glands.
- Poor posture.
- Inco-ordination of head, arm, trunk, neck, tongue, lips, and jaw.

2 The oral stage

Normal requirements

Food or liquid enters the oral cavity. Tight lip closure prevents loss of material. The tongue and mandible function to move the food bolus later-ally onto the teeth for mastication. Saliva containing digestive enzymes assists in softening and moistening the bolus, begins the digestive process and helps to provide taste. Typically, breathing is nasal and the velum (soft palate) is lowered. The food or liquid bolus is then squeezed by the tongue against the hard palate and moved posteriorily towards the hypopharynx. The velum then begins to elevate to close off the nasopharynx.

Problems

- Ineffective lip seal results in drooling, an inability to suck, take food from a spoon/cup, or initiate a swallow.
- Poor tongue movement (e.g. following glossectomy) results in inability to position food between teeth for chewing, form a bolus or control liquid and propel food into the pharynx. This leads to pooling/stasis of food in the oral cavity, particularly on the side affected by surgery.
- Cleft palate or reduced velopharyngeal seal results in nasal regurgitation.
- Loss of bolus into pharynx or larynx results in aspiration.
- Poor chewing as a result of poor alignment of teeth, dental extraction, soreness, swelling and inability to wear dentures.
- Xerostomia or excessive drooling (ptyalism)

3 The pharyngeal stage

Normal requirements

This stage triggers the swallow reflex as the bolus or liquid comes into contact with the pillars of the fauces. The velum elevates, contacts the posterior pharyngeal wall and closes off the nasal cavity. The larynx is pulled upwards and the epiglottis tips down over it to protect the airway. Closure of the laryngeal valve system occurs with the false and true vocal folds closing simultaneously. The bolus or liquid moves over the closed airway and passes through the cricopharyngeal sphincter at the top of the digestive tract.

Problems
- Delayed or absent swallow reflex due to post-operative swelling or reduction in sensation from cranial nerve injury. Mis-timing of the swallow results and the bolus or liquid falls into the pharynx and then into the unprotected airway resulting in aspiration.
- Restricted laryngeal elevation results in unsatisfactory closure of the larynx and aspiration.
- Vocal fold paralysis following cranial nerve injury results in aspiration.
- Reduced pharyngeal motility results in food and liquid pooling in pockets either side of the larynx. Food residue can build up on the pharyngeal walls so food and liquid spill over into airway causing aspiration.
- The presence of a tracheostomy tube can restrict laryngeal elevation. Food particles can pool on top of the inflated cuff so bacterial colonisation can occur. Since inflated tracheostomy tube cuffs do not always prevent aspiration there is a risk of aspiration pneumonia

4 The oesophageal stage
Normal requirements
The bolus and liquid enter the oesophagus and are propelled towards the stomach by peristalsis.

Problems
- Ineffective peristalsis hinders the passage of food to the stomach.
- Incomplete or constricted cricopharyngeal and cardiac sphincters hinder passage of food to stomach.

NB Gag reflex does not provide significant information about the swallow reflex.

Cough reflex. This is a protective reflex triggered when food/fluid enters the larynx and touches the vocal folds. It may be absent in neurologically impaired patients and silent aspiration may occur.

Signs of aspiration
Acute:
- distress;
- coughing, choking, and gasping;
- respiratory difficulty—wheezing or gurgling;
- loss of voice or gurgling 'wet' sounding voice;
- change of colour (greyness);
- tachycardia and sweating.

Chronic:
- respiratory problems/chest infections;
- coughing and choking;
- excess oral secretions;
- loss of weight;
- hunger;
- refusal to eat.

Silent aspiration—patients with loss of sensation in the larynx may aspirate without coughing and without awareness of the problem. Nasogastric tubes may also be easily passed into the trachea without obvious signs.

Speech disorders
Normal speech is dependent upon normal:
- nervous system;
- hearing;
- respiratory system including both lower (trachea, bronchi, and lungs) and upper nasal cavity;
- oropharynx including lips, cheeks, tongue, dentition, and larynx.

Assessment of dysphagia
Objective assessment
These are required if aspiration or a pharyngeal stage deficit is suspected.

Fiberoptic nasendoscopy
By inserting the fiberoptic scope into the nares and over the velum, it is possible to view the pharynx and larynx before, during and after the swallow. A blue dyed bolus or milk are often swallowed. Patient tolerance will naturally vary. The advantages are a comprehensive and objective picture of the pharyngeal stage of swallow, which does not expose the patient to radiation.

Videofluoroscopy (modified barium swallow)
Videofluoroscopic assessment of swallowing is a radiographic evaluation documenting the passage of a bolus through the oral, pharyngeal and oesophageal stages of the swallow and identifying the therapeutic manoeuvres for safe and adequate oral intake. A teaspoon of barium liquid and a small quantity of paste of biscuit consistency is taken. Following each swallow the oral cavity and pharynx are kept in view rather than following the bolus into the oesophagus. The procedure is viewed on a monitor and videotaped.

Management of dysphagia
Alternative feeding methods
- The naso-gastric tube—this is usually only used in the short term. It can cause the patient discomfort and has care is required in placement and confirming its position. It is usually not retained for more than one month.
- The percutaneous endoscopic gastrostomy (PEG)—patients' often find this method more comfortable and recent research shows that patients' weight and nutritional parameters are maintained or improved on PEG feeds

Swallowing rehabilitation
A variety of exercises may be given to a patient. Full range of motion exercises will not be attempted until the surgeon agrees that is safe to do without interfering with the healing process.

1 Posture
It is always helpful for patients to sit in an upright and straight position. Keeping the head up and discouraging the head dropping forward greatly reduces drooling and aids swallowing.

Postural variations:

- **Tilting** head to the *unaffected* side—useful in patients with unilateral tongue dysfunction. The bolus should be placed on the side which has most movement and sensation. The head should be *tilted* before the bolus is presented otherwise it will fall onto the damaged side and cannot be retrieved.
- **Turning** head to the *affected* side—useful in patients' who have undergone more extensive resections, possibly involving the pharynx and or larynx. The patient *turns* his head to the affected side before placing the bolus in the mouth. This closes the pyriform sinus on that side and helps reduce the amount of pharyngeal pooling, which may be occurring.
- **The flexed head position**—useful when the patient is unable to hold the bolus effectively and/or there is a delay in triggering the swallow. The chin is placed down whilst food is presented thus preventing leakage into the hypopharynx.
- **Tipping the head backwards**—caution must be taken using this position. Useful in patients with total glossectomy as it allows gravity to help speed up oral transit. Aspiration is increased especially if there is a problem in the pharyngeal stage. To increase safety this technique can be combined with the supra-glottic swallow.
- **The supra-glottic swallow**—useful with most neurological dysphagias and with patients who have both oral stage difficulties and reflexive airway protection. It can be practiced without a bolus. Make sure the patient is sitting upright.
- Take a breath and hold it tightly (this encourages vocal fold closure).
- Take a sip/mouthful of food and keep holding breath.
- Swallow hard, still holding breath.
- Cough out hard or clear throat.
- Pause before next swallow.
- Remain seated in upright posture for 20 min after eating.

2 Prosthetics

Prosthetic devices can greatly aid the rehabilitation of swallowing after oral surgery. They help by narrowing the space between the hard palate and remaining tongue. They are known as 'palatal augmentation prosthesis', 'palatal lowering devices' and 'obturators'. They are of particular use when masticating food. The oral cavity is made smaller so residual tongue movement is more efficient, and they can aid in the raising of the velum to prevent nasal regurgitation of liquids and food.

3 Food presentation

Close liaison with the dietitian, catering department, and nursing staff is essential when recommending suitable textures and consistencies of desirable foods. Usually recommended are pureed, thickened liquids, and a soft diet, but the levels of consistency must be correct to help the patient swallow successfully. The presentation of puréed food in particular is often the deciding factor in whether a patient perseveres with their swallowing or not. Puréeing the individual vegetables and meat separately and using commercially available food moulds to shape the purée into pleasant appetizing food shapes, greatly enhances presentation making the food far more palatable and attractive to the patient. Both the dietitian and speech and language therapist will have lists and recipe books of suitable foods.

4 Feeding aids

There are a variety of commercially available feeding spoons, dysphagia cups, and mugs. They help the manoeuvring and propulsion of food and liquid. The spoons have small bowls and long handles for ease of placement. Because they are made of strong, smooth plastic they are less irritating and abrasive in sore mouths and without the metallic taste often experienced after irradiation. The therapist will advise on the appropriate aid.

5 Oral hygiene

Close liaison is required to help promote the best oral hygiene regime possible for post-surgical patients. These patients often need careful guidance and much encouragement to remember to keep their mouths clean. Swelling, soreness and xerostomia can make this difficult for them.

⑦ Tracheostomies

Indications include:
● upper airway obstruction;
● prevention of aspiration of fluids (cuffed tube);
● retention of secretions (access for suctioning);
● respiratory insufficiency (respiratory, cardiac or neurological disease).

This should be an *elective* procedure. Tracheostomy tubes are placed through a small incision midway between the cricoid cartilage and suprasternal notch. Tissues are separated keeping to the mid-line of the neck. Meticulous haemostasis is essential at all times. Often the thyroid isthmus obstructs access to the trachea and needs to be securely ligated and divided. The thyroid is a highly vascular organ and carelessness in doing so can result in profound bleeding post-operatively. Once the anterior part of the trachea is defined it is opened, the endotracheal tube withdrawn and the tracheostomy tube inserted into the lumen. Several different access openings in the trachea have been described—a verticle slit, cutting a small hole or the 'Bjork' flap, which is U-shaped and remains attached inferiorly. Each has its own merits and which is chosen is down to the operating surgeon. Once in place the flanges of the tube need to be securely fastened to the patient and the wound closed.

Complications include:
● displacement of the tube;
● tube obstruction from secretions or crusting;
● bleeding;
● tracheal stenosis;
● local tissue injury;
● vocal cord paralysis (the recurrent laryngeal nerve runs alongside the trachea);
● emphysema and pneumothorax;
● chest infection;
● difficulty in re-intubation.

Although providing direct access to the lower respiratory tract for suction by by-passing the larynx, many patients find it difficult to produce an 'explosive' cough, useful in clearing secretions from the lungs. However they can be taught to expectorate, physiotherapists encouraging 'huffing' using the diaphragm. With a cooperative and well humidified patient, very little suction is required; most patients can effectively clear their lungs on their own.

Facial pain and palsy

⑦ Anatomy and physiology of pain

There are two types of pain fibres:
- A-delta ('fast' pain) fibres—these conduct quickly and are responsible for the acute sense of pain (sharp, pricking);
- C-type (slow pain) fibres—these conduct slowly and are associated with a dull aching, nagging pain.

Following noxious stimuli (heat, pressure, cuts, etc.), receptors sensitive to these, release metabolites such as bradykinin, prostaglandins, and H^+ ions. These act on neural receptors initiating impulses in the nerve.

Regulation of pain

Pain fibres initially synapse in the dorsal horn of the spinal cord where impulses are relayed via the spinothalamic and anterolateral tracts to the midbrain and thalamus. Inhibitory impulses also pass down to the dorsal horn, while other fibres activate encephalin release, inhibiting transmission.

In addition, transmission of pain impulses is influenced by the **'gating mechanism',** located in the substantia gelatinosa of the dorsal horn. This gate 'opens' in response to pain peripherally. However stimulation of large sensory non-pain fibres is thought to inhibit pain transmission by 'closing' the gate. Pain impulses from peripheral nerves can therefore be prevented from reaching the brain by other non-pain nerve fibres. This explains why we rub injured areas and also the basis of TENS.

The cortex can also discriminate the site of the pain, its distribution, possible cause, and, together with adrenaline, can exert an inhibitory influence—sports injuries are often not apparent until after the game.

⑦ Anatomy and physiology of oro-facial pain

The **upper cervical nerves** carrying pain impulses from the cervical spine, back of the head, and the neck, converge with **trigeminal** sensory neurons in the dorsal horn—the 'trigeminocervical complex'. This convergence is the basis for referred pain from the neck to the face and head. Facial sensation is principally from the trigeminal nerve, although there is some contribution from the **facial** and **vagus** nerves.

The posterior aspect of the tongue, tonsils, tympanic cavity, and the pharynx are innervated by the **glossopharyngeal** nerve. The cornea and dental pulp are predominately innervated by pain fibres.

There is a large representation of the oro-facial region in the cerebral somatosensory system, accounting for the exquisite sensibility of the oro-facial tissues.

Types of pain
- 'Somatic' pain, i.e. arising from structures that one is generally aware of (skin, oral mucosa, joints, etc.), often subsides following healing. It is usually described as sharp or sore.
- 'Neuropathic' pain is due to injury to the nociceptive (pain) pathway and may persist long after healing has taken place. It is often described as burning, shooting, or like an electric shock. Injury may occur peripherally or centrally, anywhere along the neural pathway. This can occur following herpes zoster infection—'post-herpetic neuralgia'.
- 'Deafferentation'. This refers to partial or total loss of sensation in a localized area following loss or interruption of sensory fibres. Instead of a decrease in pain sensation in the affected area, spontaneous pain may develop. This is referred to as 'dysaesthesia'. It is occasionally seen following inferior alveolar or lingual nerve injury (e.g. after wisdom tooth removal)
- 'Allodynia' is pain caused by stimuli that would normally not produce pain, e.g. bedclothes producing a burning sensation.

Psychology of pain
The complex nature of pain is highlighted by anecdotes of severely wounded soldiers who do not complain of pain, or of athletes who are injured but do not experience pain until the contest is over. The way we perceive and react to pain is highly subjective and dependent upon the individual, current situation, and changes over time.

⑦ Oro-facial (idiopathic) pain syndromes

Trigeminal neuralgia and **atypical facial pain** are among the most challenging pain conditions in the oro-facial area. It is not always easy to distinguish between these and other diagnoses, but it is important to do so, as treatments and prognoses differ.

All forms of idiopathic facial pain syndromes should remain a 'diagnosis of exclusion', that is all other causes of facial pain should be considered and if necessary investigated for. Every now and then patients with odd pains turn out to have significant underlying disease, notably tumours.

Idiopathic facial pain makes up a significant portion of out-patient attendances. Four symptom complexes are described:

- **facial arthromyalgia** (FAM, temperomandibular joint dysfunction syndrome);
- **atypical facial pain** (non-joint or muscle pain);
- **atypical odontalgia;**
- **oral dysaesthesia** (oral sensory disturbances).

It has been suggested that these symptoms may form part of a whole-body pain syndrome involving the neck, back, abdomen, and skin. Adverse life events and impaired coping ability are the strongest known aetiological factors.

The aetiology of idiopathic facial pain is still unknown. It has been suggested that stress-induced neuropeptide inflammation within the tissues (e.g. TMJ) causes pain and local production of free radicals. Eicosinoids have been suggested as responsible for unexplained pain in non-joint areas including the teeth.

⑦ Overview of oro-facial pain

In 1994, the International Association for the Study of Pain revised its classification of chronic pain: This framework enables us to identify different diseases and syndromes and facilitate uniformity of information essential to research.

Odontalgia (toothache 1)

- Short-lasting diffuse pain due to exposed dentine. Evoked by local stimuli.
- Sharp or dull, mild to moderate pain lasting less than a second to minutes.

Protect defective area with a dressing or restoration, simple analgesics.

Pulpitis (toothache 2)

- Pain due to pulpal inflammation, evoked by local stimuli.
- Sharp, poorly localized, dull ache, or throbbing pain, moderate to severe, lasting minutes or hours, with episodes that may continue for several days.

Extirpation of the pulp, extraction, combination analgesics, e.g. NSAIDs and paracetamol.

Periapical periodontitis and abscess (toothache 3)

- Severe throbbing pain arising from the periodontal tissues.
- Continuous, well-localized, mild to intense aching, especially after hot or cold stimuli—may last a few minutes to several hours.

Extirpation or extraction, antibiotics, NSAIDs.

Atypical odontalgia (toothache 4)

- Severe throbbing pain in the tooth *without* major pathology.
- Often described as severe continual throbbing in teeth and gingivae. May vary from mild pain to intense pain, especially with hot or cold stimuli. It may be widespread or well localized, frequently precipitated by a dental procedure and may move from tooth to tooth. It may last a few minutes to several hours.
- May be a symptom of hypochondriacal psychosis or depression and there is often excessive concern with oral hygiene.

Counselling, avoidance of unnecessary pulp extirpations and extractions, anti-depressants, phenothiazines.

Glossodynia and sore mouth (also known as 'burning mouth' or 'oral dysesthesia')

- Burning pain in the tongue or mucous membranes.
- Burning, tender, nagging pain, usually constant, but may be variable, and increases in intensity from morning to evening. Occasionally associated with iron, vitamin B12, or folate deficiency.

Treat deficiency states. Often responds to tricyclic anti-depressants.

Cracked tooth syndrome

- Brief sharp pain in a tooth, due to cusp flexion and 'microleakage'.
- Moderate pain on biting, lasting a few seconds.

Repair cracked portion of the tooth. Simple analgesics.

Trigeminal herpes zoster
- Acute herpetic infection in the Vth cranial nerve.
- Burning, tingling pain with occasional lancinating components felt in the skin. Pain may precede or follow herpetic eruptions and last from one to several weeks.

Spontaneous permanent remission is common, although patient may progress to chronic (post-herpetic) neuralgia. In the acute phase, stellate ganglion blocks using local anaesthetic, such as bupivacaine, are indicated for severe pain. Transcutaneous Nerve Stimulation (TENS), capsaicin cream, and tricyclic anti-depressants are useful.

Post-herpetic neuralgia
- Chronic pain with skin changes in the distribution of the Vth cranial nerve following acute herpes zoster.
- Burning, tearing, itching dysaesthesias and crawling dysaesthesias in skin of affected areas of moderate intensity. Exacerbated by mechanical contact. May last for several years, spontaneous subsidence is not uncommon.

Combination therapy including capsaicin cream, TENS, tricyclic anti-depressants, supportive counselling.

Trigeminal neuralgia (tic douloureux)

Secondary neuralgia from central nervous system lesions
- Pains in the distribution of one or more branches of the Vth cranial nerve, due to recognized lesion (e.g. tumour, multiple sclerosis, aneurysm).
- May be indistinguishable from trigeminal neuralgia, or a constant, severe dull pain.

Treatment of the underlying cause. A combination of centrally-acting drugs such as carbamazepine, phenothiazines, tricyclic anti-depressants is useful.

Glossopharyngeal neuralgia (IXth cranial nerve)
- Sudden severe recurrent brief stabbing pains in the distribution of the glossopharyngeal nerve.
- Sharp, stabbing bouts of severe pain felt deep in throat or ear, often triggered by touch or swallowing and by ingestion of cold fluids. Episodes may interfere with eating and can last for weeks to several months and subside spontaneously. Recurrence is common.

Application of local anaesthetic to trigger point relieves the pain.

Temporomandibular pain and dysfunction syndrome

Rheumatoid arthritis of the temporomandibular joint

Dry socket

⑦ Assessment and measurement of pain

Simple methods of measuring pain rely upon assessing intensity. This should be assessed at regular intervals using a rating scale that the patient understands. Several scales have been developed to measure and document pain intensity and its response to therapy. By far the simplest tools that rely upon the patients report of pain are Visual Analogue Scales, where the patient marks on the line the intensity of their pain (see Fig. 7.1).

These scoring systems facilitate measurement and recording. They also proved useful in measuring and assessing the effectiveness of management of other symptoms such as nausea and vomiting.

For more complex assessment, the McGill Pain Questionnaire explores the sensory, affective, and evaluative dimensions of pain. This questionnaire is lengthy and dependent upon the patients level of understanding of the vocabulary. It is particularly useful in the assessment of chronic pain.

Consider also:

- Site of pain—this must be documented with reference to trigger points and/or referred pain. Use a body diagram and date each assessment to determine changes.
- Description of pain—terms include constant, intermittent, dull, aching, throbbing, sharp, burning, or shooting. Comparison to previous experience, e.g. like a knife, is helpful.
- Periodicity—speed of onset, duration, frequency, seasonality.
- Influences—does anything affect the pain e.g. movement, heat, or cold. Does the pain fluctuate during the 24-h period.
- Associated symptoms—swelling, jaw dysfunction, numbness or dysaesthesia, pain anywhere else.
- Previous therapies—has anything to date influenced the pain (analgesics, position, movement, time)?
- Past medical history.
- Social history—occupation, family situation, living conditions, smoking, alcohol consumption, employment, hobbies.

Visual Analogue Scale (VAS)

no pain -- worst pain imaginable

and Verbal Rating Scales which enable staff to demonstrate the intensity of the pain.

Verbal Rating Scale

0----------------   --1------------------2----------------3--------------------4
none   mild   moderate   severe   excruciating

0 = none
1 = mild
2 = moderate
3 = severe
4 = excruciating

Fig. 7.1 Visual analogue scales.

Assessing pain in children

Several tools are available for children, although difficulties arise in deciding which to apply for each age group. An adolescent can report and describe their pain as well as an adult, yet a baby cannot. It uses mainly vocal expressions, especially crying.

Physiological measures, such as tachycardia, reliably occur in infants who are in acute pain and therefore have been suggested as a way of assessing pain in infants. However, this response is non-specific and not sustained, making physiological indicators an unreliable method of recording chronic pain.

Other scales include the Children's Hospital of Eastern Ontario Pain Scale (CHEOPS), and the Princess Margaret Hospital Pain Assessment tool (PMHPAT), in assessing and measuring chronic pain in children. The CHEOPS scale was designed for 1–5-year-olds and consists of six groups of behaviour patterns: cry; facial expression; verbalizing; movements of torso and legs; and touching of the wound. The PMHPAT was designed for 7–14-year-olds and comprises of five elements indicative of pain: facial expression; nurse's assessment; position in bed; sounds; and self-assessment.

In order to assess children's pain effectively, it is necessary to measure more than one dimension of pain. The King's Healthcare Pain Assessment Tool for Children (PATCH) evolved in this way. It combines elements from five existing varieties of paediatric pain assessment scales: faces scale; body outline; numeric analogue scale; descriptive words; and a behavioural scale.

Post-operative pain

- Prevention is better than cure.
- Post-operative pain has inflammatory, nociceptive, neurogenic, and psychological components. Each will contribute to varying degrees and may need to be assessed individually.
- NSAIDs are good in relieving bone pain. They may be given peri-operatively as 'pre-emptive' analgesia and then continued post-operatively to minimalize pain.
- Short-acting opioids, such as intravenous fentanyl, are commonly used for peri-operative analgesia. A longer acting opioid, such as morphine, may be used for extension into the post-operative period. Traditional regimens include 4-hourly intra-muscular or subcutaneous opioids, as required. However, a common mode of administration is now via continuous intravenous infusion or 'patient controlled analgesia'. This allows the patient to titrate the analgesia to their pain. In doing so, they are more likely to remain within the 'therapeutic window'. Small pre-set doses can be given, reducing time delay in administration, but by limiting the amount given, preventing overdose.

Other techniques of pain control

These include:
- topical capsaicin;
- transcutaneous nerve stimulation (TENS);
- cryotherapy;
- acupuncture;
- sympathetic neural blockade;
- cognitive behavioural therapy;
- local heat (*not* extra-orally in infection);
- local or regional anaesthesia;
- splinting of fractures;
- radiotherapy;
- hypnosis;
- nitrous oxide.

Capsaicin is the active principle of hot chilli pepper and is a substance P depletor. This reduces the transmission of painful stimuli to higher centres. It is applied topically, in very small amounts, four times a day to the painful area and does not seem to be associated with any adverse side-effects. However, initial burning or stinging is often reported by patients.

Transcutaneous nerve stimulation (TENS) is thought to work via the gate control theory. Rubbing or massaging a painful area, or the application of pads through which an electrical current is passed, stimulates A-delta fibres. These are placed over the region of the pain or the associated dermatome Stimulation of the *non*-pain fibres closes the 'gate' by releasing inhibitory neurotransmitters. The result is that the patient feels less or no pain. TENS and some types of acupuncture are also thought to promote endogenous opiate release thereby reducing the pain sensation.

While the exact benefits of this treatment remain unclear, it has few side-effects and is best used in conjunction with medical therapy, such as previously described. In the head and neck it can be effective in post-herpatic neuralgia and other forms of deep seated facial pain.

Use of TENS is contra-indicated in patients with pacemakers and should be avoided over the carotid sinus. Safety in early pregnancy has not been established.

⑦ Temporomandibular dysfunction (TMJPDS)

An overview

- Although up to 70% of the general population may have at least one clinical feature of this disorder, only about 5% of those with one or more will actually seek treatment.
- Temporomandibular dysfunction is not always progressive or destructive. It is a complex disorder involving many interacting factors such as stress, anxiety, and depression.
- Non-surgical treatments, such as counselling, pharmacotherapy, and occlusal splint therapy, continue to be the most effective way of managing over 80% of patients.
- The three most common temporomandibular dysfunction disorders are myofascial pain and dysfunction, internal derangement, and osteoarthrosis.

Myofascial pain and dysfunction are by far the commonest. This is primarily a muscular problem resulting from 'parafunctional' habits, such as clenching or bruxism. Stress, anxiety, and depression are also commonly associated.

Internal derangement describes a temporomandibular disorder in which the articular disc is in an abnormal position, resulting in mechanical interference and restriction of the movement.

Osteoarthrosis is a localized degenerative disorder that affects mainly the articular cartilage of the temporomandibular joint. It is usually seen in older age groups.

Applied anatomy

The temporomandibular joint (TMJ) is the joint between the mandible and the skull base, located in the pre-auricular region. It is a synovial 'ball and socket' type joint, the 'ball' portion being the mandibular condyle, and the 'socket' the glenoid fossa of the temporal bone. A fibrous sleeve encapsulates the joint, and between the condyle and fossa there is a fibro-cartilaginous disc, or 'meniscus', which is attached peripherally to the deep surface of the joint capsule. The four muscles of mastication (the masseter, the temporalis, and the medial and lateral pterygoids) act directly across the TMJ to effect mandibular movements. Of note, the insertion of the lateral pterygoid is into both the condylar neck, and through the fibrous capsule, into the anterior aspect of the articular disc.

Movement across the joint is complex. On opening the mouth from the closed position initially a hinge-type movement occurs for the first 1 cm. After that a forward translation is added in which the condyle moves forward and downwards along the slope of the eminence. Very little movement occurs side to side. Appreciation of TMJ anatomy and function helps understand the clinical picture associated with fractures of the condyle.

Aetiology

This is a controversial area. Temporomandibular dysfunction/disorders is a **collective term** used to describe a number of related conditions affecting the joints, muscles of mastication, and associated structures.

These all result in common symptoms such as pain and limited mouth opening. No *single* condition has been found to cause temporomandibular dysfunction syndrome (TMJDS). Approximately 70% of the general population have at least one sign of TMJDS, yet only around 5% will actually seek treatment. Females outnumber male patients by at least four to one. Patients most commonly present in early adulthood.

Various aetiological factors have been suggested to contribute, but in reality it is likely that the condition is multi-factorial, with one cause exacerbating the effects of another.

Suggested aetiologies

Parafunction such as tooth clenching and grinding 'bruxism' (often subconsciously or during sleep), or abnormal movements of the jaw in function (e.g. a swing from left to right, reversed on closing—'chewing the cud'). Such movements often exert unbalanced forces on the joints, with one condyle translating further than the other, resulting in painful muscle spasm.

Occlusal anomalies are a common feature of patients with TMJ dysfunction and there is *may* be a higher frequency of TMJ problems in patients with heavily restored dentitions. However, there are plenty of patients who have abnormal bites yet do *not* have TMJ symptoms. Some studies have also suggested that poor dentures can contribute to TMJ dysfunction, especially in patients with loss of posterior support and those with reduced vertical facial height (short anterior face).

Trauma either directly from a blow, or indirectly from wide opening (e.g. for dental treatment). In these cases it is suggested that trauma may cause tears or adhesions affecting the disc, or a synovitis resulting in pain and altered function.

Stressful life events and impaired coping mechanisms are more frequent in patients with TMJ dysfunction compared to non-affected control patients. Anxiety neuroses, affective disorders (particularly depression), and somatoform disorders are also more common. These psychogenic factors are often considered as exacerbating factors rather than the primary cause of temporomandibular disorders.

However, it is well known that very few patients with malocclusion, mandibular trauma, or psychogenic illnesses actually go on to develop temporomandibular pain and dysfunction. It seems therefore, that only those who are vulnerable, will develop symptoms after an exacerbating event such as trauma.

Diagnosis

It has been suggested that up to 70% of the population have, at some time, experienced at least one episode of painful symptoms that can be attributed to TMJ dysfunction.

Three 'cardinal' features exist:

- pain;
- joint noise;
- restricted movement.

Pain is the most common presenting complaint and is by far the most difficult component to assess. It is characterized clinically by pain in and around the jaw joint, involving the muscles of mastication, and often radiating to the temple, jaw and into the neck. Patients often describe a dull, deep ache around the joint, which they may call 'earache', along with a superimposed sharper component, which may radiate over the side of the face. Patients may also report **clicking** of the joints with **limitation of the range of mouth opening**. Joint noise, however, is quite common in asymptomatic people in the general population, and is of little clinical importance in the absence of pain. When *mechanical* symptoms predominate the term 'internal derangement' is sometimes used, implying that there is a problem with the meniscus. However clicking is a common finding in the normal population and in the absence of other symptoms does not need treatment.

Clinical examination

Assess for tenderness in the muscles of mastication. Areas of tenderness, trigger points, and patterns of pain referral should be noted. Place the finger tips in the pre-auricular region just in front of the tragus of the ear and ask the patient to open and close their mouth—the finger tip should fall into a depression left by the translating condyle. Listen for joint sounds.

Assess mandibular function by noting whether the mouth opens in a straight line or deviates with jerky movements. Normal painless maximal opening should be around 40–55 mm, between the tips of the incisor teeth.

Diagnosis is essentially based on clinical grounds. A history of limited mouth opening, which may be intermittent or progressive, is a key feature of temporomandibular disorders.

Investigations

These are often required to rule out other conditions that may mimic temporomandibular disorders. These include:

- **Plain radiographs**—these are generally undertaken to exclude any primary joint disease, bony pathology, trauma, or possible dental cause for the patient's symptoms. Of course any of these may co-exist and should be treated appropriately. The view taken is often an orthopantomogram (OPG), although it poorly demonstrates the joint position or surfaces. Serial sagittal tomograms are more useful.
- **Magnetic resonance imaging**—most clinicians now consider MRI the investigation of choice. It is a non-invasive procedure, which involves no radiation and is certainly more favourable in the young. MRIs can accurately show disc morphology and internal derangements of the TMJs, along with excellent imaging of the muscles of mastication and the local vasculature.
- **CT scanning**—this is particularly useful for imaging the bones and can therefore demonstrate destructive disease and loose bodies.
- **Arthroscopy** may be both diagnostic and therapeutic.

Myofascial pain and dysfunction generally presents with diffuse cyclical pain found in several sites in the head and neck, particularly the muscles of mastication. It is often worst in the morning, and the patient may also describe sore teeth from clenching. There is often a history of stress and difficulty in sleeping. There may be diffuse muscle tenderness and a decreased range of mandibular movements, with wear facets on the teeth.

Internal joint derangement presents with continuous pain that is *localized* to the temporomandibular joint and is exacerbated by jaw movement. Mechanical interferences in the joint, such as clicking and locking, will often result in restricted opening or deviation during opening and closing.

Crepitus or grating sounds emanating from the joint is highly suggestive of osteoarthrosis in the elderly. Computed tomograms of the temporomandibular joint will often show degeneration and flattening of the condylar head. In younger patients with similar appearances on CT, other arthridities, such as rheumatoid arthritis, should be considered and investigated further.

Differential diagnosis
- Dental pain.
- Disorders of the ears, nose, and sinuses.
- Neuralgias.
- Headaches.
- Diseases of the major salivary glands.

Treatment
Many treatments are available, none of which have been consistently shown to be better than the others. Because the clinical course does not reflect a progressive disease, the main goals of treatment are to reduce or eliminate pain, joint noises and to restore normal function. This is best achieved when contributing factors such as stress, depression, and oral parafunctional habits (such as bruxism) are also addressed. Psychogenic factors are mostly found in patients with myofascial pain and dysfunction. These patients may need psychotropic medication and psychotherapy, described below.

Non-surgical
- **Explanation and reassurance**—this is probably one of the most important components of treatment. Explain to the patient the cause and nature of the disorder, and reassure them of its benign nature.
- **Lifestyle changes**—advise a soft diet and avoid heavy chewing, wide yawning, chewing gum, and any other activities that would cause excessive jaw movement. Patients should also be advised to identify the source of any stress, and try and change their lifestyle accordingly (which is easier said than done).
- **Massaging** the affected muscles and applying moist heat will promote muscle relaxation and help soothe aching or tired muscles.
- **Biofeedback techniques and jaw exercises**—these are indicated in cases of parafunction and may prove useful for clicking joints, restricted mouth opening and recurrent anterior dislocation of the condyle.
- **Analgesia**—simple non-steroidal anti-inflammatory (NSAIDs) analgesics will relieve the pain and certainly reduce inflammation around the TMJ.
- **Restorative and prosthetic rehabilitation**—to provide occlusal balance, posterior support, and correct vertical discrepancies.
- **Soft bite guard** ('gum shield')—worn at night may be effective in reducing symptoms caused by muscle spasm secondary to night grinding of the teeth and may lessen TMJ dysfunction related headaches and clicking.

- **Hard acrylic splint**—muscle and joint pain may be reduced but they are unlikely to have an effect on joint clicking and limitation of opening.
- **Psychiatric support**—psychiatric referral for assessment and consideration of suitable therapy should be considered in those patients where a psychogenic element may be present. Dothiepin, amitryptyline and nortryptyline have all been shown to be useful but close monitoring and appropriate patient selection is essential.
- **'Alternative therapies'**—few, if any, controlled studies exist to support the benefit of such treatment modalities, but in refractory cases other possible treatment options include:
  - **ultrasound**
  - **laser**
  - **transcutaneous electrical nerve stimulation**
  - **acupuncture**
  - **relaxation therapy**
  - **hypnosis**.

Surgical

Around 5% of patients require surgery. A range of surgical procedures is currently used ranging from arthrocentesis and arthroscopy to more complex open joint procedures. These are more useful in patients who have internal derangement where there is severe chronic pain or significant mechanical symptoms.

! Atypical facial pain

Atypical facial pain has many distinguishing features that make it a clinical entity in its own right and not just a 'catch all' diagnosis for seemingly unexplained facial pains. It is, however, essentially a **diagnosis of exclusion** that should only be made after all other possible organic causes have been excluded.

Clinical features

Patients often have a 'flat affect' and the more they are questioned about the pain the more vague their answers become. The pain is typically described as being a deep, dull ache, sometimes fluctuating, sometimes continuous, with intermittent severe episodes that the patient can find no causative factor for. Often the pain has been present for several years and analgesics rarely affect its nature. It is most commonly bilateral, but ill defined, and its **distribution cannot be explained on an anatomical basis**. The patient may say they are kept from sleeping by the pain but look well-rested. When they do admit to sleeping, the pain does not wake them. A proportion of these patients certainly do show symptoms of depressive illness or anxiety states, and patients often complain of other symptoms such as back and neck pain and irritable bowel syndrome. The patient's mood often does not correlate to the description of their symptoms and they may show exaggerated responses to examination and report an excess of adverse stressful life events.

Management

Often the ill-defined nature of the patient's pain results in unnecessary dental work being carried out. In light of the association of atypical facial pain with the neuroses (particularly depression), and the belief that it essentially has a psychogenic basis, emphasis has been placed on the use of anti-depressant therapeutic agents as the main treatment option.

Dothiepin, a tricyclic anti-depressant, has been shown to be effective in reducing the painful symptoms as it has in temporomandibular joint dysfunction. It is thought that these drugs alter the sensory discrimination component of pain independently of its anti-depressive effect. The possibility of the use of selective serotonin re-uptake inhibitors (SSRIs) to interfere with serotonin metabolism in the brainstem (a known effective treatment of mono-polar depression) has yet to be clarified by any trials.

① Trigeminal neuralgia ('tic douloureux')

Trigeminal neuralgia is most commonly a disorder seen in middle aged and elderly patients. It is more common in women with a peak incidence between 50 and 60 years of age and a reported incidence of 4 per 100 000 persons. **In young patients it may be an early feature of multiple sclerosis, HIV disease, or as a consequence of a lesion in the distribution of the trigeminal nerve (either centrally or peripherally).**

Patients complain of a sharp, intense, lancinating pain induced by a specific trigger point that radiates across the distribution of a branch of the trigeminal nerve. The pain is almost always unilateral, with over 30–40% of patients showing a distribution affecting both the maxillary and mandibular divisions. In approximately 20% of patients, the pain is confined to the mandibular division, and the ophthalmic division in 3%.

Repetitive bursts can be triggered with refractory periods of 30 seconds to several minutes. Episodes may last up to several hours with a major affect on normal lifestyle, and the pain is so severe patients may admit to feeling suicidal. It is not unusual for attacks to become more frequent and of increasing intensity.

The aetiology of trigeminal neuralgia may be multi-factorial with currently accepted evidence suggesting local nerve microcompression within the skull base, altered neuronal processing, along with a possible demyelinating process.

Management

Medical

The mainstay of treatment remains medical, typically with anticonvulsant agents. Usually, trigeminal neuralgia responds well to carbamazepine and/or amitriptyline, and a muscle relaxant such as baclofen. Carbamazepine remains the drug of choice with an initial regime of 100 mg three times daily being gradually increased to a maximum of 1200 mg daily titrated against effect. 20% of patients may develop side-effects such as tremor, dizziness, double vision and vomiting, which will obviously limit its use. Patients should be carefully titrated to the lowest dose required to control the pain and have regular monitoring of liver function and plasma carbamazepine concentration. Haematological monitoring of patients on long-term therapy is essential, as it has been reported that up to 17% can develop folic acid deficiency with megaloblastic anaemia, and hyponatraemia (low sodium) in the elderly. It is also advisable to withdraw therapy slowly to prevent acute psychosis associated with abrupt withdrawal.

Alternative agents: phenytoin, sodium valproate, lamotrigine, baclofen.

Surgical

- **Peripheral**—local surgical procedures may be considered in trigeminal neuralgia not responsive to medical management. Such procedures include:
  - **cryotherapy**—good response, but often there is the need for repeated episodes of surgery;

- **alcohol/glycerol injections**—permanent anaesthesia (which the patients often find preferable to the pain) and the risk of local tissue damage should not be forgotten;
- **nerve avulsion**—may be considered when other local procedures have failed.
- **Central**—a major undertaking considered for those patients in whom other forms of treatment modalities have failed and who are significantly affected by their symptoms of trigeminal neuralgia.

① **Glossopharyngeal neuralgia**

This is a rare condition characterized by a sharp, lancinating pain in the tonsillar region of the oro-pharynx and ipsilateral ear, which may be precipitated by swallowing or talking. It is 100 times less common than trigeminal neuralgia, usually occurring in middle to late age and affecting the sexes equally. Bouts of attacks may last for weeks or months with a tendency to recur.

The management of glossopharyngeal neuralgia parallels that of trigeminal neuralgia with carbamazepine being the drug of choice. Local surgical procedures are more difficult although surgical-sectioning of the glossopharyngeal nerve may prove beneficial. Central surgical procedures are not without significant risk although microvascular decompression has been reported to produce complete cure in 75% of patients treated.

⑦ Burning mouth

'Burning mouth syndrome' is a recognized clinical entity that presents in a variety of guises. Prevalence ranges from 2 to 5% and the condition is three times more common in females than males. Patients are usually in their 50s and 60s.

Many of the patients diagnosed with burning mouth syndrome have no underlying organic cause. In such idiopathic cases there is often a psychogenic background, such as depression or an anxiety state (e.g. cancer phobia), the burning mouth simply being a somatization of the underlying mental condition. Some patients may respond to simple reassurance, others may need formal psychiatric assessment and management.

Patients complain of burning or itching of the mouth, and may often describe pain of varying types. The site of symptoms may be localized to just one area such as the tongue (glossodynia), or lips, or may involve the whole of the oral mucosa. The frequency of symptoms may also vary from being persistent throughout the day, to being intermittent often unrelated to any particular activity.

Examination of these patients rarely elicits anything other than a normal, healthy mucosa, although a **thorough examination is important to exclude any obvious local causes such as trauma or infection**. Patients often report recent dental treatment and may express concerns relating to possible 'mercury poisoning' or 'allergy' to denture materials. Such concerns are only rarely proven.

Several systemic conditions have been implicated in burning mouth, notably certain haematological and hormonal deficiencies (vitamins B1, B2, and/or B6, vitamin B12, folate and iron, and female sex steroids). In the few studies that have looked at the results of replacement therapy outcomes seem very variable, and indeed only a small proportion of patients with burning mouth have proven deficiencies.

Management
- Reassurance.
- Difflam mouth rinse.
- Topical anaesthetics.
- Occasionally anti-depressants.

ⓘ Facial palsy

The VIIth cranial nerve supplies:

- **motor** fibres to muscles of facial expression, post belly of digastric, and a branch to the stapedius muscle in the middle ear;
- **taste** sensation from the anterior two thirds of the tongue via the chorda tympani;
- **secretomotor** fibres to the submandibular, sublingual salivary glands, and to the lacrimal glands.

Clinical picture

- Varying degrees of weakness of the muscles of facial expression:
  - **Upper motor neurone** pathology will cause a unilateral facial palsy with sparing of the muscles of the upper face (frontalis and obicularis). The upper face receives innervation bilaterally from both motor cortices. All facial muscles may also *still move with emotional responses.*
  - **Lower motor neurone** palsy will show a unilateral paralysis of *all* muscles of facial expression, both voluntarily and to emotional stimulus.
- Facial asymmetry is exaggerated by attempting to show the teeth, whistle, or close the eyes tightly (the eyes roll upwards—Bell's phenomenon).
- Food collects in the vestibule because of buccinator paralysis.
- Loss of the naso-labial fold/commisure of the mouth drops.

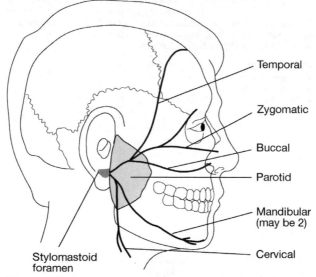

Fig. 7.2 Extra-cranial course of the facial nerve.

- Epiphora—tears overflow to the cheek.
- Reduced lacrimation (lesions above the geniculate ganglion).
- Hyperacusis: loss of stapedius reflex (lesions above nerve to stapedius).

Aetiology

- Supranuclear:
  - cerebro-vascular accidents CVAs
  - **cerebral tumours.**
- Infranuclear—Bell's palsy:
  - infection
    - acute/chronic otitis media;
    - Ramsay Hunt syndrome (herpes zoster infection of the geniculate ganglion);
  - trauma
    - surgical (iatrogenic—possibly intentional);
    - temporal bone fracture;
    - birth injury;
  - **neoplastic**—malignant disease of the middle ear
  - extra-temporal/miscellaneous:
    - parotid tumours;
    - sarcoidosis;
    - multiple sclerosis;
    - Guillain–Barre syndrome (acute idiopathic polyneuritis).

Underlying disorders

Head injury

Facial weakness following a head injury usually indicates a fracture involving the temporal bone. Diagnosis is usually clinical with a history of significant trauma. In addition there may be:

- bleeding from the ear;
- haemotympanum;
- vertigo;
- nystagmus,
- deafness.

Herpes zoster infection (Ramsay Hunt syndrome)

This is a viral infection, usually chickenpox, affecting the geniculate ganglion. In addition to facial weakness, vesicles are visible on the ear canal, pharynx and face. Management requires the use of systemic anti-viral agents (acyclovir).

Bell's palsy

Idiopathic facial palsy (Bell's palsy) should be a 'diagnosis of exclusion'. All other causes must be eliminated clinically or following investigations. Thorough examination of the head and neck especially the cranial nerves, is essential before the diagnosis can be made with any degree of confidence. High dose intravenous steroids may be of use, although this is controversial and if the diagnosis is wrong (e.g. herpes zoster) this will lead to rapid spread and deterioration in the patient. The prognosis for Bell's palsy is generally good.

Clinical features
- Unilateral facial paralysis.
- Possibly loss of taste and hearing, or occasionally hyperacusis.
- Often preceding mastoid pain.

Bells palsy can sometimes be confused with Ramsay Hunt syndrome (in which steroids are contra-indicated). To differentiate between the two consider the history and carefully examine for vesicles in the external meatus.

Parotid tumours
Acoustic neuroma

Management of facial palsy

This is dependent on the cause and so an accurate history, examination and investigation is imperative to finalise a diagnosis—treatment is then targeted.
- **Infection**—appropriate antibiotic or antiviral therapy.
- **Trauma**—identification of the site of injury: if peripheral, microscopic anastamosis or insertion of a nerve graft may be considered.

General supportive measures include:
- **Eye care**—inability to close the eyelid in severe weakness may lead to drying of the conjunctiva and corneal damage. Ophthalmic opinion should be sought to ensure the cornea is protected and to prevent the possibility of corneal abrasion. Prophylactic measures: regular eye drops/lateral tarsorrhaphy/gold weights in the upper eyelid.
- **Dental care**—regular hygiene support and advice in techniques to clear food from the bucco-gingival sulcus. Denture build up to disguise cheek hollowing.
- **Cosmetic/functional**—improvements may be considered with innervated muscle transfer (either cross-facial or as free flaps).

Chapter 8

Injuries to the face, nose, and ears

:☻: General points in facial trauma

In trauma care **time is of the essence**. A useful working approach is needed, in order to rapidly identify those patients that need immediate care, from those that can wait.

Facial 'emergencies' following maxillofacial trauma can be regarded as those that are **life- and sight-threatening**. These may occur following isolated injuries, or they may be associated with significant injuries elsewhere. They may even present following what would usually be regarded as a minor injury (highlighting the need to maintain a high index of suspicion), or after some delay. In the context of emergencies following facial trauma, the objectives are therefore to **safeguard life first and vision second**.

Assessment therefore needs to be systematic and repeated, with the establishment of clear priorities in the patient's overall care.

In many respects parallels can be drawn with orthopaedic surgery. Management of facial trauma can arguably be regarded as 'facial orthopaedics', as both specialties share common surgical principles in trauma care.

What is an 'emergency'?

In this text, any clinical problem requiring *immediate* identification and/or management, constitutes an emergency. Many conditions may be considered 'urgent' (i.e. contaminated, mucky wounds, open fractures), but these can be left until the patient is fully stabilized, with little or no increase in mortality or morbidity. **In the *face*, emergency care effectively means airway control, control of profuse bleeding, and the management of vision-threatening injuries (VTI)**. Failure to rapidly recognize and manage these conditions can result in loss of life or sight.

Head and neck injuries resulting in life-threatening conditions

- Facial injuries resulting in airway compromise (e.g. pan-facial fractures with gross mobility or swelling, comminuted #s of the mandible, gun-shot, profuse bleeding, foreign bodies, burns, etc.).
- Anterior neck injuries resulting in airway compromise (e.g. penetrating injuries, circumferential burns, laryngeal injuries).
- Injuries resulting in profuse blood loss (e.g. penetrating neck, pan-facial fractures).
- Intracranial injuries.

ATLS and the maxillofacial region

In over 29 countries worldwide, management of trauma is now based on Advanced Trauma Life Support (ATLS) principles. This is now generally accepted as the 'gold standard' of trauma care, and many of its principles are equally important in the management of facial injuries. However, it is important to remember that every case is unique and on occasions, strict adherence to guidelines may result in some difficulties. It is therefore important to be mindful of potential complications when dealing with severe facial injuries and be aware of early warning signs. **If in doubt, re-assess the patient from the start**.

All clinicians involved in trauma care need to be able to assess and maintain airway problems and control obvious bleeding during the primary survey. Be alert also to possible vision-threatening injuries during the primary survey, i.e. retrobulbar haemorrhage. Although the aim of the primary survey is to identify and treat life-threatening problems, the early identification of a sight-threatening condition may be possible during 'D' when the pupils are assessed. This enables early referral to an 'appropriate' specialist. When dealing with acute sight-threatening conditions, 'appropriate' may refer to an on-site speciality with expertise in peri-orbital trauma care.

Airway, bleeding, and sight-threatening conditions may initially be subtle and may not become apparent until the secondary survey is under way. This reminds us of the two well-known principles in trauma care:

- **the need for a high index of suspicion;**
- **the need for frequent re-revaluation.**

Preliminary assessment of multiple injured patients—the primary survey

The sequence in which the primary survey should proceed is related to those conditions that would lead to loss of life quickest:

- **A**irway (whilst protecting the cervical spine to prevent any neurological damage).
- **B**reathing (all trauma patients should be given 100% oxygen to breathe on arrival).
- **C**irculation with control of haemorrhage.
- **D**isability (brain function).
- **E**xposure—this must be complete so a full examination, front and back, can be undertaken. However, the patient needs to be covered to prevent hypothermia.

Any problem discovered is corrected **at the time of identification.** This is preferably done by a team approach where different team members carry out the above simultaneously. In such cases, a 'team leader' ensures that everything is done. If team numbers are not sufficient for this, the above sequence is followed. It is also vital to enlist the help of any speciality not on the team early, if a problem or potential problem is identified that requires their input, e.g. neurosurgery.

☻ Maxillofacial (trauma) emergencies

Airway

- Obstruction can be caused by dentures/teeth or severely displaced fractures of the mandible or mid-face. The commonest cause is bleeding and/or saliva, notably when the patient is intoxicated or supine.
- Mid-face fractures may displace downwards and backwards along the skull base, impinging on the posterior pharyngeal wall, resulting in obstruction. Bilateral anterior ('bucket handle') or comminuted mandibular fractures can similarly displace backwards allowing the base of the tongue to fall back. Both of these are much more likely when patients are supine and there is alteration in the conscious level. Both can be dealt with by pulling the fractured part forward to relieve the obstruction. This provides only temporary relief and a definitive airway will probably be required.
- Saliva and blood should be cleared by suction. If the bleeding is ongoing from an identifiable source, which can be stopped, it should be. However, it is usually generalized from multiple sites. Displaced fractures should be manually reduced as this often helps slow the bleeding. Nasal packs may be necessary (remember the possibility of skull base #). If bleeding continues the airway should be protected with a definitive airway.
- Direct trauma to the airway will probably require a definitive airway to be placed.

Beware the patient who keeps trying to sit up—they may be trying to clear their airway.

Bleeding

- Bleeding from maxillofacial injury is common but not usually life-threatening. **If the patient is in shock, look for another cause.** Actively consider facial bleeding, as supine patients will be swallowing blood, which will go unnoticed.
- If obvious and significant, bleeding is controlled in the primary survey by **pressure**. Bleeding from lacerations can usually be controlled by pressure applied either with a swab (care with scalps if risk of skull fracture) or by placement of **sutures**. These are used to apply pressure and not intended as definitive closure.
- Mid-face bleeding can be troublesome as the bleeding is from multiple sites from comminuted bones and torn mucosa. Pressure can be applied to the nose with anterior and posterior nasal packs. Bleeding from **displaced/mobile mid-face fractures should be reduced**. Gentle pressure can be applied antero-superiorly on the maxilla and maintained by placing mouth props bilaterally against an intact mandible. Surprisingly, this is not as painful as one might think. In selected cases, use of external fixators from skull to maxilla, may be necessary but this requires transfer to an operating theatre and considerably more time.

- Bleeding from a 'hole' (e.g. following a gun-shot) can sometimes be stemmed by placing a **Foley catheter** in the hole and inflating it. Obviously be careful and think what may be in the depths of the hole!
- If local pressure is not sufficient to stop haemorrhage from either soft or hard tissue injury, the use of **angiography and embolization or ligation of external carotids should be considered**. This is rare.

Vision-threatening injuries

(See also The Eye.)

Following trauma, vision can be threatened anywhere along the visual pathway from globe to cortex. The main (potentially treatable) causes to consider are:

- direct globe injury;
- retrobulbar haemorrhage;
- optic nerve compression;
- loss of eyelids;

direct injury to the globe requires urgent ophthalmic referral.

Retrobulbar haemorrhage

Bleeding behind the globe is a form of compartment syndrome. **This is a surgical emergency.** It can lead to an increase in pressure that results eventually in irreversible ischaemia of the retina and optic nerve. Key symptoms are:

- severe pain;
- progressive loss of vision;
- the eye becomes proptosed with ophthalmoplegia;
- development of a fixed dilated pupil as the vision deteriorates.

Treatment requires immediate relief of pressure. In the emergency department the following should be given intravenously:

- acetazolamide;
- mannitol;
- steroids;

during which arrangements are made for surgery. Under LA, a lateral canthotomy may be possible, but these measures really only buy time while preparation for surgery is made. Definitive treatment involves drainage of the haematoma. Decompression should lead to an improvement in visual acuity if undertaken early enough.

Traumatic optic neuropathy

Traumatic optic neuropathy occurs when there is disruption around the optic canal resulting in either compression of the optic nerve, shearing forces to the nerve as it passes through the canal, or haematoma formation within the nerve itself. Untreated it can render the patient blind; the diagnosis needs to be made early to allow the best chance of visual recovery. The signs that suggest an optic nerve injury include **poorly reactive pupil, afferent papillary defect, and decreased colour vision, decreased visual acuity with relatively normal ocular examination**. This is an ophthalmic emergency and should be referred accordingly.

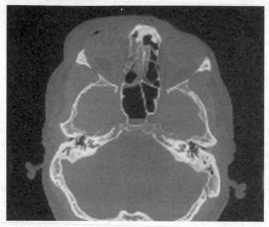

Fig. 8.1 CT scan showing compression of the right optic nerve at the optic foramen following blunt trauma. This required urgent decompression.

Treatment of optic nerve compression is controversial and again may be either medical or surgical. The options include observation, IV corticosteroids, and optic nerve decompression. The latter option is carried out via either a craniotomy approach or lateral facial approach.

One steroid regime is:
- methylprednisolone 30 mg/kg STAT;
- followed by methylprednisolone 15 mg/kg every 6 h.

Of course others exist—always check local policy.

Time is of the essence, best results are obtained if steroids are given within 8 h of the injury.

⑦ Facial trauma—general considerations

Minor injuries to the maxillofacial region are very common in the UK, around 80% occur in children. Major facial disruption is less frequently seen and motor vehicle crashes (MVC) now accounts for about 5% of facial trauma. This is partly due to seat belt and drink-driving legislation. However, whereas patients would have previously died at the scene as a result of their head injuries, many are now surviving having sustained major facial injuries. Sporting injuries and assaults account for most of the remainder.

In assessing the multiple-injured patient, the first step is to determine whether any life-threatening injuries exist and to deal with them first. The advanced trauma life-support system—ATLS—is one approach to assessment and initial management of the multiply injured patient. It recognizes that identification of life-threatening injuries needs to be prioritized (primary survey) and treated at the time of identification (resuscitation). Most maxillofacial injuries can wait treatment, and in the multiply injured patient, the first step is keeping the patient alive.

Once the primary survey and resuscitation have been carried out, attention can then be focused on the maxillofacial region.

Facial skeleton

The arrangement of the facial bones may be considered as comprising three areas:
- upper-third (frontal bone);
- middle-third, between the supra-orbital ridges and the upper teeth (2 maxillae, 2 zygomas, 2 lacrimal bones, 2 nasal bones, 1 vomer, 1 ethmoid);
- lower-third (mandible).

Some of these bones, such as the ethmoid and those comprising the orbital roof, are extremely delicate and so thin that on a dry skull light can easily pass through. The remainder vary in thickness but often remain quite delicate (nasal, zygoma). The mandible is the strongest of the facial bones. It is a U-shaped bone comprised of an outer dense cortical layer and delicate trabecular bone inside. The face is not solid but contains several 'cavities', such as the sinuses, orbits, oral and nasal cavities. Around these the bones form a series of vertical struts known as 'buttresses' As a result, these bones are very good at resisting vertically directed forces (e.g. during chewing) but are weak when it comes to resisting horizontal forces (i.e. during most injuries).

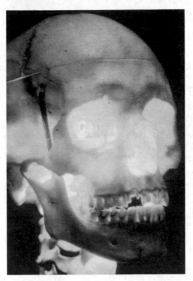

Fig. 8.2 Transilluminated skull demonstrating the thinness of many of its bones.

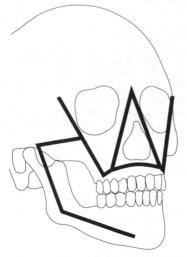

Fig. 8.3 Diagrammatic representation of the 'butresses' of the face.

⑦ Useful clinical signs and their significance

The usefulness of clinical signs can vary from those that only suggest an underlying pathology (*) to those that are almost pathognomonic (***). Their interpretation must be taken in conjunction with the history and likelihood of the condition being present.

General

Facial burns***

When associated with soot in the nose and mouth, singeing of the nasal vibrissae, and sooty sputum, this represents a potential airway problem. There is also the risk of inhalation of carbon monoxide and other toxins.

Facial nerve palsy**

Following head injury—fractured base of skull.

Horse voice/bovine cough**

Following a direct blow to the anterior neck, may indicate disruption of the larynx. A bovine cough is where the vocal cords do not meet in the mid-line prior to the explosive expulsion of air. As a result the cough is relatively weak and ineffectual.

Wry neck*

Following trauma is due to muscle spasm. May occasionally be associated with dislocation of the posterior facet joints.

The face

Intercanthal distance**

Separation of the eyes. If greater than 30–32 mm (female) or 32–34 mm (male) the patient may have detached canthi secondary to an underlying naso-ethmoidal fracture. As well as an increased intercanthal distance, the medial canthus loses its pointed shape becoming rounded. This can occur uni- or bilaterally. If unilateral the distance from mid-line to canthus will be greater on one side. The interpupillary distance should be within normal limits. There may also be depression at the root of the nose.

Anterior open bite and elongated face**

If not pre existing, is suggestive of posterior and inferior displacement of the maxilla following a Le Fort fracture. This results in posterior gagging of the molar teeth. If the maxilla is stable, then the teeth should be percussed. If the note is dull ('cracked cup' sound), the maxilla is likely to be fractured and impacted—hence the stability. If the percussion note is normal, the anterior open bite may be due to bilateral fractured condyles.

Septal haematoma*

Seen as a blue/reddened swelling on the septum on direct examination. Needs drainage, as failure to do so can result in septal perforation, abscesses, and intra-cranial infection.

Numbness of the cheek*

Suggests a cheek or blow-out fracture.

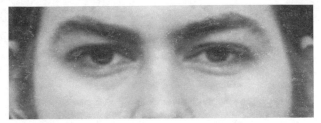

Fig. 8.4 Normal intercanthal distance.

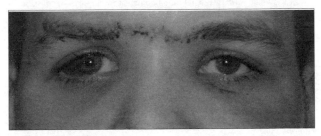

Fig. 8.5 Increased intercanthal distance.

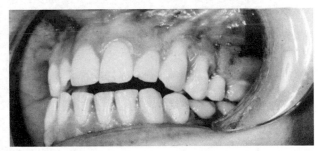

Fig. 8.6 Anterior open bite—when biting together the front teeth do not overlap (try it on yourself, have you got one?).

*Numbness of the lower lip**
Suggests a mandibular fracture.

*Anosmia**
Loss of smell due to tearing of olfactory nerves secondary to an underlying anterior cranial fossa floor fracture. Not reliably detectable in acute phase of injury.

*'Bow-string' test***
Assess for medial canthal detachment in nasothmoid injuries—the lateral canthus is pulled laterally, if there is detachment medially this will also move away.

Within the mouth

*Dysphagia**
Many causes. When related to submandibular, pharyngeal, or other posterior oral swellings, it is a significant finding often requiring admission. Is often painful **(odynophagia)**.

*Inability to protrude the tongue***
When related to submandibular, sublingual, or other oral swellings, it is a significant finding often requiring admission.

*Trismus***
Limitation of mouth opening due to muscle spasm (usually masseter or medial pterygoid). May be seen following a direct blow. When related to submandibular, pharyngeal, or other posterior oral swellings, it is a significant finding often requiring admission.

*Guerins sign****
Palatal bruising of the hard palate—underlying fracture involving palatine foramen.

*Upper buccal sulcus bruising***
Fractured zygoma or unilateral Le Fort I or II.

*Sublingual haematoma****
Bruising/bleeding under the tongue—fractured mandible (body/symphysis/parasymphysis).

*Peri-odontal bleeding**
May indicate an associated fracture of the tooth or bone.

*Change in the patients bite****
In either the mandible or maxilla may indicate a fracture.

*'Cracked cup' note**
When percussing the maxillary teeth, suggests a fracture.

*Malocclusion**
If the occlusion has changed it is likely that there is an underlying fracture of maxilla, mandible, or alveolar bone. Subluxation of teeth may also produce a malocclusion, although usually much more minor. If none of the above are present a malocclusion may be a result of a TMJ effusion/haemarthrosis.

The eyes

Visual acuity

This is the single most sensitive indicator of visual impairment. It must be recorded in all patients with mid-facial trauma. In patients who wear spectacles to correct short sight, the recording must be done with the spectacles on or through a pinhole. Acuity is expressed as a distance in meters from which a chart being read is usually $6/X$ where X is the line on the chart the patient can read, usually 6. If less than 6, e.g.12 or 60, this means the patient can read at 6 m from the chart that which a person with normal vision could read at 12 or 60 m from the chart. A visual acuity of 6/18 or worse should be referred for an ophthalmological opinion.

If the patient cannot read the chart at all at 6 m, the distance at which they can read the top line is recorded as $Y/60$. If they are not able to do this, whether they can count fingers, see them moving, or perceive light, are recorded as the visual acuity, in that order.

If the patient is unconscious, pupillary responses to light must be checked.

All patients must have a documented visual acuity. Any decrease in visual acuity requires an ophthalmic opinion.

Pupillary responses**

Check direct response to light and consensual response. Responses should be equal on both sides and to direct and consensual stimulation. A pupil that reacts poorly to direct stimulation but briskly to consensual has an afferent pupillary defect.

Swinging flashlight test***

Detects subtle defects to the optic nerve. Light is shone in one eye, then swung to the other, and back and forth. If the right eye has a problem, on shining the light in the right eye, both pupils will constrict, as the light moves to the left they will constrict further. As the light is brought back to the right, the pupils will not respond or dilate a little.

Peri-orbital haematoma***

When *well-defined* this represents a fracture involving the orbit. Usually this means a fractured zygoma but can also include a blow-out fracture, fractured base of skull (anterior cranial fossa), unilateral naso-ethmoidal, or nasal bones.

Racoon (panda) eyes***

Bilateral well-defined 'black eyes'—fractured base of skull (anterior cranial fossa), Le Fort III or naso-ethmoid fracture.

Lateral subconjunctival haemorrhage**

This indicates a fracture involving the orbit usually the cheek or naso-ethmoid region. There is no posterior limit.

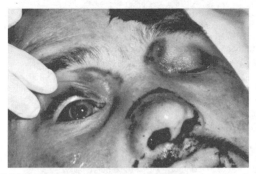

Fig. 8.7 RAPD. When the eye is opened the pupil does not react. When the contralateral eye is opened it does—this patient is blind.

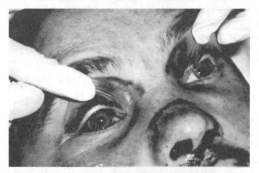

Fig. 8.8 RAPD. When the eye is opened the pupil does not react. When the contralateral eye is opened it does—this patient is blind.

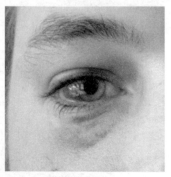

Fig. 8.9 Well-defined 'black' and 'red' eye.

Chemosis*

Swelling of conjunctiva often seen in significant trauma, looks a bit like frog's spawn. If no tear of conjunctiva present, it will resolve. If tear present, then you need to rule out globe injury.

Hyphema**

Blood in anterior chamber seen as fluid level when patient is standing. Needs ophthalmic assessment probably require admission and observation.

Iridodialysis*

The iris is detached from its root leading to a distorted pupil shape.

Dilated pupil (traumatic mydriasis)*

Spasm of the dilator pupillae. Can be seen following a direct blow to the eye. Not to be confused with a third nerve palsy.

Diplopia*

Double vision may be neurogenic, myogenic, or bony in origin. It may be temporary or permanent and should be reviewed. Depending on possible cause, refer to ophthalmics or maxillofacial.

Unilateral restricted upward gaze**

Often a sign of a 'blow-out' fracture, occasionally due to injury to ocular muscle or its nerve. **Painful diplopia** from a blow-out may require urgent release.

Retraction sign***

When looking from the side of the patient, as they look up, the globe is seen to move posteriorly. This is a good sign for a blow-out fracture. Entrapment of the fat and restriction of the inferior rectus muscle results in a shift of the axis of rotation of the globe from its centre to the point of entrapment. Thus the pull of the superior rectus results in a backward rotation of the globe.

Hypoglobus*

Inferior displacement of the globe seen in cheek complex fractures, where the bone and Lockwood's ligament drop down. May also be seen in large blow-out fractures.

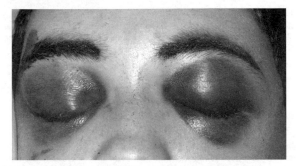

Fig. 8.10 'Panda' or 'Racoon' eyes. Often not as obvious as this example.

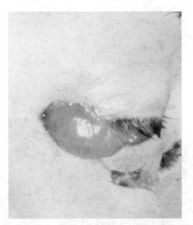

Fig. 8.11 Chemosis.

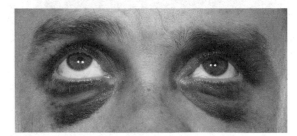

Fig. 8.12 Unilateral restricted upward gaze.

Enophthalmos*

Posterior displacement of the globe due to increased orbital volume. Seen in blow-out fractures of the orbit and cheek fractures. Globe appears 'sunken in' with a deep supra tarsal groove.

Third nerve palsy***

Dilated pupil, the eye looks down and out, and ptosis. In severe head injuries this represents third nerve compression from an expanding intra-cranial lesion. The patient has a reduced GCS.

Aqueous leakage***

A penetrating injury of the cornea.

Superior orbital fissure (SOF) syndrome**

Ophthalmoplegia, fixed dilated pupil, and ipsilateral forehead numbness—fracture extending into the SOF, or possible carotid anuerism. This is usually part of a significant injury.

Orbital apex syndrome**

As in the SOF but here the patient has reduced visual acuity.

Peri-orbital oedema*

When infective in origin represents significant spread of infection. If the eye is closing the patient may probably need admission.

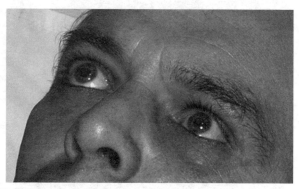

Fig. 8.13 Enophthalmos.

The ears

Haemotympanum**
Blood visualized behind the eardrum. Indicative of a fracture of the middle cranial fossa.

Battles sign***
Bruising around the mastoid region—fractured base of skull (middle cranial fossa).

CSF rhinorrhea/otorrhea***
'Tramlining'—fractured base of skull. Blood mixes with CSF and leaks out. Along the edges the blood clots while centrally the CSF leak washes it away to form two parallel lines (like tramlines).

Bleeding from the ear**
Fractured base of skull or mandibular condyle. If the tympanic membrane is intact the bleeding is local to the EAM, usually the anterior wall, often secondary to an underlying condylar fracture. If the tympanic membrane is perforated the blood may be from a middle cranial fossa fracture.

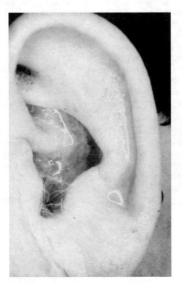

Fig. 8.14 CSF otorrhea.

① Mandibular fractures

Applied anatomy

The mandible forms the lower third of the face and facial skeleton. It is the only mobile bone of the face (excluding the ossicles) and has numerous muscle insertions. It plays an important role in:

- speech;
- mastication (chewing);
- deglutition (swallowing);
- maintaining the airway.

Patients with mandibular injuries, therefore, have difficulty in talking, and are unable to eat and drink easily. In severe injuries the airway may be at risk.

Osteology

Morphologically the mandible is a U-shaped 'long bone' (e.g. femur, radius, etc.). It can be divided anatomically into:

- symphysis
- parasymphysis
- body
- angle
- ramus.

The almost vertical ramus carries two processes, the condyle, which articulates with the glenoid fossa of the temporal bone to form the temporo-mandibular joint, and the coronoid process, which receives the insertion of temporalis. The condyle is supported on a slender condylar neck, a frequent site for fracture.

On the medial or inner aspect of the ramus the inferior alveolar neurovascular bundle enters the bone via the mandibular foramen and runs through a bony canal within the mandible providing nutrition and sensory innervation to the lower teeth. An important branch of this bundle, the mental nerve, leaves the bone via the mental foramen in the premolar region and provides sensation to the lower lip and anterior gums

Muscle attachments

The muscles of mastication (temporalis, masseter, medial and lateral pterygoid), together with the suprahyoid muscles (digastric, geniohyoid, and mylohyoid) are the principle movers of the mandible. In addition the mandible receives the insertion of genioglossus, which forms the main bulk of the tongue. Note that genioglossus and geniohyoid are attached to the mid-line genial tubercles. A fracture in this region may, therefore, lead to loss of anterior support for the tongue, leading to posterior displacement and airway compromise.

Dentition

The full complement of adult teeth in a mandible is 16 comprising of:

- 4 incisor teeth;
- 2 canines;
- 4 premolars;
- 6 molars.

The canine teeth have long roots and the third molar (wisdom) teeth are often partially erupted, these factors tend to weaken the bone locally and account for the frequency of fractures in these regions.

Age-related changes

In the child, the dentition will be at various stages of development and developing tooth germs are present within the bone. While these lead to a structural weakening of the bone, this is compensated for by increased elasticity and pliability of the young mandible, compared with mature bone. As a result, relatively higher forces are required to fracture the bone in children. Furthermore, the facial skeleton is less prominent in children and hence mandibular fractures are somewhat rare in this age group. In the edentulous elderly jaw, loss of the 'alveolar bone', which would normally support the teeth, leads to a gradual reduction in bone height. This feature, together with age-related conditions such as osteoporosis, weaken its structure and, as a result, the bone is more vulnerable to fracture.

Common fracture patterns

The **periosteum** is an important structure in determining the stability of a mandibular fracture. In young patients it is generally a strong unyielding membrane. Gross displacement of fragments cannot occur if it remains intact and attached to the bone. However, once the periosteum has been breeched (by injury or surgical exposure), **displacement of the bones can occur under the influence of the attached muscles.**
   Common fracture patterns include the following.

Angle fractures

Fractures of the angle are affected by the medial pterygoid and masseteric muscles. Fractures in this region have been classified as **vertically and horizontally favourable or unfavourable**. The medial pterygoid muscle may pull the posterior fragment lingually or together with the masseter in an upward direction. This is only important when the periosteum has been ruptured or stripped from the bone allowing displacement to occur.

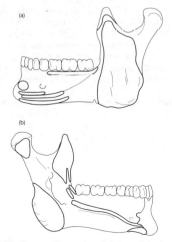

Fig. 8.15 (a) and (b) Outer and inner view of the mandible showing muscle attachments.

Fractures at the symphysis and parasymphysis

The mylohyoid muscle has been described as the 'diaphragm' of the mouth, passing between the hyoid bone and the inner aspect of the mandible. With mid-line fractures of the symphysis, the mylohyoid and geniohyoid muscles can act as a stabilizing force. However, oblique fractures will tend to overlap due to the pull of these muscles. With bilateral parasymphyseal fractures (which result from considerable force), the periosteum is often torn and the fragments can displace posteriorly under the influence of the genioglossus—so called **'bucket handle'** fractures.

Condylar fractures

The hinge joint of the mandible is a common site of fracture and often occurs in association with fractures elsewhere in the jaw. The classical history is a blow or fall onto the point of the chin, where one or both condyles are fractured, often associated with a symphyseal or parasymphyseal fracture (so called 'gaurdsmans' fracture). **Beware the laceration over the chin following a fall—check the condyles.** On mouth opening, the jaw deviates *towards* the site of injury.

Condylar fractures in adults tend to occur outside the joint, although transmitted forces can still damage the joint and cause long-term problems. Effusion or bleeding into the joint space can occur in the absence of a fracture, the space is distended and the patient complains of an abnormal bite. Intra-capsular fractures in children are more common and can result in growth disturbances in the condyle later on.

Injuries to related structures

- The **inferior alveolar nerve** is often damaged in fractures of the body and angle causing paraesthesia of the lower lip on the same side.
- Medial displacement of the condyle can compress the trigeminal nerve leading to loss of **facial sensation.**
- The **facial nerve** may be damaged by a direct blow over the ramus and needs to be assessed especially if a laceration is present. Rarely, the mandibular condyle may impact upon and fracture the temporal bone through which the facial nerve runs. Facial nerve injury leads to variable paralysis or weakness of the facial muscles.
- Injury to major **blood vessels** is unusual, although the facial artery and vein may be damaged where they cross the lower border of the mandible.
- **Temperomandibular joint.** Condylar fractures in adults tend to occur outside the joint, although transmitted forces can still damage the joint and cause long-term problems. **Effusion** into the joint space can occur in the absence of a fracture, the space is distended and the patient complains of an abnormal bite. Intra-capsular fractures in children are more common and can result in growth disturbances in the condyle later on.

Assessment

Secondary survey

History

Most patients will give a history of blunt injury to the face, the most common mechanism being interpersonal violence. Sports, falls, and accidents are other common causes. Common symptoms include:

- pain;
- swelling;
- altered bite;
- numbness of the lower lip;
- difficulty in opening and closing of the jaw;
- pain on swallowing with drooling.

The hallmark of a mandible fracture is a *change* in the bite (occlusion); however, normal occlusion does not rule out a mandible fracture.

Other physical findings include:

- loosened teeth;
- facial deformity;
- mobility of fractured segment;
- bleeding (= tear) in gingival tissue;
- sublingual haematoma;
- trismus;
- numbness of the lower lip (ID nerve).

Examination

This must be undertaken in good light, having cleansed the face of blood and debris. Suction must be immediately available. Look for:

- facial swelling;
- asymmetry;
- bruising;
- palpate the lower border for any step deformity;
- feel the condyles and assess their movements—this is done best by placing a gloved finger in each auditory meatus;
- document the dentition, any occlusal derangement, or steps in the occlusal plane;
- gently manipulate across the suspected fracture site feeling for abnormal movement or crepitus;
- look for gingival lacerations; and
- mucosal bruising, in particular, for a sublingual haematoma.

Remember

- Mental parasthesia is both an important diagnostic sign and an important **medico-legal observation** prior to treatment.
- **Missing teeth must be accounted for.** If unable, get a chest and soft tissue view of the neck. Similarly, if associated with a lip laceration, a soft tissue radiograph of the lips is essential.
- A **sublingual haematoma is pathognmonic** of a mandibular fracture and may also compromise the airway.
- **Bleeding from the external auditory meatus** may be a result of tearing of its anterior wall by a condylar fracture. However, it may also be a sign of a fractured skull base—be careful in your assessment.

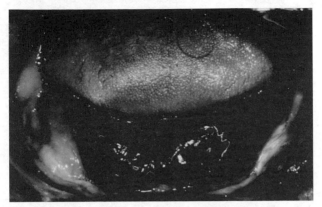

Fig. 8.16 A sublingual haematoma in a toothless mandible.

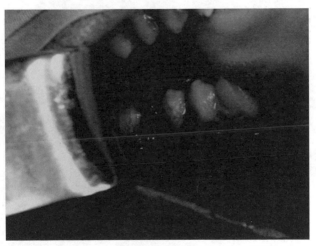

Fig. 8.17 A displaced fracture resulting in a gap. This was misinterpreted as a missing tooth—count the teeth and assess for fracture mobility.

Radiographs

The principle of radiology for any fracture is to take two views at 90 degrees to each other. This minimizes the risk of missing a fracture that may be minimally displaced. For the mandible, this is most simply achieved by ordering:

- ortho-pantomagram (OPG, OPT, DPT), or lateral obliques, together with a PA view of the mandible.

It is essential that both views include the entire bone from lower border to the condylar processes. For anterior fractures, if facilities exist, a true lower occlusal view is also very helpful. These will often provide sufficient information, but supplementary views include:

- reverse townes for the condylar neck;
- CT scans are useful for further evaluation of condylar fracture/ dislocations but are not necessary in A&E.

The mandible is usually fractured in two places—if you see one fracture, look for another (cf. pelvic fractures). Fractures sites include:

- condyle (36 %);
- body (21 %);
- angle (20 %);
- parasymphyseal (14%);
- ramus (3 %);
- alveolar (3%);
- coronoid (2%);
- mid-line symphysis (1 %).

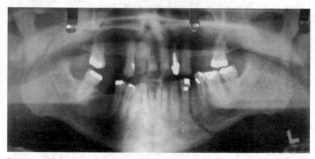

Fig. 8.18 OPG.

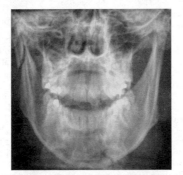

Fig. 8.19 PA mandible.

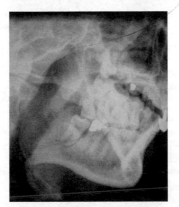

Fig. 8.20 Lateral oblique.

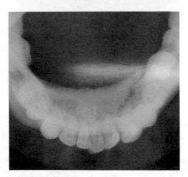

Fig. 8.21 Lower occlusal view anterior mandible.

Treatment

First-aid measures

A mandibular fracture is often painful and if it occurs through the tooth socket, it is by definition a compound or **open fracture**. **Pain relief** is a priority and may be simply achieved by infiltration of local anaesthesia or, if possible, by an inferior dental nerve block. It is important to **minimize movement** across the fracture site, not only for pain relief (as for all long-bone fractures) but also to reduce bleeding and contamination from oral bacteria. A simple method is to apply a **soft neck collar** but this should only be done after the cervical spine has been formally cleared. A common procedure is to apply a **bridal wire** across the fracture site. This is a loop of stainless steel wire encircling the teeth either side of the fracture. Clearly this is only relevant if the fracture is in a tooth-bearing segment and care must be taken not to avulse the teeth by applying too much force. Any loose dento-alveolar fractures should be splinted.

Treatment principles

In general, fracture treatment has traditionally been classified as conservative or operative. Today the preferred terminology is **closed** or **open** to avoid ambiguity.

Indications for closed treatment (soft diet, antibiotics, review)
- No or minimal displacement of stable fracture.
- No or minimal mobility across fracture line.
- No impairment of function.
- Ability to obtain pre-trauma occlusion with or without analgesia and instructions.
- Absence of evidence of infection.
- Absence of haemorrhage requiring immobilization to control.
- Good patient co-operation and follow-up.

Indications for open treatment

When conservative treatment is inappropriate or has failed.

Closed treatment

In its simplest form, closed treatment would be:
- analgesia;
- antibiotics in open fractures (1 week);
- soft diet until a firm callus forms (usually around 4–6 weeks).

This is often suitable for a **firm, minimally or un-displaced fracture with a normal bite**.

Intermaxillary fixation (IMF)

For painful or more displaced fractures this may be applied. Here the upper and lower teeth are fixed together using wires or elastics. This uses the upper teeth as both a splint and a mandibular positioning device, ensuring a normal bite and immobilization of the fracture for healing. However, reduction is not anatomical. Various devices are available to achieve intermaxillary fixation including eyelet wires, Leonard buttons, arch bars, and splints. These are ligated or cemented to the teeth thereby enabling the two jaws to be fixed to each other. If the patient has no teeth (edentulous patients), modified dentures (Gunning splints) can be ligated to the jaws to achieve a similar goal.

A further variation is to use elastic bands instead of wires between the jaws to allow some degree of movement.

Closed treatment is known to work and has remained a main method of treatment. However, it is not risk free. Disadvantages include:
- airway risk (asthmatics, COAD, epileptics, reduced conscious level);
- loss of weight;
- patients need to tolerate it (beware alcoholics and mentally ill);
- injury to tooth structure, restorations, and the periodontal tissues.

Relative contra-indications to IMF are:
- inadequate post-operative monitoring of airway during recovery from general anaesthesia;
- need for prolonged oral/nasal airway post-operatively;
- possibility of convulsions;
- head injury (GCS 8 or less).

Open treatment
Closed treatment does not produce *anatomical* reduction of the fracture (hence the term closed *treatment* as opposed to closed *reduction*). With open treatment, surgical exposure of the fracture site and (hopefully) anatomical reduction is carried out. Exposure is most commonly carried out through the mouth, but occasionally may be done through a skin incision or an existing laceration. Once exposed, the fracture is accurately reduced and fixed. Common fixation techniques use titanium 'mini' plates or screws. This is now the preferred approach to most mandibular

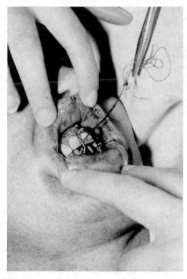

Fig. 8.22 Wire IMF—rarely used now (note no gloves).

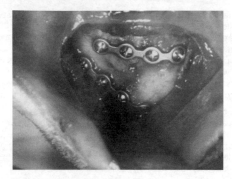

Fig. 8.23 'ORIF' parasymphyseal fracture.

fractures resulting in faster recovery and rehabilitation. However, there is potentially more morbidity, especially injury to the inferior alveolar nerve and tooth roots. The patient still requires a soft diet for the same period of time.

Treatment of condylar fractures

Particular concerns with these fractures are long-term joint dysfunction, ankylosis, and, in children, abnormal growth of mandible

Undisplaced condylar fractures, where the occlusion is normal, are generally managed with rest, soft diet, and simple analgesics. These are not compound fractures and so antibiotics are not necessary. Regular review is essential in the early stages of healing to ensure that the fracture does not 'slip' and derange the bite. Fractures that are **displaced with an associated malocclusion**, however, need to be reduced. This is often carried out using rigid or elastic IMF, the latter encouraging dynamic realignment of the fragments. IMF is applied for 7–14 days to avoid ankylosis. Following IMF early mobilization and physiotherapy are required.

Alternatively, and where IMF is contra-indicated, fractures may be openly **reduced and fixed** using mini plates, interosseous wires, screws. These are approached via a skin incision just behind the angle of the jaw below the ear. There is a small risk of facial nerve injury, although with careful surgical technique, this can be kept to a minimum. **Bilateral condylar fractures** may be managed similarly. However, these fractures must be kept under close review until healed. 'Telescoping' of the condyles with loss of jaw height posteriorly can lead to the occlusion being propped open at the front—an anterior open bite. This would require surgical correction at a later date.

Rarely, the condylar head may dislocate out of the articular fossa. This usually requires open reduction

Special considerations

Tooth in the fracture site

For angle, body, parasymphyseal and symphyseal fractures, usually a tooth is present in the fracture site. This is especially common in angle fractures, where an unerupted third molar may weaken the bone locally. While it may be tempting to remove the tooth (especially in open treatment), this may make reduction of the fracture more difficult and unstable. For anterior fractures, the loss of a tooth has obvious aesthetic consequences. Consequently, unless the tooth itself is fractured, grossly decayed, has associated periapical infection, or is interfering with fracture reduction, it may be preferable to leave it *in situ*. Opinions may differ.

Analgesia/antibiotics/tetanus

Mandibular fractures are painful. The use of local anaesthesia (LA) and bridal wires has been described in the first-aid section. LA can also be repeated with a long-acting local anaesthetic, such as bupivicaine. Analgesia requirements often dramatically reduce following fracture reduction and fixation; useful agents include NSAIDS or paracetamol-based compounds.

Antibiotic therapy is generally required for compound (open) fractures and should give appropriate cover against anaerobic organisms and streptococci. Many policies exist and may include metronidazole with benzyl penicillin or a compound agent such as co-amoxyclav. Antibiotic treatment may be continued for 5 days.

Tetanus status should be checked and the patient given tetanus toxoid, if appropriate.

Fractures in children

Similar principles apply and early mobilization is desirable, as there is an increased risk of ankylosis. Consideration must be given to the unerupted teeth, if plating is necessary. Long-term follow-up during growth is recommended, as some fractures (especially condylar) are associated with disturbances of growth.

Post-operative care

Closed treatment without intermaxillary fixation is usually treated on an out-patient basis with regular review to ensure the occlusion remains normal. Post-operative radiographs are necessary to confirm a correct position of the bone fragments. Hospital dieticians are a valuable resource and will give nutritional advice and provide supplements.

Closed treatment with intermaxillary wire fixation requires very close observation in the immediate post-operative period. Prior to discharge, the patient must be provided with wire cutters, which must be with him/her 24 h a day, and they must be instructed on their use. More recently there has been a swing in favour of using elastics rather that wire. This enables quicker release and a degree of flexibility in the immobilization enabling 'micro-movement'.

Following open treatment, the occlusion should be assessed the following day. It is not uncommon for this to be slightly deranged due to muscle spasm or a joint effusion; this should settle with appropriate analgesia or light elastic IMF. The position of the fragments should be confirmed with post-operative radiographs (OPT and PA mandible) and arrangements made to review the patient weekly. A soft diet is needed for the next 4–6 weeks.

ⓘ Dislocated condyle

The temporomandibular joint (TMJ) is the joint between the mandible and the skull base, located in the pre-auricular region. It is a synovial 'ball and socket' type joint, the 'ball' portion being the mandibular condyle, and the 'socket' the glenoid fossa of the temporal bone. A fibrous sleeve encapsulates the joint. Between the condyle and fossa there is a fibro-cartilaginous disc, or 'meniscus', which is attached peripherally to the deep surface of the joint capsule. The four muscles of mastication (the masseter, the temporalis, and the medial and lateral pterygoids) act directly across the TMJ to effect mandibular movements. Of note, the insertion of the lateral pterygoid is into both the condylar neck, and through the fibrous capsule, into the anterior aspect of the articular disc.

Movement across the joint is complex. On opening the mouth from the closed position, initially a hinge-type movement occurs for the first 1 cm. After that a forward translation is added in which the condyle moves forward and downwards along the slope of the fossa. Very little movement occurs side-to-side. Appreciation of TMJ anatomy and function helps understand the clinical picture associated with fractures of the condyle.

Displacement of the mandibular condyle from the glenoid fossa is termed dislocation of the condyle. This may be unilateral or bilateral, solitary or recurrent. Following significant trauma, it can be associated with a fracture of the condylar process (fracture dislocation).

Dislocation is usually in an anterior direction so that the condyle comes to lie in front of the articular eminence. Following major trauma it may occur in other directions, including intra-cranially.

Patients present with a sudden inability to close the mouth, which is painful and held **wide open**. This is in distinction to 'open lock', where the mouth is held open only a few millimeters due to meniscal entrapment.

Reduction of a dislocation can often be accomplished with simple analgesia alone or in combination with local anaesthetic. LA can be injected into lateral pterygoid and masseter muscles and, if necessary, into the periarticular tissues (possible temporary VII palsy). This weakens those muscles that keep the condyle dislocated and reduces capsular pain, which stimulates spasm. Oral or intravenous sedation may also be necessary. Entonox has the advantage of being rapidly excreted afterwards, so the patient can go home. General anaesthesia may be required if the previous methods fail. Manual reduction of an anteriorly displaced condyle requires downward pressure on the retromolar (wisdom tooth) region and simultaneous upward pressure on the chin. This can be accomplished either by standing in front or behind the patient. (Protect your thumbs from being bitten if reduction is successful!) In long-standing cases, prolonged traction on the mandibular ramus under general anaesthesia or open reduction may be necessary.

Management of *fracture-dislocation* is either closed (intermaxillary fixation) or open (surgical repositioning of the displaced condyle with internal fixation)

Recurrent dislocation may also be treated conservatively with a barrel bandage, injection of sclerosant solutions into the capsule (to produce tightening), or by a variety of surgical procedures (capsular plication, eminectomy, or articular augmentation).

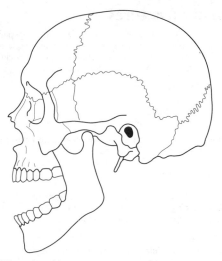

Fig. 8.24 Dislocated condyle.

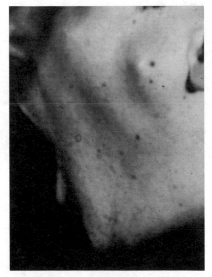

Fig. 8.25 Dislocated condyle—the mouth is *wide* open and the condyle can easily be seen displaced.

⊙ Alveolar fractures

This term relates to fractures of the **tooth-bearing part of the mandible and maxilla.** Where there is minimal displacement and minimal mobility, and the patient can obtain a pre-injury occlusion, these tend to be managed conservatively, as for mandibular fractures.

Indications for treatment

- Disruption of the bite.
- Physical evidence of fracture.
- Evidence of fracture from imaging—plain radiographs.

Closed, non-surgical treatment is required when there is:

- no or minimal displacement of fracture;
- no or minimal mobility of fracture line;
- ability to bite normally;
- absence of infection;
- no or minimal soft tissue loss from the bone segment;
- absence of bleeding requiring immobilization;
- good patient co-operation and follow-up.

Closed treatment

- Soft diet, analgesia, antibiotics, and close monitoring.
- Indirect fixation using arch bars or splints.
- Intermaxillary fixation may be required for large segments.

Operative treatment

- Removal of bone segment—indicated where segment is severely comminuted or significant soft tissue loss (loss of blood supply to the fragment).
- Open reduction and fixation with wires or plates. However this may compromise the blood supply.

If the teeth on the fragment are damaged, these need appropriate attention. If they need to be removed, this is sometimes delayed until the alveolar fracture has healed to maximize the blood supply to the segment.

⚠ Dental trauma

(See also the Mouth, lips, and teeth.)

This includes injuries to the teeth or their supporting structures. Despite continuing improvements in oral health, one in four children in Britain suffer some form of injury to their front teeth. Injuries range from chips off the enamel to crown/root fractures involving the tooth pulp.

The periodontal ligament and surrounding 'gum' support the teeth in their sockets and cushion the forces of mastication. These structures may be concussed (periodontal injury without loosening). Alternatively, intact teeth may be intruded (driven into the bone), displaced, or avulsed (pulled out the socket). Fractures of the teeth and/or supporting alveolar bone may also occur.

Treatment

This is required when there is:
- pain (pulp exposure);
- sensitivity to hot and cold (dentine exposure);
- recent avulsion;
- mobility (fracture or displacement);
- alveolar bone fracture;
- retention of part of the tooth;
- cosmetic deformity.

Principles of treatment

These include:
- pain relief;
- control of bleeding;
- dressing of exposed dentine or pulp;
- repositioning/replantation of the tooth—this is then splinted for a variable time depending on the nature of the injury;
- reduction and fixation of alveolar bone;
- cosmetic repair.

The avulsed tooth

Immediate action is required when one or more adult teeth are knocked out of the mouth. If these teeth are put back into the socket, there is a good chance they will take. **The primary aim of treatment is to replant an avulsed *adult* tooth as soon as possible**. This does not apply to baby teeth, if one is knocked out, it should not be pushed back into the socket because the underlying developing adult tooth may be damaged. The chances of success depend on how long it has been out of the mouth. Ideally, encourage an adult at the scene of the accident to replant it. Unfortunately, many lay people (and a few doctors) are worried about pushing a tooth back into a socket and getting it the right way round. If unable to do this, store the tooth in an appropriate solution and refer as quickly as possible. The main reason why avulsed teeth do not re-attach is that the periodontal cells on the root dry out. **The tooth must be kept moist**. Milk is good storage medium. Provided that the tooth is kept moist in milk, it can be replanted up to 24h later.

You therefore have two options when confronted by a patient with a tooth in his hand:

- re-implant the tooth back into its socket and refer the child immediately to a dentist for splinting;
- make sure the tooth is safe (in milk or physiological saline) and arrange for immediate dental treatment.

Consider antibiotics and, if appropriate, a tetanus booster. Treatment is often prolonged, usually requiring endodontic treatment (root filling) at a later stage.

Premature loss of an adult tooth can be particularly disfiguring, as the bone around the margins of the socket becomes resorbed. This compromises the success of replacement bridge work.

① Zygomatic and orbital fractures—applied anatomy

Fractures of the orbit and cheek often go hand in hand. Hence both will be considered together.

The cheek is predominently formed by the zygomatic bone. More correctly, it is made up of a complex of bones known as the zygomatico-maxillary complex or 'malar' bone.

The zygomatic bone links with the frontal bone at the fronto-zygomatic suture under the eyebrow; the maxilla medially and the temporal bone posteriorly. The body of the zygoma provides the **aesthetic prominence of the cheek** and forms part of the inferior and lateral rim of the orbit. The orbital rim supports the lower eyelid. The face is constructed of a series of buttresses that allow the transmission of force from the maxilla to the skull base (during chewing). The zygoma forms part of the **lateral buttress** and **protects the eye** by forming part of the orbital rim. It also projects a more delicate bony bar posteriorly towards the temporal bone forming the zygomatic arch.

The temporalis muscle passes beneath the zygomatic arch to insert into the coronoid process of the mandible. Fracture of the zygomatic arch can therefore produce limitation of mouth opening by interfering with the coronoid process or temporalis muscle. The temporalis muscle is invested in temporal fascia, which arises from the superior temporal line of the skull and passes down to insert into the zygomatic arch. This is an important surgical landmark (Gillies approach).

The orbit—applied anatomy

In essence, each orbit is a pyramidal-shaped structure. Its primary function is to contain, protect, and support the globe of the eye enabling binocular 3D vision. The walls of the pyramid are made up of a number of different bones and are of varying thickness and strengths. The orbital floor and medial orbital wall are particularly delicate and are prone to damage (blow-out fractures). The orbital floor carries the infra-orbital nerve, which supplies sensation to the majority of the cheek and one half of the nose and upper lip. Under the floor lies the maxillary sinus. The medial wall is predominately made up of the ethmoid bones and the ethmoidal air cells. The ethmoidal vessels pass through the orbit, into the nose, and may bleed profusely following trauma.

Numbness of the cheek and upper lip is an important sign that should generate a high index of suspicion for orbital or cheek bone fracture.

Peri-orbital fat fills the gaps in orbit and contains a radiating pattern of fine but strong septa that are the principal method of support for the eye. Damage to the bony orbit can result in herniation of peri-orbital fat and associated trapping of the septa. This prevents the co-ordinated action of the ocular muscles and results in restricted eye movements and double vision (diplopia).

Co-ordinated movements of the eye are achieved by the extra-ocular muscles—four recti and two oblique. The recti muscles have a common point of attachment at the tendinious ring at the orbital apex. They form a

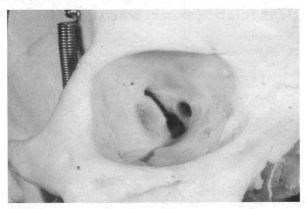

Fig. 8.26 Fissures and foramina of the orbit.

muscular cone before inserting into the sclera. This cone is important in that it can act as a closed compartment containing blood following surgery or trauma (see Retrobulbar haemorrhage).

Terminology

Many terms are used including zygomatic, zygomatic complex (ZC), zygomatico-maxillary complex, zygomatico-orbital, tripod and malar fractures. They all mean the same thing.

Epidemiology

- ZC fractures are the second most common facial fracture after nasal bone fractures.
- Most occur in males in their 2nd to 3rd decades.
- Inter-personal violence is the commonest cause.
- When fracture is caused by assault, the left side is affected more often than the right.
- Most are unilateral fractures.

① Zygomatic (malar) fractures

Assessment

Fractures involving the 'zygomatic complex' (ZC) involve the zygoma and adjacent bones (maxilla, frontal, and temporal bones). They are, therefore, not just zygomatic fractures. Strictly speaking they should be termed 'zygomatico-maxillary complex' fractures.

Practically, fractures can be considered as:
- isolated:
  - zygomatic arch;
  - infra-orbital rim (uncommon);
- minimally displaced malar;
- displaced fractured malar;
- comminuted fractured malar;
- fractured malar with associated mid-facial or orbital floor/wall injury.

All zygomatico-maxillary fractures, by definition, have a fracture line running through the orbit. Patients should therefore be assessed for ocular injury, diplopia, and entrapment. **The eye takes priority**. Associated ocular problems include:
- globe/muscle injury;
- retrobulbar haemorrhage;
- superior orbital fissure syndrome;
- orbital apex syndrome.

Symptoms
- Pain;
- Swelling;
- Depressed cheek bone;
- Altered sensation of cheek/upper lip;
- Double vision;
- Restricted jaw movements;

Examination

Signs of ZC fractures may include:
- ocular injury (check visual acuity);
- peri-orbital bruising and swelling;
- subconjunctival haemorrhage;
- surgical emphysema;
- numb cheek;
- flattening of malar prominence (often masked by swelling immediately after injury);
- palpable infra-orbital step;
- antimongaloid slant;
- unilateral epistaxis (due to bleeding into maxillary sinus);
- limitation of eye movements with diplopia;
- enophthalmos;
- exophthalmos;
- hypoglobus (vertical ocular dystopia);
- restricted mouth opening;
- malocclusion (premature contact on molar teeth).

Radiographs and other useful investigations
- Visual acuity.
- Orthoptic assessment (Hess chart).
- Plain radiographs—occipitomental (OM), lateral face and submental-vertex (SMV)—look carefully, sometimes the only clue is a fluid level in the antrum.
- CT scan-axial and coronal.
- Ultrasound scan.
- Maxillary sinus endoscopy for orbital floor fractures.

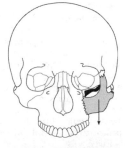

Fig. 8.27 Vertical displacement of the zygoma can drag the lateral canthus and lateral attachment of the globe with it. This can result in diplopia, hypoglobus, and an anti-mongoloid slant to the eye.

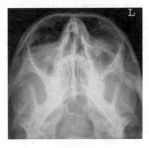

Fig. 8.28 OM view of the mid-face, showing a fractured zygoma.

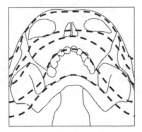

Fig. 8.29 'Campbell's' lines aid identification of midface fractures.

Indications for CT scan
- Suspected orbital floor fracture.
- Comminuted or severely displaced fractures.
- Injuries associated with other facial fractures.

Fractures
These are classified according to:
- degree of comminution;
- whether or not they are compound (open);
- the site of fractures;
- the direction and degree of displacement.

(At present no universally accepted classification system exists.)

Treatment
First aid and warnings

These fractures do not require urgent intervention and can be assessed as an out-patient. **The eye takes priority**—a high percentage of injuries to the orbit are also associated with injuries to the eye itself. **Check visual acuity and consider ophthalmic opinion if abnormal**. Also refer to maxillofacial team on-call. Advise the patient **not to blow their nose**. If they do this, it can result in peri-orbital surgical emphysema. Pressurized air passes through the nose and antrum into the orbit through the fracture. If it gets infected this can result in **orbital cellulitis**, which can be devastating. Many hospitals advise prophylactic **antibiotics**. Tell the patient to return if they have increasing swelling, pain, or change in visual acuity.

Remember—a high percentage of injuries to the bony orbit are also associated with injuries to the eye itself. **Always check visual acuity to identify rare sight-threatening emergencies that can occur**.

Indications for operative treatment
- Clinical signs consistent with displaced zygomatic fracture.
- Radiological evidence of displaced fracture.
- Sensory nerve deficit.
- Limitation of mandibular opening.
- Ocular dysfunction.
- Facial deformity.

The timing of surgical intervention depends on the degree of swelling and general medical/surgical considerations—in particular, head or ocular injury. Surgery is usually carried out either immediately or about 5–6 days following injury. Acceptable results can still be obtained at 3 weeks, but reduction becomes more difficult.

Surgical reduction
This depends on the degree and nature of displacement of the fracture sites.

Isolated arch or simple fractures, which are incomplete at the fronto-zygomatic suture, are those most suitable for simple elevation by the Gillies approach. Closed reduction techniques include:
- Temporal approach (Gillies).
- Percutaneous hook.
- Eyebrow approach—zygomatic elevator.
- Carroll–Girard screw.
- Intra-oral approaches (upper buccal sulcus).

Most fractures are now treated by **open reduction and internal fixation (ORIF)** with titanium miniplates. Surgical access for reduction and fixation is commonly through the mouth to avoid facial scars. Access to the fronto-zygomatic suture and infra-orbital rim may be necessary to assist reduction and fixation. The more displaced or comminuted the fracture the more fracture sites need to be exposed.

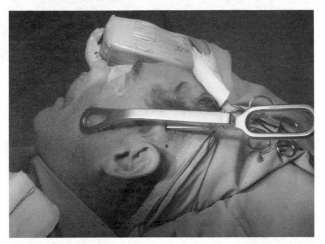

Fig. 8.30 Gillies approach.

Gillies' approach

This consists of a temporal hairline incision, which is deepened to expose the temporalis fascia overlying the temporalis muscle. This is incised and an elevator is slid *beneath* the fascia over the underlying muscle. The fascia acts as conduit to guide the elevator under the body of the zygoma. The zygoma can then be elevated into its correct position with care taken not to use the temporal bone as a fulcrum. (Iatrogenic temporal skull fracture is an embarrassing complication!)

⊙ Orbital fractures (isolated)

This refers to fractures affecting the bony orbital walls or orbital margin but not involving the surrounding complexes, e.g. naso-ethmoid, zygomatic, anterior cranial fossa.

Blow-out fractures

The classical isolated injury to the orbit is the orbital floor 'blow-out' fracture, which occurs as result of a direct blow to the globe (e.g. squash ball to the eye). This increases pressure within the bony orbit. It may also follow a blow to the prominence of the cheek, where the bone 'buckles', resulting in fracture propagation. The floor of the orbit is relatively weak and is fractured with herniation of orbital contents into the maxillary sinus. The injury can also occur on the medial wall in association with other localized facial fracture (fractured malar or Le Fort fracture) or in any combination.

Clinical features

Early assessment of the eye is essential, as management takes priority over the fracture itself. Very often the eyelids become closed due to painful swelling. However, gently pressing on the eyelids (*not* the globe) for a few minutes reduces this sufficiently to assess visual acuity, pupillary size, and reaction and visualize the anterior chamber for hyphema. Contact lenses and superficial foreign bodies can be removed. **If a penetrating injury to the eye is suspected, pressure should be avoided.** A dilated pupil may often be due to traumatic midryasis but its significance in relation to head injuries must be remembered.

   Look for:
- peri-orbital bruising;
- subconjunctival haemorrhage;
- numb cheek;
- restricted eye movements (usually upwards);
- retraction sign;
- diplopia;
- enopthalmous (may not be apparent immediately unless severe injury—may occur late, >3 months).

Consider also the following:
- naso-lacrimal dysfunction;
- presence of foreign bodies;
- motor and sensory nerve deficit;
- other peri-orbital soft tissue injuries.

Remember—a high percentage of injuries to the bony orbit are also associated with injuries to the eye itself. **Always check visual acuity to identify rare sight-threatening emergencies that can occur. Associated ocular problems include:**
- globe/muscle injury;
- retrobulbar haemorrhage;
- superior orbital fissure syndrome;
- orbital apex syndrome.

Assessment and initial investigations

- Visual acuity.
- Examination of globe.
- Plain radiographs If possible get occipitomental (OM), and lateral facial views (for associated malar or mid-facial injury). Look for a 'hanging drop': this represents the herniation of orbital contents into the maxillary sinus. It may not be easily seen. A fluid level in the sinus suggests a fracture somewhere.
- Coronal/axial CT of orbits.
- Orthoptic assessment—Hess chart, measurement of globe projection and fields of binocular vision (to assess restriction of ocular movement).

Treatment

Where an injury to the globe or associated nerves is suspected an ophthalmic opinion should be sought. In all cases advise the patient **not to blow their nose**. If they do this, it can result in peri-orbital surgical emphysema. Pressurized air passes through the nose and antrum into the orbit via the fracture. If it gets infected this can result in **orbital cellulitis** which can be devastating. Many hospitals advise prophylactic **antibiotics**. Tell the patient to return if they have increasing swelling, pain or change in visual acuity. Chloramphenicol ointment may be applied to any conjunctival injury.

Further management

This is controversial. Some fractures can be treated conservatively. Indications for surgery include significant diplopia, a retraction sign, dystopia (displacement of globe), enopthalmous or a 'large' blow-out on CT—said to predispose to the late development of enopthalmous. The aim is to release entrapped soft tissues and restore orbital volume. This should release any restriction of eye movement and restore globe position.

Surgical treatment

The timing of surgery is controversial and dependent on multiple factors. If there is minimal displacement and no evidence of enophthalmos or significant orbital volume change (which might result in late enophthalmos), it is common practice to delay surgery for up to 10–14 days post-injury. This allows any swelling to settle and gives an idea of any deformity. **If there is evidence of ischaemic incarceration of the orbital soft tissues or muscles *immediate* intervention may prevent scar contraction**.

There are a number of cosmetically acceptable local approaches to the orbit. Extensive injuries, particularly of the medial wall, may need a bicoronal approach. The orbit can be reconstructed with a number of allogenic or autogenous materials. Bone can be used and may be harvested from the maxillary antral wall, cranium, rib, or iliac crest. Allogenic materials are numerous and include specially formed titanium plates or mesh, polymers and newer resorbable materials.

☼ Mid-facial ('middle-third') fractures—applied anatomy

The bones of the mid-face consist of:
- 2 maxillae;
- 2 zygomas;
- 2 zygomatic processes of the temporal bones;
- 2 palatine bones;
- 2 nasal bones;
- 2 lacrimal bones;
- 2 inferior conchae;
- sphenoid pterygoid plates;
- ethmoid;
- vomer.

The arrangement of these bones, together with the presence of the air-filled sinuses, essentially converts the mid-face into a **series of vertical bony struts, or buttresses**, passing upwards from the teeth to the skull base. The lateral buttresses are formed by the lateral orbital margins and the zygomatic complex. The medial butresses are formed by the frontal processes and medial body of the maxillae.

Anatomy of the buttresses

The mid-face has three paired buttresses that are the 'pillars' that take the load of any vertically applied force. These are
- **anterior**, which runs up from the piriform fossa lateral to the nose, up to the fronto-nasal process, which is made up by the articulation of the maxilla with the frontal bone;
- **middle**, which is formed by the buttress of the zygoma articulating with the maxilla anteriorly and inferiorly, and the frontal bone above;
- **posterior**, which is made up by the pterygoid plates attaching the maxilla to the base of skull.

The mandible can be thought of as being indirectly buttressed through the maxilla by the above buttresses when the teeth are in occlusion.

As a result of these butresses, the face is very good at resisting vertically directed forces (i.e. chewing). However, there are very few strong, horizontally directed butresses and consequently the face is not good at resisting horizontally directed forces (i.e. a significant vector in most trauma). It has been argued that the **sinuses effectively convert the face into a 'crumple zone'**, thereby absorbing kinetic energy and protecting the brain from injury.

Because the mid-facial skeleton sits on an inclined skull base at 45 degrees to the horizontal plane, mid-face fractures can result in the middle-third being sheered off the cranial base, and forced downwards and backwards along this inclined plane. Clinically this results in an elongated face and deranged bite (anterior open bite).

☼ Le Fort mid-face fractures

Fracture patterns

The terms used to describe these mid-facial fractures, **refer to the level of the fracture** related to the skull base.

Le Fort I ('low level')

The fracture lies horizontally at a level just above the nasal floor, passing backwards from the piriform aperture, above the alveolus, to below the zygomatic buttress. From the mid-line it passes along the lower-third of the nasal septum and lateral walls of the nose to join the lateral aspects of the fracture across the lower third of the pterygoid plates. **This is essentially the tooth-bearing part of the mid-face (think of a denture).**

Le Fort II ('pyramidal')

From the mid-line, through the nasal bones, this fracture crosses the frontal processes of the maxillae to the medial orbital walls. The fracture passes through the lacrimal bones and crosses the inferior orbital margin at the level of, or just medial to, the infra-orbital foramen. The fracture continues in an infero-posterior extension across the lateral wall of the antrum below the zygomatico-maxillary suture. Infero-posteriorly the fracture passes through the mid-point of the pterygoid plates. Supero-medially the fracture passes through the nasal septum and may involve the cribriform plate of the anterior cranial fossa.

Le Fort III ('high transverse' or 'cranio-facial dysjunction')

From the mid-line the fracture passes from the fronto-nasal suture backwards through the ethmoid bone involving the cribriform plate. Laterally the fracture runs within the orbit below the level of the optic foramen to the posterior aspect of the inferior orbital fissure. From here the fracture passes laterally through the lateral wall of the orbit and fronto-zygomatic

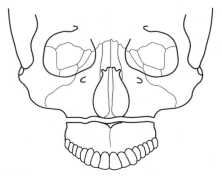

Fig. 8.31 Le Fort I.

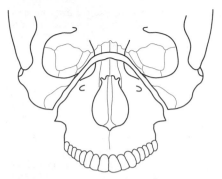

Fig. 8.32 Le Fort II.

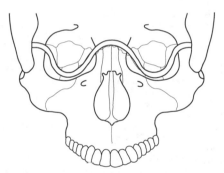

Fig. 8.33 Le Fort III.

process and posteriorly it crosses the pterygo-maxillary fissure to separate the base of the pterygoids. **This separates the entire facial skeleton from the skull base**.

Le Fort II and III both
• **Involve the orbit (risk to the eyes).**
• **Potentially involve the anterior cranial fossa (associated head injury/CSF leakage).**

Often these fractures occur in various combinations ipsilaterally and bilaterally.

The type of Le Fort fracture can usually be determined by examination. This consists of holding the head stable and rocking on the upper front teeth (or the alveolar ridge, if the patient is edentulous).
- If the teeth and palate move but the nasal bones are stable, it is a Le Fort I.
- If the teeth, palate and nasal bones move but the inferior orbital rims are stable it is a Le Fort II.
- If the whole mid-face feels unstable, it is probably a Le Fort III.

Assessment
(See also Pan-facial fractures below.)
   Consider serious facial injuries in anyone with gross swelling.

Clinical features and associated problems
Clinical features may be a direct result of the force of trauma, or as a consequence of the effects of this force on disruption and displacement of the mid-facial skeleton.

General features
- **Airway** compromise (uncommon).
- **Haemorrhage**—associated with mucosal tears in the naso-pharynx or facial wounds/lacerations. Rarely torrential, although may require nasal packing or fracture reduction to stem the flow. If the patient is shocked, look for another cause.
- **CSF rhinorrhoea**—CSF leak from the nose (anterior cranial fossa #).
- **CSF otorrhoea**—CSF leak from the ear (middle cranial fossa #).
- **'Tramlining'** may be seen when blood mixes with CSF and leaks from the nose or ear. Along the edges of the flow the blood clots while the CSF washes it away centrally forming two parallel lines: hence 'tramlining'.
- **Complications of CSF leaks** (meningitis, aerocele or fistula formation with significant CSF loss).
- **Facial swelling.**
- **Massive facial oedema**.
- **Abnormal mobility** of the mid-face—checked by holding the anterior maxillary alveolus and gently attempting to mobilize the maxilla; the other hand is held at sites of suspected fractures, e.g. the nasal bridge or the inferior orbital margins.

Eye signs
- Bilateral peri-orbital ecchymoses **('panda faces' or 'racoon eyes')**. These are often associated with the gross degree of facial oedema as seen in the Le Fort II and III fractures.
- Bilateral **subconjunctival ecchymoses** (bright red). This is bruising within the conjunctiva adjacent to fractures that pass through the orbit (Le Fort II and III).
- **Enophthalmus**—sinking in of the eyes—may initially be masked by oedema.
- **Diplopia**—caused by swelling , orbital displacement, or tethering of ocular muscles within fracture lines and hence lack of stereoscopic vision.
- **Traumatic mydriasis** (dilated pupil)—spasm of dilator pupillae secondary to a direct blow.

Features related to the displacement of the mid-face skeleton

The mid-face may be forced downwards and backwards along the skull base at 45 degrees to the maxillary occlussal plane. This can result in:

- **obstructed airway**—this results from the soft palate resting on the dorsum of the tongue and the posterior oro-pharyngeal wall;
- **anterior open bite;**
- **apparent trismus** caused by gagging of the occlusion due to premature contact in the molar region;
- **lengthening of the mid-face;**
- **'dish-faced' deformity**—comminution of the mid-facial bones (naso-ethmoid complex/anterior maxilla) may result in a central collapse rather than a posterior displacement of the whole mid-face: this will produce the classic dish-face deformity;
- **pain and crepitus**;
  - over the nasal bridge and palpable fracture sites; step deformities may also be elicited;
  - inferior orbital rims (Le Fort II);
  - upper buccal sulcus (Le Fort I and II);
- **upper buccal sulcus bruising;**
- **anaesthesia**—commonly in the distribution of the infra-orbital nerve—may be as a result of direct trauma, or the widespread compressive effects of facial oedema.

Radiographs and other useful investigations

Except for the CXR and Head CT these can wait.

- **Chest radiograph**. Remember the possibility of inhaled foreign bodies, e.g. from dental trauma.
- **Occipito-mental**. One or two projections (15 and 30 degrees) together with a good clinical examination will usually show most Le Fort fractures adequately. Campbell's 'search' lines provide a system of assessing these views.
- **True lateral projection**. This may demonstrate the postero-inferior displacement of the maxilla responsible for gagging on the posterior dentition and an anterior open bite. It is also useful for assessment of the frontal sinuses (fluid levels, posterior wall fractures) and visualizing the pterygoid plates (an indication of the level of the fracture).
- **Peri-apical and upper occlusal views**. These are useful for assessment of dento-alveolar fractures and identification of a palatal mid-line split.
- **Panoral tomography (OPG)**. Very useful if a mandibular fracture is suspected. It may also show low level Le Fort I fractures, dento-alveolar fractures, and dental injuries.
- **Computed tomography (CT scans)**. These are particularly useful in associated head injuries and in assessing fractures of the naso-ethmoidal complex, frontal sinus and orbit.
- **Magnetic resonance imaging**. May be of value in the diagnosis of CSF leaks and in the assessment of soft tissue injury, particularly the orbit.

Treatment

(See also Pan-facial fractures below.)

Maxillofacial trauma should be integrated into **Advanced Trauma Life Support—ATLS**. ATLS dictates:

...maxillofacial trauma, not associated with airway obstruction or major bleeding, should be treated only after the patient is stabilized completely and life threatening injuries have been managed.

Consider first:

- airway with c spine;
- breathing;
- circulation;
- head injuries;
- ocular injuries.

Beware the patient who keeps trying to sit up—they may be trying to clear their airway. If there is no spinal injury let them sit up, if unsure log roll or tip the table head down. This is at variance with ATLS guidelines but facial bleeding will continue unrecognized in the supine position until the patient vomits and possibly aspirates.

First aid

Le Fort fractures can present with prolonged **epistaxis** (nose bleed). Definitive treatment may involve reduction of the fracture or cautery/ ligation of appropriate vessels. As a first-aid measure nasal packs may tamponade the flow. If posterior nasal packing is required, urinary (Foley) catheters may be inserted beyond the soft palate prior to inflating the balloon and then withdrawn until the balloons wedge in the posterior naso-pharynx; anterior nasal packing with ribbon gauze may also be required. Custom devices are available (Epistat™) with dual balloons that will occlude the entire nasal airway and hence tamponade haemorrhage.

Wounds and haemorrhage—'assess, arrest, and replace'

Remove any dressings to fully assess wounds, remembering that they may have been placed as pressure dressings to stem initial blood loss. Ideally careful exploration under LA should be carried out before closure to clean and remove any debris or foreign bodies, and to identify any underlying fractures. If the patient obviously requires to go to theatre, then formal wound closure should be delayed (although ideally no longer than 24 h) but judicious placement of a few sutures along with simple dressings should help to stem a steady venous ooze.

Replace lost fluids—any patient with Le Fort fractures must have adequate intravenous (IV) access and appropriate fluid resuscitation. Assessment must be made of any losses, as well as ongoing needs.

Prevent infection

Le Fort fractures are almost always compound injuries via communications with the sinuses or facial wounds.

- **Antibiotics**—intravenous and broad spectrum. Many regimes exist and include augmentin, or benzyl penecillin + metronidazole.
- **Tetanus**—ensure tetanus prophylaxis is up to date.

Analgesia

Remember, pain is a potent stimulus for the release of catecholamines. However, facial fractures are often not as painful as one may think.

- **Local**—regional nerve blocks: bilateral infra-orbital blocks may be particularly useful in the Le Fort I and II fractures. Consider supra-orbital blocks for the Le Fort III pattern.
- **Systemic**—avoid opiates until the patient is cleared of a head injury:
  - **IM (intramuscular)**, a possibility but avoid in the shocked patient;
  - **IV (intravenous)** rapid onset, and easy to titrate. Ideally, if the patient's conscious level is appropriate, establish a PCA (patient controlled analgesia) in liaison with anaesthetic colleagues.

Definitive management—'reduction and fixation' (See also Pan-facial fractures below.)

Indications for treatment
These include:
- disruption of the occlusion of the teeth;
- displacement of the maxilla;
- fractured or displaced teeth;
- cerebrospinal fluid leak (controversial);
- abnormal eye movement or restriction of eye movement;
- occlusion of the naso-lacrimal duct;
- sensory or motor nerve deficit.

Reduction
Anatomical reduction is the key to successful treatment of mid-face fractures. However, mobilization of the fractures varies greatly and is dependent on fracture pattern, comminution, and impaction. Surgical reduction and fixation of the maxilla is usually required in the majority of cases. Where the maxilla is undisplaced and stable or if the patient if unfit for an operation non-operative treatment may be appropriate.

Manual reduction involves reduction by digital pressure. Sometimes disimpaction forceps (Rowe's) are required. These are two forceps with upper blades, which pass into the nostril to grip the nasal floor above, and lower blades to grip the intra-orally against the palate. **Open reduction** involves visualization of the fracture sites via incisions for mobilization.

Fixation
A variety of fixation techniques may be used either by an open or closed approach. In some cases no fixation is necessary (undisplaced, immobile fractures).

Internal fixation is achieved by the application of plates to the main bone buttresses of the mid-face via intra-oral incisions. The teeth are usually wired together (IMF) during the operation to help guide the fragments into position, although this is usually removed at the end of the procedure. In the edentulous patient, Gunning splints may be appropriate. Fixation uses semi-rigid mini-plates and mono-cortical screws. Under direct vision the fractures are reduced and plated. For complete fixation of Le Fort II and III fractures access may be gained via peri-orbital incisions or a coronal flap.

Indirect fixation and external fixation may be indicated for rapid immobilization of Le Fort fractures. In such cases the bite is used to align and stabilize the fracture or the fracture is immobilized by fixing it to the stable cranium/frontal bone. **External fixation** is generally carried out using supra-orbital pins or a halo frame connected to the maxilla with a bar. However, this method has largely been superseded by internal

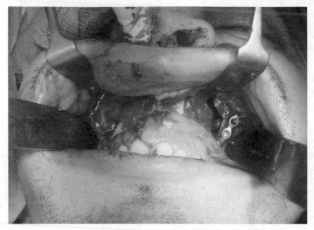

Fig. 8.34 'ORIF' of a butress in Le Fort I fracture.

fixation using plates. It may still be useful when rapid fixation is required, there are infected wounds (rare), in extensive comminution, or in children. Associated skull or frontal bone fractures is a relative contra-indication to external fixation.

Internal suspension involves suspending the maxillary fracture from the skull with wires and placing the patient in IMF.

Surgical approaches
Exposure of fracture sites is the key to accurate reduction and fixation. This can be:
- **via wounds;**
- **intra-orally;**
- **peri-orbital incisions:**
  - lateral brow;
  - supra-tarsal fold ('upper blepharoplasty');
  - mid-tarsal;
  - subciliary ('lower blepharoplasty');
  - trans-conjunctival +/− lateral canthotomy;
- **through the skin in the fronto-nasal area:**
  - 'H' (converse);
  - mid-line vertical;
  - 'W';
  - bilateral medial canthal incisions;
- **Coronal flap ('bicoronal flap')**—an incision is placed in the coronal plane across the scalp from left to right preauricular regions. The scalp is reflected forwards to give excellent exposure of the upper cranio-facial skeleton, including the zygomatic complexes and the fronto-naso-ethmoidal region. This also enables harvesting of cranial bone grafts if required.

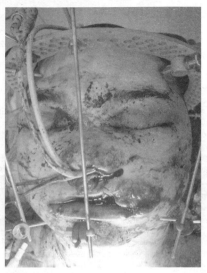

Fig. 8.35 External fixation.

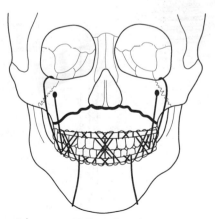

Fig. 8.36 Internal suspension and IMF in Le Fort 1 fracture.

① Nasal fractures

This refers to disruption of the normal **bony and cartilaginous** skeleton of the nose. The nose is the most commonly fractured bone in the face. **Diagnosis is clinical not radiological**. The pattern of injury depends on the magnitude and direction of the force applied (lateral or frontal direction).

Three levels of frontal directed injury can be distinguished:

- **plane one** injuries do not extend beyond a line joining the nasal bones and the anterior nasal spine and therefore involve the **cartilaginous nasal skeleton only**;
- **plane two** injuries are limited to the **external nose** and do not transgress the orbital rims;
- **plane three** injuries are more serious and involve orbit walls and possibly the cranium—this corresponds to a **naso-ethmoidal fracture.**

Indications for treatment

- Nasal deformity.
- Obstructed nasal airway.
- Epistaxis.
- **Septal haematoma**—this forms between the septal cartilage and its perichondrium. It must be ruled out in every patient, and appears as a dark swelling on the septum with narrowing of the nasal airway. This requires urgent incision and drainage. If missed it can lead to a septal abscess with intra-cranial complications or a delayed 'saddle nose' following necrosis and cartilage loss.

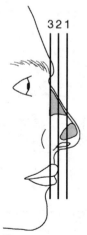

Fig. 8.37 Classification of nasal fractures.

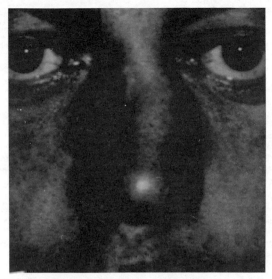

Fig. 8.38 Nasal fracture (predominantly the nasal bones).

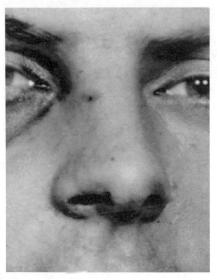

Fig. 8.39 Nasal fracture (predominantly the cartilagenous septum—compare tip position).

Conservative management

This is indicated if there is no significant deformity, airway obstruction, or haemorrhage.

Septal haematoma may be aspirated but may require open drainage under local or general anaesthesia.

Anterior **nasal packing** may be required if there is any nasal bleeding. For more serious bleeding, post-nasal packs may be required. For torrential haemorrhage, uncontrollable by packing, surgery or embolization may be necessary.

Closed manipulation (MUA) of nasal bones with nasal packing and external splinting (POP) is usually carried out to correct simple deformity. If undertaken very early (on the sports field), this often requires no anaesthesia. Cases must be selected carefully, as manipulation may start bleeding. Nasal manipulation and packing otherwise requires general anaesthesia. If the septum is significantly damaged, closed manipulation **with SMR or septoplasty** may be undertaken.

Open reduction

Naso-ethmoidal fractures require open surgery to correct fronto-nasal dysjunction and associated frontal and orbital fractures. Correction of traumatic telecanthus may be necessary.

Beware nasal fractures with associated black eyes—they may be naso-ethmoid injuries.

☼ Naso-ethmoid (naso-orbital-ethmoid) fractures

(See also Pan-facial fractures below.)

Consider serious facial injuries in anyone with gross swelling.

This refers to injuries to the **nose, orbits, and ethmoid sinuses (NOE)**. Naso-orbital-ethmoid fractures are among the most challenging facial injuries to diagnose and treat. Fractures of this region are often complex and comminuted. When assessing these fractures **consideration of the frontal sinus should also be made**. This is because the drainage apparatus of the sinus may be blocked as it passes through the ethmoid region or it may be communicating with the CSF.

Clinical features

NOE fractures occur following a direct blow to the bridge of the nose. The ethmoid sinuses act as a crumple zone absorbing the impact. This results in a 'pushed-in' look to bridge of the nose—a 'Miss Piggy nose'. Clinically there can be:

- severely comminuted nasal fracture;
- detachment of the medial canthal tendons resulting in pseudotelecanthus;
- fracture of the anterior cranial fossa;
- fracture of the frontal sinus;
- CSF leak.

The **'bow-string' test** assesses for canthal detachment—the lateral canthus is pulled laterally, if there is detachment medially the medial canthus will also move laterally.

Consider also concomitant injury to:

- the head/neck;
- the eye;
- frontal sinus;
- canthal ligaments;
- naso-lacrimal apparatus.

The severity of the injury may vary considerably in this region. The degree of bone displacement and comminution is difficult to visualize on plain radiographs, and computerized tomography is necessary. Usually there is extensive comminution of the involved bones with associated soft tissue injuries. This makes reduction and fixation difficult, particularly when there are other facial bone fractures.

Indications for treatment

- Cerebrospinal fluid leakage (controversial).
- Traumatic telecanthus.

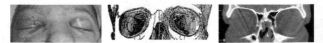

Fig. 8.40 (a) and (b) Nasoethmoid (naso-orbital-ethmoid) fractures.

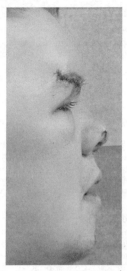

Fig. 8.41 Flat face and 'Miss Piggy nose' in NOE fracture.

- Orbital dystopia.
- Abnormalities of eye movement.
- Naso-lacrimal duct obstruction.
- Deformity of the nose.
- Functional abnormality of the nose including nasal airway obstruction.
- Deviation of the nasal septum, and septal haematoma.

Reduction is indicated in the majority of cases. Non-operative treatment may be appropriate where the fracture is undisplaced or when the general condition of the patient makes surgery inadvisable. Simple **closed reduction** of the nasal bones may be carried out under a day case general anaesthetic or even local anaesthesia. More complex fractures may require **open reduction and internal fixation**. Accurate repositioning of the canthal ligaments is essential for a good cosmetic result. A number of surgical techniques may be employed using either an open or closed approach. An open approach (usually via a bicoronal flap) is indicated for complex fractures or when frontal sinus treatment is required.

In general, the best cosmetic result is obtained when a definitive anatomical reduction of the bone fragments and soft tissue reconstruction is carried out at the primary operative procedure.

☼ Pan-facial fractures

(See also Le Fort fractures above.)

The term 'pan-facial' is used when multiple fracture patterns are seen in the patient. Commonly this means a mid-face and mandibular fracture, but can include any of the previously described fracture patterns. Fractures of the face can be considered as those involving the **upper-third, mid-face, and lower face**. Some of these bones, such as the ethmoid and those comprising the orbital roof, are extremely delicate and so thin that on a dry skull light can easily pass through. The remainder vary in thickness but often remain quite delicate (nasal, zygoma). The mandible is the strongest of the facial bones.

The face is not solid but contains several 'cavities', such as the sinuses, orbits, oral, and nasal cavities. Around these the bones form a series of vertical struts known as 'buttresses'. As a result, these bones are very good at resisting vertically directed forces (e.g. during chewing) but are weak when it comes to resisting horizontal forces (i.e. during most injuries).

Upper facial fractures

These involve the frontal bone, fronto-naso-ethmoidal region, orbits- and associated sinuses. The important points to note are whether there is a displaced fracture and/or any fracture of the posterior wall of the frontal sinus, fronto-naso-ethmoidal region- or orbit. These will be seen following CT scans.

Mid-face fractures

These are classically those described by Le Fort as I, II, and III.

- **Le Fort I** runs above the apices of the teeth from the nasal aperture back to and across the lower end of the pterygoid plates, it also runs down the lateral nasal wall; these two are connected by a fracture running across the posterior wall of the maxilla.
- **Le Fort II** runs from the nasal bridge down across medial orbital wall and floor, and across the anterior maxilla under the zygomatic buttress. From there it passes across the lateral wall of the maxilla to the pterygomaxillary plates. It also runs down the lateral wall of nose and across the posterior wall of the maxilla.
- **Le Fort III** runs across the bridge of the nose into the orbit, down the medial orbital wall, across the orbital apex, and up the lateral orbital wall. There is also a fracture along the arch of the zygoma. This results in disruption at the fronto-nasal zygomatico-frontal and zygomatico-temporal sutures leading to cranio-facial disruption.
- **Le Fort II and III both:**
  - **involve the orbit (risk to the eyes);**
  - **potentially involve the anterior cranial fossa (associated head injury/CSF leakage).**

Fractures may be **unilateral or bilateral**—more commonly the latter. If it is unilateral and is displaced, there must be an associated palatal fracture. It is not uncommon to find one or more of these fracture patterns present. The bones are often comminuted and the fracture lines rarely run as neatly as described from one point to another.

Lower facial fractures

Mandibular fractures in pan-facial trauma are of the same pattern as isolated mandibular fractures but are more often multiple and comminuted.

Associated problems

- Associated problems from the pan-facial trauma relate to the **airway**. These are usually secondary to swelling and haemorrhage but can occasionally be secondary to posterior displacement of the facial bones, obstructing the airway.
- Although **blood loss** from facial wounds can look dramatic, in a shocked patient with facial injuries it is wise to look for other causes of the shock, as often there is more significant blood loss elsewhere (chest, abdomen, pelvis, or long bones, etc.) that is responsible for the shock.
- All pan-facial trauma patients have suffered a significant degree of trauma and have a high risk of **injury elsewhere**. In particular, they are at risk of having sustained a head injury and/or cervical spine injury. A careful and repeated evaluation of the neurological status must be made. Particular care must be taken, in those patients who have ingested alcohol prior to the injury, not to assume that drowsiness or poor co-operation is secondary to the effects of the alcohol.

Assessment

Consider serious facial injuries in anyone with gross swelling.

These should be elicited after completion of the primary survey. If the patient is intubated, some aspects cannot be undertaken at this stage but must be recorded in the notes as requiring completion later.

Inspection

All patients with pan-facial fractures will have **considerable facial swelling**, unless seen almost immediately after injury or several days later. The face should be cleaned of blood to enable a clear inspection.

Look for:

- tramline or clear fluid suggestive of **CSF leak**;
- **facial swelling**;
- presence of **lacerations**;
- obvious **asymmetry** despite swelling;
- check **visual acuity;**
- **diplopia**;
- **inter-canthal distance**;
- shape of **medial canthus** (does it come to a sharp point angled slightly downward at the insertion or is it rounded?);
- inter-pupillary distance;
- **pupillary levels**;
- **nasal deviation/air entry and septal haematoma**;
- how far can the patient **open their mouth**? is there any pain or deviation on opening any reduction of lateral movement?;
- **auroscopy**—looking for tears in external auditory meatus and blood behind the tympanic membrane;
- examine **VII nerve** function;
- **missing teeth**, crowns, dentures, etc. (if any are missing where are they?);
- any evidence of **palatal or sublingual haematoma**.

Palpation

Be systematic start at the top and work down (or bottom and work up).
Feel for:
- **Examine lacerations for depth and underlying fractures**. If the laceration overlies the course of the parotid duct, look for saliva in the wound. Remember the **lacrimal system, facial nerve, and canthal attachments of the eye**.
- **Palpated bony margin** for tenderness or steps.
- Palpate **nasal bones** for mobility.
- **Assess sensation** in if the patient is awake.
- **Assess the medial canthus** by displacing the lateral canthus posteriorly. If the medial canthus is detached it will move laterally; if not, the point of the medial canthus will sharpen.
- **Assess maxilla for mobility**. If there is mobility assess the level. When the maxilla moves, is there any movement of the bone at the infra-orbital and or zygomatico-frontal level? Mobility can also be due to isolated dentoalveolar fractures.
- **Assess the palate for a split**.
- Palpate the **mandible** for mobility and assess the occlusion if possible.

Investigations

- Baseline **biochemical and haematological** investigations should be undertaken, and patients **grouped and saved or cross-matched**, depending on blood loss. Other blood investigations should be determined by specific features of the medical history, e.g. diabetes.
- Imaging is the most useful investigation to ascertain the presence and location of bony fractures. Generally these will either be **CT scan or plain radiographs**. Patients with pan-facial fractures frequently have an associated head injury and will have a brain CT. If it does not compromise the patient's overall well-being, scan the facial bones at the same time; if possible, generating axial of the facial skeleton and coronal views of the orbits. Occasionally **angiography** may be required to indicate the source of persistent or major haemorrhage.
- If it is not possible to obtain images as part of a head series of scans, imaging is likely to be required prior to definitive treatment. Alternatively, good quality plain radiographs are valuable. An **OPG, PA mandible, OMs, and lateral facial bones** should be obtained. If good plain views are not obtainable, or there are condylar, orbital, frontal sinus, or NOE fractures present, coronal and axial CTs should be obtained.
- Determining the position of foreign bodies relative to vital structures will require two images at 90 degrees to one another. Occasionally angiography may be needed to establish the position of a foreign body to major vessels. If foreign bodies may be present that are radiolucent, e.g. wood, **ultra sound** scans can be useful to demonstrate their presence.
- **Impressions for study models** can often be invaluable in planning to establish pre-operatively the desired occlusion and enable an occlusal wafer to be constructed pre operatively
- Ask relatives to bring in any **pre-injury photographs** of the patient.

Treatment

Maxillofacial trauma should be integrated into **Advanced Trauma Life Support—ATLS**. ATLS dictates:

...maxillofacial trauma, not associated with airway obstruction or major bleeding, should be treated only after the patient is stabilized completely and life threatening injuries have been managed.

Consider first:
- airway with c spine;
- breathing;
- circulation;
- head injuries;
- ocular injuries.

Beware the patient who keeps trying to sit up—they may be trying to clear their airway. If there is no spinal injury, let them sit up; if unsure, either let them lay on their side or tip the table head down. This is at variance with ATLS guidelines but facial bleeding will continue unrecognized in the supine position until the patient vomits and possibly aspirates.

First aid

Haemorrhage is usually due to displacement of fractured bones or lacerations. Displaced mandibular fractures can be reduced and if teeth are present on either side of the fracture, a bridle wire placed This provides some stability to the fracture thereby reducing bleeding and making the patient more comfortable. Ideally the bridle wire should include two teeth on each fractured segment.

Associated Le Fort fractures can present with prolonged **epistaxis** (nose bleed). Definitive treatment may involve reduction of the fracture

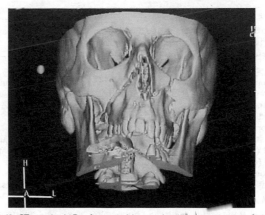

Fig. 8.42 CT scan (and 3D reformatting) has revol utilized assessment in facial trauma.

or cautery/ligation of appropriate vessels. As a first-aid measure, nasal packs may tamponade the flow. If posterior nasal packing is required urinary (Foley) catheters may be inserted beyond the soft palate prior to inflating the balloon and then withdrawn until the balloons wedge in the posterior naso-pharynx; anterior nasal packing with ribbon gauze may also be required. Custom devices are available (Epistat™) with dual balloons that will occlude the entire nasal airway and hence tamponade haemorrhage.

Replace lost fluids—any patient with Le Fort fractures must have adequate intravenous (IV) access and appropriate fluid resuscitation. Assessment must be made of any losses as well as ongoing needs.

Dento-alveolar fractures can be reduced and stabilized with splints. If teeth have been avulsed or subluxed, they are best **re-implanted or repositioned** as soon as possible and splinted.

Lacerations should be inspected for **contamination** and foreign bodies (do not do this with your fingers if glass could be involved). This is particularly important to prevent tattooing of the skin, which can be difficult to eradicate. Bites should be thoroughly **irrigated** to minimize the risk of infection. Assess the **viability of the soft tissues**. Due to the extremely good blood supply of the face, loss of viability is unusual, so tissue should not be discarded unless it is certain that it is not viable.

Assess **facial nerve** function. If this is disrupted, repair should be undertaken prior to definitive closure, which should be done as soon as possible. However, if a large laceration is present, and other more urgent problems need attention, tack the wound with a few large sutures, and close it definitively later. If a laceration gives access to an underlying fracture, which may not be addressed for several days, it is probably best to close the wound definitively and accept that it may be re-opened later, than leave definitive closure until fixation of any fractures.

Prevent infection
- Le Fort fractures are almost always compound injuries via the sinuses or facial wounds.
- **Antibiotics**—intravenous and broad spectrum. Many regimes exist and include augmentin, or benzyl penecillin + metronidazole.
- **Tetanus**—ensure tetanus prophylaxis is up to date.

Analgesia
Remember, pain is a potent stimulus for the release of catecholamines. However, facial fractures are often not as painful as one may think.
- **Local**—regional nerve blocks: bilateral infra-orbital blocks may be particularly useful in the Le Fort I and II fractures. Consider supra-orbital blocks for the Le Fort III pattern.
- **Systemic**—avoid opiates until the patient is cleared of a head injury.
- **IM (intramuscular)**, a possibility but avoid in the shocked patient.
- **IV (intravenous)**—rapid onset, and easy to titrate. Ideally, if the patient's conscious level is appropriate, establish a PCA (patient-controlled analgesia) in liaison with anaesthetic colleagues.

Definitive treatment
Optimal results requires careful pre-operative assessment and planning. This should result in a comprehensive list of the problems and objectives

of treatment. This can be summarized as restoration of normal form and function without producing complications. Broadly speaking definitive management can be broken down into **non-operative or operative** management. The benefits of each needs to be weighed against the risks, taking into account all aspects of the patient, particularly other injuries and pre-existing medical conditions.

Planning should be undertaken in collaboration with other specialities that may be involved, e.g. anaesthesia, neurosurgery, or ophthalmology. Consideration should be given to whether there is any need for primary bone-grafting of orbital walls or expected bony defects

Anaesthetic

Because IMF is usually required, avoid an oratracheal tube if possible. Given also that patients also require nasal reduction, thought may need to be given to either a tracheostomy or submental tube.

Access

This can be via wide exposure of the facial skeleton via a bicoronal approach or through localized incisions. In the presence of naso-ethmoid, frontal sinus, anterior cranial fossa fractures, or Le Fort III fractures, **wide exposure is usually required to get the best results**. This allows direct visualization of fractures, while hiding scars in the scalp. Localized incisions in the infra-orbital area may still be requires as will intra oral incisions.

Surgery aims to:
- exposure and sealing of cranial floor fractures;
- restore:
  - facial width;
  - orbital volume;
  - orbital rim;
  - occlusion;
  - nasal projection;
- repair of VII nerve;
- precise neat closure of lacerations.

If the mandible has bilateral condylar fractures, then, if possible, at least one condyle should be fixed to **restore mandibular height. Mandibular width** must not be increased. This can occur with parasymphyseal fractures.

Often all fractures are exposed before fixation. Fixation starts peripherally, at the junction with uninjured bone. In the mid-face this usually means either starting laterally and working medially, restoring the orbital rims and arch. Restoration of orbital volume may require grafting. Nasal projection can then be addressed. If cranial floor repair is required this should be done after reduction of fractures to prevent disruption of repair.

When mid-face and mandibular fractures are present, the mandible should be fixed and the occlusion established with IMF prior to the Le Fort fractures being fixed.

Any soft tissue repair must be undertaken last. Facial sutures should be removed at 4–5 days, scalp sutures/clips at 7–10 days.

⑦ General principles in management and terminology

- Debridement—thoroughly clean any open wounds.
- Reduction—open/closed.
- Fixation—IMF/internal/external.
- Care of soft tissues.
- Functional rehabilitation.

Debridement

All wounds need to be thoroughly cleaned as soon as possible, as often there may be some delay in surgery. Skin wounds need to be gently cleaned and kept from drying out with saline or antiseptic-soaked swabs. Oral hygiene is particularly important with fractures of the mandible and maxilla, as these often communicate with the oral cavity, which, due to pain, is hard for the patient to keep scrupulously clean. In such cases regular use of antiseptic mouthwashes (e.g. corsodyl) and hot salt-water mouthwashes is recommended. Remember the possible need for tetanus prophylaxis. Once in theatre, dead tissue is excised but this is kept to a minimum. Wounds are thoroughly irrigated and if grit is ingrained, scrubbed.

Open reduction and internal fixation (ORIF)

This involves exposing and reducing the fracture(s) under direct vision. Whenever possible (e.g. mandible, maxilla, and some zygomatic fractures) this is done via the mouth so as to avoid incisions on the face and scars. However, if there are associated lacerations these may be used instead. Although the mouth is heavily colonized with numerous organisms, infection is surprisingly uncommon. This is in part due to the excellent blood

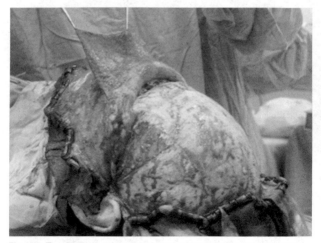

Fig. 8.43 The 'Coronal' or 'Bicoronal' flap provides excellent access with minimal morbidity.

supply to the face and its capacity to fight infection. By directly visualizing the fracture, more precise anatomical reduction is possible when compared to indirect methods (e.g. IMF). Methods of fixation include transosseous wiring, intra-medullary pins, and rigid/semi-rigid plates and screws. Plates used for internal fixation may be adaptional plates (semi-rigid), compression plates (rigid), or mesh. For some overlapping fragments a 'lag screw' technique may be possible.

Rigid internal fixation

This form of 'ORIF' uses heavy metal plates and screws to rigidly immobilize fractures. This facilitates precise anatomical reduction and increased mechanical stability, enabling early return of function. Intermaxillary fixation is not needed and the patient can eat soon afterwards. However, this technique risks damaging the inferior dental nerve or teeth. Plates may become infected and the wound may dehisce.

Intermaxillary fixation (IMF)

This form of immobilization uses the patient's bite to reduce and stabilize fractures and therefore can only be used for those fragments firmly attached to healthy teeth (usually the mandible or dentoalveolar fractures). It is also commonly used in the treatment of condylar fractures. Fracture reduction is not directly visualized and can result in non-precise alignment. Examples include eyelet wiring, arch bars, cast cap silver splints, and gunning splints (edentulous fractures). Caution with post-op airway problems, COAD, head injury, epileptics, patients likely to vomit, psychiatrically unwell. IMF needs to be in place for two to three weeks and patients can lose weight.

External pin fixation

This involves inserting rigid pins into the bone fragments via the skin, which are then joined by universal joints and connecting rods or splints. This method is particularly useful where tissue has been lost ('continuity defects', e.g. gun-shot injuries), infected, severely comminuted, and pathological fractures. Fixation can be applied rapidly. However, reduction is 'blind'—the pins may damage the inferior dental nerve or teeth, patient activity is restricted, and the pin sites may become infected and scarred.

Timing of surgery

Early repair (within 5–10 days) gives the best results; immediate surgery is only required for life-threatening injuries, or sometimes if the patient is going to theatre for some other reason. Most maxillofacial injuries can wait, although late repair (once the fractures have united) is difficult to carry out well. By delaying surgery for several days:

- observation for head or 'missed' injuries is possible;
- facial swelling will settle, enabling better assessment;
- quality radiographs can be obtained (face, teeth);
- further investigations can be carried out, e.g. CT scan, study models, vitality testing;
- further details including pre injury photographs can be obtained from relatives, GP, etc.;
- aids to surgery can be fabricated, e.g. custom-made arch bars, gunnings splint.

Antibiotics, steroids, and tetanus prophylaxis

Protocols may vary between different units. Antibiotics are usually given for fractures that are compound (open) into the mouth or through the skin (e.g. mandible). Oral bacteria of a mixed anaerobic type, and a combination of a penicillin and metronidazole, is one suitable choice. Prophylactic antibiotics when there is CFS leakage is controversial and the opinion of a neurosurgeon should be sought. Tetanus prophylaxis should be considered, especially in mucky wounds, which should be thoroughly cleaned as soon as possible. Steroids, e.g. dexamethasone, may be given to reduce facial swelling.

Reduction of and fixation of fractures

If untreated, displaced facial fractures may result in significant disfigurement and functional problems, such as diplopia and malocclusion. Inadequate treatment can also result in poor aesthetics or function requiring further surgery to correct these. However, not all displaced facial fractures need anatomical reduction. Poor results may occur for several of reasons, for example:

• coexisting medical problems (e.g. head injuries, multi-organ failure, sepsis- etc.) may delay definitive repair making it difficult to get good reduction;
• inadequate work up, particularly with radiographs, may miss bony injuries resulting in inadequate repair;
• fractures may be treated by inadequately trained surgeons;
• patients refuse or fail to attend for treatment.

Reduction—open vs. closed

Terminology can be confusing. 'Closed' treatment is preferable to 'conservative' treatment. Intermaxillary fixation (IMF) for instance is often referred to as 'conservative', but still has reported morbidity and even mortality.

Facial fractures 30 years ago were commonly managed by closed techniques, since it was thought that open reduction would lead to infection and severe osteomyelitis. Open reduction was reserved for compound fractures or certain unstable mandibular fractures.

Nowadays, many fractures are treated by **open reduction**, allowing direct access for fixation. This involves exposure of the fracture, either through the skin or mucosa. It can then be *anatomically* reduced and directly fixed through the incision. **Closed reduction**, however, is a 'blind' procedure relying on the fragments 'locking' together. Fixation normally occurs without direct visualization of the fragments in their final position. Examples of closed reduction include nasal manipulation (MUA), fixing the teeth in occlusion (IMF), or using an arch bar to support dento-alveolar fractures. IMF relies on the teeth to guide the bones, and then fixing them to provide adequate stabilization.

Closed reduction—advantages

In the UK, particularly in the Second World War, this technique was widely used. Custom-made silver splints were constructed, and sectioned at the fracture site. These were then cemented on to the teeth and inter-maxillary fixation slowly applied via the splints. This enabled gradual reduction followed by fixation, often without the need for anaesthetics.

Closed reduction worked well in missile injuries, stabilizing continuity defects. Today in Third World countries with inadequate resources or surgical skills, these simple techniques still have a place. Cast silver splints have been replaced by arch bars, which are a lot easier and cheaper to manufacture.

Closed treatment may be an acceptable compromise in a patient with medical problems precluding a general anaesthetic. IMF may be used to treat simple, minimally displaced, 'crack' fractures relatively easily. However, those very conditions that prevent a general anaesthetic may also contra-indicate IMF (e.g. uncontrolled epilepsy, chronic respiratory disease).

Closed reduction—disadvantages

Since the fragments are not directly visualized, 'closed' techniques mean that only the teeth, palpation, or X-rays are used as a guide to the accuracy of the reduction. The commonest problem with closed reduction, therefore, is poor fracture alignment. Errors in reduction are tolerated much less in the face than in long-bone fractures.

IMF relies on positioning the teeth correctly, assuming that this will correctly orientate the bony fractures. However, the teeth *per se* have only limited control over the positioning of the bones. The attached muscles may also displace fragments, despite firm location of the teeth. Control significantly diminishes with fractures further from the occlusion. This becomes compounded in patients with pre-existing malocclusions or missing teeth.

The choice between 'open' and 'closed' reduction may be clear in some cases, but there are many in which both are equally acceptable. Nowadays, with good outcomes from surgery and anaesthesia, open reduction offers the chance of better reduction and fixation. In most cases this means a safer post-operative recovery and earlier return to normal function.

Timing of reduction

Timing of surgery is not clearly defined in the literature. For compound (open) fractures, it is generally assumed that the longer the delay the more likely the wound will become contaminated. However, it is not clear what is considered to be an *excessive* delay. Some studies have failed to show any differences in complications whether treated within or after 24 h following injury.

However, after long delays (around 14 days), initial healing is well-established and this makes mobilization and reduction difficult. Soft tissues become adherent to the displaced bones and this makes reduction even harder to achieve. This is particularly important in the upper mid-face, especially the canthal region of the eye. Once displacement is established, the canthal ligament will never settle into its correct position. This is especially difficult to correct at a later date.

Life-threatening conditions often take precedent, and in patients with associated head injuries, fears over long reconstructions leads to delay in definitive surgery. However, some studies have shown that early intervention is possible without any significant morbidity. Close working relations with neurosugeons is essential.

Dynamic compression osteosynthesis

Compression plates have had an enormous impact in orthopaedics and have become established practice in most trauma units. This has not been the case in maxillofacial surgery. There are a number of reasons for this:

- only mandibular fractures can be treated in this way;
- the complex curvature of the mandible creates difficulties in plate placement;
- the teeth and the inferior alveolar nerve are at risk with bicortical screws;
- precision of reduction is much more than in orthopaedic surgery;
- skin incisions are required (scarring and a small risk of damage to the mandibular branch of the facial nerve);
- dynamic compression plating is an unforgiving and a difficult technique;
- fears exist that the plates are so rigid that stress shielding delayed healing strength;
- there is normally a need for a second, often extra oral, operation to remove these thick bulky plates.

Miniplates

Animal models have shown that some *micro* movement, using semi-rigid fixation, encourages prompt healing. Rigid fixation is, therefore, not essential to fracture healing. Non-compression, smaller sized plates ('miniplates') have now become the standard method of internal fixation in many units. Furthermore, these plates can be placed orally with much less morbidity.

The principle of this technique is to identify a 'zone of tension' within the mandible at the site of the fracture. The plate is then applied across the fracture along this line. In a way analogous to suspension bridges, huge loads can be controlled by relatively small structures, relying on the tensile strength of the materials. Relatively large loads can be controlled by small plates—'miniplates'. In additon, the plate can be fixed by monocortical screws and, as a result, can be placed where it is biomechanically desirable. Monocortical screws can be safely placed over dental roots and the inferior alveolar nerve.

Miniplates have reduced the risks of malocclusions, compared with the very rigid compression plates. Fine-tuning of the bite is possible with elastic IMF. The technique is carried out entirely through the mouth, with no need for skin incisions. The plates are small and can be left *in situ* if desired.

Other methods of fixation

External fixation was, prior to plating, an important method of fixation. It is used in two main ways.

In mid-face fractures, it can be used to immobilize upper and/or lower arch bars by fixing the frame usually to the cranium. This involves the use of a halo frame around the skull. This is mechanically very stable and was initially developed for traction of unstable cervical injuries.

Alternatively, it can be used as a direct fixator across a fracture, commonly the mandible or zygoma. Fixators placed across fractures have several attractions: they can be quickly applied, there is minimal exposure, and stripping of the periosteum around the fracture. Stability can be adjusted and modified during healing (dynamization), thereby reducing the potential effects of stress shielding. The position of the fractures can be adjusted if post-operative radiology shows inadequate reduction.

Unfortunately the bulky apparatus is disliked by patients, and care is required not to injure themselves. Placement normally involves skin punctures and these can leave unsightly scars.

Nowadays, its main role is to provide 'first-aid' stabilization in the multiply injured patient or where there are limited facilities prior to transfer to a definitive care centre. In those areas where gun-shot wounds are common, this method of fixation provides good 'long-term' temporary fixation, until the contaminated wounds have healed. The external fixator is also particularly useful in maintaining space and orientation in continuity defects.

⑦ Special considerations for children and the elderly atrophic mandible

Both these groups respond to treatments differently.

Fractures in **children** are marked by *rapid healing and rapid remodelling*. In most fractures, reduction and fixation is not necessary. However, there is a risk of ankylosis in intra-capsular mandibular joint fractures and early mobilization is necessary. If fixation is required, microplating systems normally are adequate.

Edentulous mandibular fractures

In the atrophic mandible, the picture is the opposite. The severely atrophic edentulous mandible often has a poor outcome, especially those in which the radiographic height of the mandible is 10 mm or less. They are characterized by poor blood supply and slow reparative efforts. In addition, the older population are frequently complicated by poor general health, sometimes precluding prolonged general anaesthesia. Patients are commonly female with osteoportic bones, making screw-fixation difficult and unreliable. The poor blood supply within the mandible places greater demands on having an intact periosteal blood supply, making use of large plates undesirable. Traditional methods of fixation are severely compromised by the lack of teeth.

Fractures of the edentulous mandible may be treated using the patients dentures (if a good fit) or customized 'gunning splints'. These are essentially modified dentures that are wired to the maxilla and mandible and then fixed together while healing takes place. In selected cases, open reduction and internal fixation using miniplates applied extra-periostally (to preserve the blood supply) may be carried out. This is preferable in the presence of respiratory disease to avoid IMF.

⑦ Wound healing

General considerations
The head and neck has a very rich blood supply, which helps fight infection and improves healing. Intact skin and mucosa also prevents infection of deeper structures, particulary bone. Skin is also essential in maintaining body fluids, as seen following extensive burns.

Despite the high bacterial count in the mouth, infected wounds are uncommon. Saliva and exudates from around the gums contain antibodies and 'growth factors', which stimulate rapid wound healing and prevent infections (which is why dogs lick their wounds). Skin infections may, however, occur secondary to commensals (normal inhabitants of the skin), or from contact with another source (e.g. MRSA).

In the head and neck, unrepaired wounds may produce functional problems with important structures, such as the eyelids, resulting in significant morbidity. Poor repair and aftercare may also result in unacceptable scarring with distortion of the surrounding structures.

Following trauma, partially avulsed skin, even if attached by a small pedicle, may still have a good enough blood supply to enable it to heal if replaced. This is highlighted in the irradiated patient in whom wound breakdown and infection is more common following surgery or injury.

If in doubt save tissue—never excise widely.

Wound closure is a most effective form of analgesia

The wound-healing environment
The wound needs the correct environment to heal. Many intrinsic and extrinsic factors (e.g. nutrition, poor dressing, infection, slough, and necrosis) can delay wound healing.

The ideal dressing should:
- be impermeable to bacteria;
- be free of particles and toxic wound contaminates;
- maintain high humidity at the wound/dressing interface;
- remove excess exudate;
- allow gaseous exchange;
- provide thermal insulation;
- allow removal without causing trauma to the wound;
- be comfortable for the patient whilst *in situ* and not cause distress or pain on removal.

Wounds, therefore, heal more effectively in a moist, warm environment, which new-generation dressings now provide. Epithelial cells can migrate easily, decreasing healing time. Pain from the wound is reduced as exposed nerve endings are not allowed to dry out. The body's natural autolytic response to deslough is increased.

Wounds heal best at a constant temperature of 37°C. It can take several hours for normal cell activity to return following a dressing change. It is, therefore, important to reduce the number of dressing changes. Historically, some dressings have been changed up to three to four times a day. This means that wound healing could potentially be delayed. Too frequent dressing changes also increase the risk of infection and cross-infection to other patients.

⑦ Types of wound healing

This can be considered as:

- Primary intention or primary wound healing. The wound is closed as soon as possible using sutures, clips or 'steristrips'. There are no gaps in the wound.
- Secondary intention (granulation) or secondary wound healing. The skin edges are not closed but left if there is infection or tissue loss. The wound granulates from its base. This is seen where tissue is lost. It is unpredictable and can be lengthy. Scarring and deformity are significant
- Exuberant granulation—overgrowth of granulation tissue prevents in-growth of surrounding epithelium.

Phases of wound healing

This involves a complex interaction between epidermis, dermis, extra-cellular matrix, angiogenesis, and plasma proteins, all coordinated by cytokines and growth factors. It is divided into several phases, which overlap—inflammation, proliferation, and remodelling. The initial stimulus is thrombus formation. Cells within the clot, notably platelets, trigger an inflammatory response by releasing vasodilators and chemo-attractants.

Four phases are described here, although there is often a large degree of overlap between them.

Inflammatory phase

Inflammation is the body's immediate response to trauma (including surgery), tissue damage, or invasion of bacteria. Initial vessel constriction occurs and a loose fibrin clot forms a 'plug' loosely uniting the skin edges. If sutured, wound strength at this stage depends on the suture and any break-down is the result of poor closure. Mast cells release histamine, resulting in vasodilation, increased capillary permeability, and swelling, and neutrophils are attracted by kinins. As the capillaries dilate, tissue fluids rich in plasma proteins, antibodies, red cells, white cells, and platelets 'leak' into the tissues. Platelets release growth factors and fibrnectin, which promote cell migration and wound healing. Macrophages are attracted and these remove any wound debris, thereby beginning the process of repair. Signs of inflammation are heat, swelling, redness, and pain.

Reconstructive phase

Macrophages stimulate the formation of fibroblasts, which migrate along fibrin threads and produce collagen. Fibroblasts are important in the production of the extra-cellular matrix (granulation tissue). They produce collagen, fibronectin, and proteoglycans, such as hyaluronic acid. Fibrin is produced from the second day and forms a weak framework for healing. Immature blood vessels develop (angiogenesis) providing oxygen and nutrients to the wound. It therefore becomes filled with capillaries and collagen fibres—'granulation tissue', which appears deep red in colour and bleeds easily. Granulation tissue is abundant in secondary intention healing, although not seen as much following primary closure. It is important in scar formation. In addition, the wound undergoes contraction. This may be responsible for 40–80% of wound closure.

Epithelialization or proliferative phase
Re-epithelializtion is usually evident within 24h. Cells at the wound edges migrate across the surface–this can only take place over a healthy moist wound. If infection or debris are present, the inflammatory phase is prolonged and migration will not take place. 'Scabs' are separated from the wound by proteolytic enzymes. Collagen continues to be produced, resulting in a red, raised, and often unsightly scars. Wound strength increases rapidly but is still relatively weak and can stretch if not protected.

Maturation phase
Remodelling takes places over several years, with a reduction of both cell content and blood flow. The vascularity of the wound decreases and the scar changes colour, fading to a silvery white appearance. Collagen fibres re-align themselves, tending to lie at right angles to the wound, increasing the strength of the scar. At one year, 70% or more of the original tissue may be regained, but scar tissue is never as strong as unwounded tissue.

Secondary intention healing
Wounds may gape following trauma or infection, coupled with the elastic pull of the dermis on each side. This defect initially fills with blood clot, which dries to form a scab. In small, uninfected wounds, re-epithelialization begins from the wound edges, passing under the scab. The scab is gradually lifted at its edges until it falls off. The wound heals from below upwards. Capillary loops and fibroblasts form granulation tissue giving a velvet appearance to the wound. Myofibroblasts in the wound contract and reduce the volume of the defect.
The difference between primary and secondary intention healing is quantitative only.

Healing chronic wounds
Because of the rich blood supply to the head and neck, most wounds heal quickly. However, when chronic wounds occur, they can be difficult to treat and, depending on their site, quite disfiguring.
In any patient with a non-healing, chronic wound, ask yourself why has it not healed?. Consider the possibility of underlying:
- **foreign body**;
- **infection**;
- **malignancy**;
- **immunosuppression**.

Management strategies
Consider any predisposing conditions (local or systemic).

Dressings
In recent years there has been the development of dressings that promote a moist environment to assist healing. In animals, re-epithelialization of partial thickness, acute wounds occurs more rapidly if it is occluded. In patients they reduce pain. As yet there is still not a dressing that can alter the healing cascade, although dressings containing hyaluronic acid seem to promote healing.

Topical growth factors
Clinical results from application of growth factors to chronic wounds have not been as good as initially hoped. To date, only platelet derived growth factor has been licensed for use, but only for treating non-infected foot ulcers in diabetic patients (becaplermin, regranex). Other factors showing some promise include granulocyte colony stimulating factor, fibroblast growth factor, and epidermal growth factor.

Skin grafts
Split thickness and pinch skin-grafting techniques are very useful, so long as there is no infection and a health bed on which to place the graft.

Synthetic 'skin'
Previously, cultured patient's epidermal cells, in which a skin biopsy was cultured to produce epidermal sheets, were used following in burns. These have had only limited success due to graft fragility, difficulty in application, poor rate of uptake, and the frequent occurrence of infection.

More recently synthetic skin equivalents have been developed, in which donor tissue with reduced immunogenicity is used.
- Alloderm is a dermal matrix without immunogenic cells.
- Integra is a combination of dermal fibroblasts and bovine collagen.
- Dermagraft consists of non-immunogenic neonatal fibroblast cultured on a polyglactin mesh.
- Apligraf contains both epidermal and dermal components.

All of these products have been used to treat burns. They are absorbed into the wound bed and are thought to alter the profile of cytokines

Future developments
Vascular endothelial growth factor and proteinase inhibitors may have a role in improving healing of chronic wounds. Gene therapy may allow genes important in healing to be delivered directly into a wound. Another potential treatment lies in embryonic stem cells.

Risk factors in wound breakdown
General
- Advanced age.
- Malnourished (protein, vitamins, trace elements).
- Anaemic.
- Uraemic.
- Jaundice.
- Malignancy (cachexia).
- Chronic steroid therapy.
- Diabetes mellitis.
- Nutritional deficiencies (vitamin C, vitamin K, hypoproteinaemia, zinc).
- Chemotherapy and radiotherapy.

Local
- Tension.
- Infection.
- Crushed tissues (forceps, tight sutures).
- Poor tissue vascularity eg after irradiation.
- Foreign body, e.g. dirt, gravel, glass.

- Necrotic tissue (crushed, excessive use of diathermy).
- Haematoma.

Non-healing
Many factors can impair healing.

Local factors
- Foreign bodies.
- Tissue maceration.
- Ischaemia.
- Infection.
- Malignancy.
- Systemic factors
- Advanced age.
- Malnutrition.
- Diabetes.
- Renal disease.
- Steroids.
- Immunosupressive drugs.

At a cellular level, tissue growth factors are reduced and an imbalance between proteolytic enzymes and their inhibitors occurs. Chronic ulcers seem to have reduced levels of platelet derived growth factor, fibroblast growth factor, epidermal growth factor, and transforming growth factor compared with acute wounds. Excessive proteinase activity (notably matrix metalloproteins) results in abnormal degradation of the extra-cellular matrix and fibroblasts have impaired responsiveness to growth hormone.

Research into newer treatments is directed at altering the imbalance by the topical application of proteinase inhibitors, or by combining proteinase inhibitors with growth factors.

Classification of early wounds
Wounds may be classified as 'clean' or 'untidy'. Clean wounds have the greatest chance of healing with minimal scar formation.

Clean
- Sharp incision.
- Uncontaminated.
- Less than 6 h old.
- Low energy trauma.

Untidy
- Ragged edge.
- Contaminated.
- More than 12 h old.
- High energy trauma.
- Crushed tissue.
- Tissue loss.
- Burns.

⑦ Wound assessment

There are many ways to assess a wound. Five types are described:
- black or necrotic;
- infected;
- sloughy;
- granulating;
- epithelializing.

Black or necrotic wounds

These are covered with a dry hard eschar, which can vary in colour (off white/yellow to brown/black). This may increase in size if not debrided (surgically, chemically, or biochemically). Dressings based on hydrocolloid or hydrogel or an enzymatic desloughing agent can be used. If a cavity wound is necrotic it can produce a heavy exudate and become very offensive. Alginate dressings may be used to control the exudate.

Infected wounds

All wounds have bacteria present but many do not have clinical evidence of infection, i.e. pus. Commensal organisms do not necessarily delay healing and cause infection. Signs of infection include:
- cellulitis/abscess formation;
- discharge
- localized heat;
- localized pain;
- oedema;
- pocketing at the base of the wound;
- delayed healing;
- wound breakdown
- offensive smell.

A wound swab should be taken. Antibiotics are not always required, some wounds can be treated topically. Flammazine is useful when *Pseudomonas* is present and iodine-based dressings have been shown to be effective against MRSA (methycillin- resistant *Staphylococcus aureus*). Hydrocolloids and hydrogels are also useful, but not when there is excessive exudate. An alginate may be appropriate in this instance but will require changing daily.

Sloughy wounds

These consist of dead neutrophils in exudate. The wound has a white /yellow appearance. Sometimes there is excessive exudate. Hydrocolloid, hydrogel, or alginate is useful in these cases.

Granulating wounds

These are red and granular in appearance. They bleed easily as the capillary loops are friable. Dressings such as hydrocolloids, hydrogels, foams, and alginates are all useful in low-exudating granulating wounds. In a more heavily exudating wound, an alginate or foam dressing can be used. Some granulating wounds develop excess granulations, silver nitrate sticks can be used to cauterize the excess.

Epithelializing wounds

These have pink/white tissue present as the epithelial cells spread over the granulating tissue. A moist, warm environment needs to be maintained, as well as one that is protective. Dressings such as hydrocolioids and foams are, therefore, appropriate.

⊙ Wound cleansing

The general aim of wound cleansing is to remove any organic and inorganic debris from the wound before applying a dressing. Debris can delay the healing process and result in infection.

A number of antiseptics are available but it is now thought that they can delay healing and harm the tissues. **Sterile saline solution or water** are not harmful to the wound and are recommended. However, swabbing a wound can damage granulating tissue and may leave small fibres in the wound, which can be a focus for infection. It is much better to irrigate wounds, where possible. A 35 ml syringe and a 19-gauge needle can be used, which should not exert too much pressure on the wound. Tap water is increasingly used to cleanse wounds. Ideally warm irrigant should be used to optimize healing.

Methicillin-resistant staphylococcus aureus (MRSA)

MRSA is a human pathogen that is resistant to a number of antibiotics, not only methicillin. Some strains show the potential to become epidemic (EMRSA). To most fit and healthy people, MRSA is not a threat. However, to those undergoing major or even minor maxillofacial surgery, it can cause serious harm.

The pathogens can colonize a particular site, e.g. nose or throat, without necessarily producing any symptoms. Staphylococci are Gram-positive organisms that grow on the surface of the skin, in the nostrils, mouth, umbillicus, and perineal areas. Since the introduction of antibiotics, *Staphylococcus aureus* has shown a history of resistance, firstly with peni-cillin then methicillin. Vancomycin is the antibiotic commonly used to treat patients with MRSA, but now there are concerns regarding resistance to it (VRSA).

Patients at risk include:
- immuno-compromised patients;
- the elderly or neonates;
- patients with wounds or skin lesions;
- patients who have had several hospital admissions in the past year;
- patients transferred from other areas where MRSA is prevalent;
- patients admitted from abroad.

The principle method of cross infection is **hand carriage**, although it can also be airborne. Other sources include clothing and bedding.

All patients with a positive result should be nursed in isolation. They should also commence a decontamination regime, which should be available in every Trust. Decontamination takes around one week followed by re-swabbing two days later. If the swabs are again positive, than the decon-tamination regime is repeated until the results are negative. If the swabs are negative, the screening process is repeated until there are three clear screens. Even then it is not advisable to nurse the patients in the same area as those patients deemed to be at risk.

⊙ Soft tissue injuries

General points

- **Consider injuries to underlying structures** (bones/eye/lacrimal gland/parotid duct/canthal attachments).
- **Consider the possibility of tattooing and scarring**—can this be managed in A&E or should I refer?
- Soft tissue injuries are best evaluated after the wound has been **cleaned** of dry blood and debris. A local anesthetic may be necessary to clean the wound so that a thorough examination can be made.
- Where applicable **assess the facial nerve prior to anesthetic use**.
- Accurately **document the injuries, ideally photographically**.
- Consider **tetanus** prophylaxis.
- Ideally **repair should be performed within 12 h**.
- Because of the rich vascular supply of the head and neck, **only minimal debridement is necessary**. Preservation of tissue is the rule—if in doubt leave.
- When suturing wounds, **alignment of key anatomic boundaries** (vermilion border, gray line of the eyelid) and alignment of the eyebrow, should be performed first. With lip lacerations, it is important to align the vermilion border for good comesis. Place the first stitch to re-approximate the vermilion border.
- **Close in layers** (mucosa to mucosa, muscle to muscle, and skin to skin). Deep sutures are used to close dead space and remove tension from the skin to prevent hematoma and scarring.
- With deep lacerations of the cheek, the wound should be explored for **injury to the parotid duct** and, if possible, the duct is repaired over a stent.
- If **facial nerve weakness** results from a laceration *medial* to a line dropped perpendicular to the lateral canthus, the nerve branches are not repaired. (The nerves are generally too fine.) If, however, paralysis results from a laceration posterior to this line, the facial nerve should be repaired. Ideally, repair should occur as soon as possible, but no later than 72 h unless the wound is heavily contaminated (e.g. gun shot). In this situation, the nerve endings are tagged and repair is performed when the wound is clean.

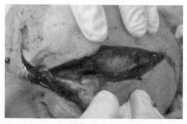

Fig. 8.44 Wound assessment—always separate the edges and assess depth before attempting to suture.

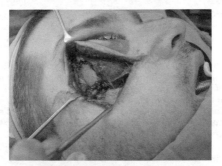

Fig. 8.45 Wound assessment—consider the possibility of underlying fractures.

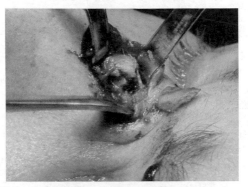

Fig. 8.46 Wound assessment—consider the possibility of underlying fractures.

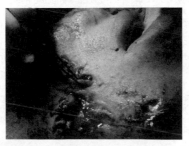

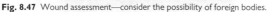

Fig. 8.47 Wound assessment—consider the possibility of foreign bodies.

- With significant tissue loss, **similar tissues should be re-approximated**: mucosa to mucosa, muscle to muscle, cartilage to cartilage, and skin to skin.
- Consider drains.

Following trauma, partially avulsed skin, even if attached by only a small pedicle, may still have a good enough blood supply to enable it to heal, if replaced. **If in doubt, save tissue—never excise widely**.

Wound closure is a most effective form of analgesia.

In addition to the obvious skin and mucosa, **assesment of soft tissue injuries must also include associated specialized structures**. These include:

- fractures;
- salivary gland and/or duct (e.g. parotid);
- lacrimal apparatus;
- nerve injury (facial, accesory, supra-orbital, supra-trochlear, infra-orbital, mental)—see Microsurgical nerve repair below.
- major vascular injury (especially in neck lacerations);
- loss of function of eyelids;
- loss of function of lips.

In penetrating injuries and lacerations, **foreign bodies and contamination** must be considered. If grit is not removed early **tattooing** can result, which is extremely difficult to remove later. **Underlying fractures** must also be considered and treated before any wounds are closed definitively. The patient's tetanus status should be assessed and managed appropriately.

Immediate primary closure with complete haemostasis and accurate restoration of anatomy should be the aim whenever possible. In most cases, head and neck wounds can be closed primarily with acceptable results. The blood supply to the tissues is a major factor in this and it is essential that the surgery itself does not damage wound edges. Provided the tissues are alive, even wounds heavily colonized with bacteria can be closed, primarily using appropriate antiseptic and antibiotics. This is seen particularly with intra-oral wounds, which are all heavily contaminated with oral bacteria.

① Bites

Whether animal or human in origin these must be considered serious and managed quickly. Both can rapidly become infected if left too long. Check for tissue loss and tetanus status (follow local protocols).

Compared to elsewhere in the body, bites on the face can be closed primarily due to its rich blood supply. However, they must be thoroughly cleaned and irrigated, and sutures placed sparingly to allow any collections to drain. Broad spectrum antibiotics should be prescribed and, ideally, take a wound swab for culture. Warn the patient about scarring.

① Abrasions

These need to be thoroughly, but *gently* cleaned to remove all traces of grit and other foreign bodies. This is the best opportunity to manage these well. Tattooing results if this is neglected, which is very difficult to deal with secondarily (excision/dermabrasion/lasers).

Specialised tissues

☼ Eyelid injuries

This requires specialist care. In the first instance, **protect and assess the underlying globe**. Assess visual acuity as soon as is practical. Consider foreign bodies and perforating injuries and therefore **avoid any pressure** on the wounds. As a temporary measure, liberally apply chlormycetin ointment (not drops) to the wound.

① Parotid injuries

Lacerations along the side of the face must be carefully assessed to exclude injuries to the **parotid gland, parotid duct**, and, most importantly, **facial nerve**. Injuries to the duct and nerve must be repaired using microsurgical techniques before the skin is closed. Failure to repair the duct may result in the formation of a 'sialocele', which will eventually drain through the wound, resulting in a salivary fistula. Failure to repair the nerve may result in various degrees of facial weakness.

Nerve injuries that may benefit from exploration and repair

These include:

- **Facial nerve**—this may be damaged following trauma (or surgery) to the parotid region. If necessary, immediate repair can be delayed and the nerve endings marked with sutures.
- **Accessory nerve**—injury to this nerve may occur following trauma (also following lymph node biopsies or neck dissection). Loss of function of the trapezius muscle results in limitations of shoulder motions.
- **Inferior alveolar nerve**—injury may occur as a result of a mandibular fracture. It can also occur following wisdom tooth removal, jaw surgery, tumour resection, fracture fixation, and placement of implants. This can result in numbness or 'dysaethesia' in the lower teeth, the lower lip, and the chin. This should be reconstructed within 3–4 weeks after injury.

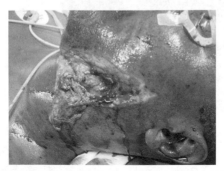

Fig. 8.48 Deep laceration over the parotid—what structures are at risk?

⑦ **Principles of initial wound care**
Decontamination and debridement
All wounds should be thoroughly cleaned and foreign bodies such as dirt and glass should be removed. However, **over-vigorous scrubbing can cause further damage**. All dead tissue should be excised and, if wound edges are ragged, trimming to form a straight line may be useful.

Wound closure
Suturing is the commonest method of wound closure. Metal clips, adhesive tapes, and glues are also available, they are more difficult to use but can be quickly applied. Accurate skin apposition is, however, difficult to achieve and, consequently, they tend to be reserved for lacerations involving the scalp. The epidermis and underlying tissues are accurately realigned to eliminate 'dead' space beneath the surface. A well-opposed everted wound edge is the aim to compensate for flattening during wound contracture.

⑦ Soft tissue injuries of the head and neck

Checklist—indications for treatment
- Presence of abrasions, lacerations and/or avulsions
- Evidence of contamination/foreign bodies.
- Penetrating wounds.
- Burns.
- Motor and/or sensory nerve deficit (5th and 7th cranial nerves).
- Vascular injury.
- Injury to salivary gland and/or duct.
- Injury to lacrimal apparatus.
- Other loss of function of eyelids and/or lips.

Factors affecting the risk
- Association with multiple injuries.
- Impairment of the airway.
- Presence of uncontrolled haemorrhage.
- Presence or absence of contamination/infection.
- Site and extent of lacerations/abrasions.
- Presence or absence of skin/mucosal loss.
- Degree of burn.
- Involvement of specialized structures.
- Presence of severe oedema/emphysema.
- Time lapse between injury and treatment.
- Co-operation of the patient.
- Propensity to keloid/hypertrophic scar formation.
- Systemic disease or treatment that will affect healing.
- Medical/surgical status.

⑦ **The closure of wounds**

This may be classified as 'primary', 'delayed primary' or 'secondary'.

Primary closure

Clean wounds are closed as soon as possible with **meticulous care, haemostasis**, and **accurate repositioning** of the tissues. Deep wounds are closed **in layers**, using resorbable sutures. In some cases, where tissue has been damaged, **trimming of the edges** may convert an untidy to a clean wound, which can then be closed primarily. However, compared to the elsewhere this is kept to a minimum. If doubt exists about viability, tissue is often left *in situ*. To widely excise tissues on the face may lead to difficulties in closing the defect cosmetically, particularly near the eyes, nose, and mouth, which may become distorted. There should be **no tension** across the wound. In cases where tension exists as a result of tissue loss, undermining of the skin, local flap closure, or skin grafts may be used.

Delayed primary closure

When doubt exists about the status of a wound, it can be maintained with moist dressings, antiseptics, and antibiotics for several days. This is useful in **heavily contaminated wounds**. Dead tissue will then 'declare itself' and can be excised, allowing primary closure. Following excision of obviously necrotic tissue, a non-adherent dressing is placed or the wound lightly packed. It is then be inspected under sterile conditions a few days later. If there is no evidence of further necrosis or infection, it can then be closed.

Secondary closure

This is the same as secondary wound healing. It is generally avoided if the face and neck because of contractures and cosmesis. If unavoidable, skin grafts are often placed on the wound bed to minimise these.

⑦ Suturing and suture removal

When carried out correctly, this provides excellent cosmetic results. Many different sutures are now available, but are generally classified as:
- absorbable—polyglactin (vicryl) and polyglycolic acid (dexon);
- non-absorbable- silk, nylon, and prolene.

They may also be classified according to structure—monofilament, twisted, or braided. Monofilament sutures minimize infection, produce less tissue reaction, and are the suture of choice for skin. Braided sutures, e.g. silk, have plated strands, which provide secure knots but may entrap material providing a focus for infection. Traditionally, silk has been used for routine suturing in the mouth, as it is easy to handle, strong, and the ends are comfortable for the patient. However, vicryl is also popular, particularly since it resorbs and does not need to be removed. Which of these is used, often depends on the preference of the surgeon.

Sutures placed in the face and neck tend to be removed at around five days, or earlier in delicate tissues. 'Cross-hatching' of a scar occurs as a result of closing the wound under tension. Ischaemia of the deeper tissues damages the skin and stimulates excess collagen formation. Such scars are difficult to improve and may require further excision and primary closure. Early removal and continued support with steristrips reduces the chances of scarring as a result of the sutures themselves. Subcuticular sutures may be kept in place for longer, as scarring is less likely. With neck lacerations, sutures are often retained for longer (7–10 days). Scalp sutures are similarly left for 7–10 days or absorbable ones used instead. In patients with poor wound healing, e.g. on steroids, with malignancy, infection, or cachexia, the sutures may need longer. Absorbable sutures are useful for deep stitches, either as part of a layered closure or for subcuticular skin closure.

'Steristrips' and 'glue'

These are particularly useful in children and those who will not co-operate. However, care is required in patient and wound selection. Only superficial and scalp wounds should be considered. The final cosmetic results are less predictable than with carefully placed sutures, as deep wounds require deep sutures. Although simpler to do, gluing can still be quite tricky—be careful not to glue your glove to the patient—although it can be removed, it is very embarrassing!

ⓘ Soft tissue injuries—tissue loss

This is relatively uncommon but may be seen, for example, following gun-shots (attempted suicides), road traffic accidents, or industrial accidents. Significant tissue loss may also occur following relatively minor injuries (animal/human bites to the ears, lips, and nose). Particularly following trauma, tissues may be displaced, rather than lost, but nevertheless result in significant problems.

With such injuries there is **often significant associated bone, brain, or ocular injuries**, and these may need to be dealt with prior to soft tissue reconstruction. However, occasionally only the soft tissues are involved, for example, following scalp avulsions. With the use of microsurgical techniques many defects can now be either reconstructed using 'free flaps' or, in selected cases (scalp avulsions), the tissues replaced and the circulation restored by vessel anastamosis.

Repair or reconstruction depends on many variables. Associated injuries may take priority. **Early repair is ideal** especially with avulsed tissue. However, if there is **gross swelling or contamination, a delayed approach may be necessary**. Following initial debridement the wound needs to be protected and dressed until reconstructed. **Local flaps** are often useful where tissue loss is not extensive and has the advantage that the tissue used is similar to that lost (e.g. Abbe flap for lip reconstruction). For elective reconstructions, **tissue expansion** can be of use. However, where the defect is extensive, larger flaps may be necessary. These can be either pedicled or free flaps depending on the defect and general condition of the patient. Where necessary, bone can also be raised with the flap in cases where bony defects are present (e.g. mandible).

Major tissue loss and gun-shot wounds

This is uncommon but may arise following assaults, industrial injuries (scalp avulsions), or pedestrian–motor vehicle collisions. The initial approach is no different to other injuries, i.e. ATLS. However, bear in mind that there can be **significant airway problems, blood loss, and a high risk of infection**. Once stabilized, gently clean the wounds and try to re-align the tissues. This prevents kinking of the veseels, which can necrose distal tissues.

Definitive management

Recent advances in biomaterials, and our understanding in microvascular reconstruction, now means that just about any defect in the cranio-facial region can be reconstructed. Unfortunately, although in most cases *functional* requirements can be met, in many patients, particularly when skin or specialized structures are involved, some stigmata of their disease persists. The eye, for instance, can not be replaced and invisible scars do not exist. However, results are considerably better than 20 years ago. It is an exciting time in deformity care.

The main choice is between using tissues from the patient (autogenous transplants) or synthetic materials. Each has its own advantages and disadvantages (risks of infection, donor site morbidity, costs, etc.) and each has its own advocates. With the recent problems of prion transmission, animal-derived products are rarely used now. The ability to grow tissues,

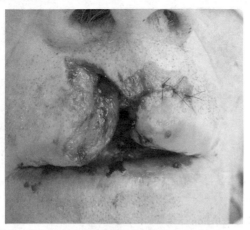

Fig. 8.49 Loss of tissue following dog bite.

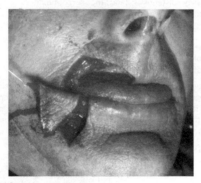

Fig. 8.50 Local flap in lip reconstruction.

either in the lab or on the patient, is the most recent of innovations and we are moving from an era of 'tissue transplantation' into one of 'tissue induction'. Bone morphogenic protein, distraction osseogenesis, bone transportation, and prefabricated 'free flaps' are such developments. Unfortunately, many of these techniques are still relatively unproven in the long term and are quite expensive.

Usually tissue loss is a mixture of both hard and soft tissues. A general principle is to 'replace like with like' wherever possible.

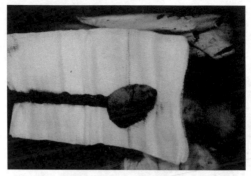

Fig. 8.51 Free tissue transfer is occasionaly required when there is extensive tissue loss.

Tissue expansion

Tissue expanders are inflatable bags with an injection port, placed under the skin, most commonly the scalp. Repeated injections of saline into the bag progressivly distends it and the surrounding skin stretches and regrows to adapt. This provides a surplus of skin, which after removal of the expander can then be used in local reconstructions. Advantages include:

- similar appearance and texture;
- retention of sensations;
- limitation of surgery and scarring to one region.

This technique has proved successful for expanding scalp skin to reduce traumatic alopecia (hair loss) and ear reconstruction. However, the procedure is not without complications; expansion of neck skin may produce pressure on the deep structures and expansion of scalp causes reciprocal depression in the underlying skull.

Local skin flaps

Where a small amount of tissue has been lost, local skin flaps may be used to close the defect. Closure of wounds under tension may not only break down or result in a stretched scar, but may also distort nearby structures such as the lips, nose, etc. Many flap designs are described. These make use of the fact that there is often excess skin on the face, which is highly vascular, elastic to a degree, and can therefore be undermined and used to close nearby defects. Well-defined 'axial flaps', e.g. glabellar flap, naso-labial flap, may be raised, based on a small pedicle through which feeding vessels pass. So long as these are preserved and not kinked during rotation of the flap, large areas of skin can be used to facilitate tissue closure. Random pattern flaps, however, require a broad attachment at the base, if necrosis is to be avoided. In contrast with the remainder of the body, the skin of the head and neck is very well vascularized and the success rate of local flaps is generally very high. These techniques are particularly usefil in the reconstruction of nasal tips, eyelids, and lips.

Parotid injuries

Lacerations along the side of the face must be carefully assessed to exclude injuries to the parotid gland, parotid duct, and, most importantly, facial nerve. Injuries to the **duct and nerve** must be repaired, often using microsurgical techniques, before the skin is closed. Failure to repair the duct may result in the formation of a 'sialocele', which will eventually drain through the wound resulting in a salivary fistula. Failure to repair the nerve may result in various degrees of facial weakness.

Microsurgical nerve repair

Repair of damaged or severed nerves is now possible with the use of the operating microscope. Both direct suturing of the cut ends or 'interpositional' nerve grafting may be carried out, depending on the type of inury. Good results have been obtained following reconstruction or repair of the accessory and facial nerves. However, reconstruction of sensory nerves has a lower success rate, but is still often of benefit to the patient. Ideally, early repair (within 24h) is preferable and should be carried out if there is no infection or significant associated soft tissue trauma. With the facial nerve, successful late repair is limited by wasting of the facial muscles, which occurs around 6–12 months after injury. In long-standing cases of facial palsy with atrophy of the facial muscles, free flaps of muscle with their associated nerves and vessels have been used.

Examples of nerve injuries which may benefit from exploration and repair include:
- **Facial nerve**—this may be damaged following trauma or surgery to the parotid region. If necessary, immediate repair can be delayed and, at the time of wound closure, the nerve endings marked with sutures. Reconstruction may also be undertaken in those cases of malignant tumours of the parotid gland, which require sacrifice of the facial nerve.
- **Accessory nerve**—injury to this nerve may occur following trauma, lymph node biopsies, or following neck dissection. Loss of function of the trapezius muscle results in limitation of shoulder motions.
- **Lingual nerve**—this supplies sensation and taste to the anterior two-thirds of the tonguue. It may be damaged during surgical removal or a lower third molar. Repair, ideally, is undertaken within 6 months following injury.
- **Inferior alveolar nerve**—injury may occur following wisdom tooth removal, orthognathic surgery, tumour resection, fracture fixation, and placement of implants. This can result in numbness of 'dysaethesia' in the lower teeth, the lower lip, and the chin. This should be reconstructed within 3–4 weeks after injury.

Since the facial and accessory nerve are purely motor nerves, and the lingual and inferior alveolar nerves mostly sensory nerves, repair can be simply carried out by alignment of the nerve stumps or by nerve grafting. Manipulation of the nerves must be kept to a minimum, as this stimulates scar tissue at the suture site, which can prevent nerve growth. It is essential that there is no tension across the repair. The least number of sutures consistent with accurate alignment are used. Where grafting is required, the great auricular and the sural nerve are often used.

⑦ Surgical drains

Drains in the head and neck are generally used:
- to provide drainage of infected material (abscess);
- to prevent the collection of blood or fluid between two large raw sur-faces (following neck dissection, coronal flap);
- where a large potential space exists for blood to collect, which cannot be closed (following removal of submandibular gland, thyroid).

Drains should not be used as a substitute for poor surgical technique and haemostasis should be established before wounds are closed. However, 'reactive' haemorrhage can occur, i.e. as the patient recovers from the anaesthetic, their blood pressure rises and previously closed vessels may open and bleeding restart. This probably happens to a minor degree in all patients and draining the small amount of blood that is released prevents the formation of haematoma, which may become infected.

Drains may be left protruding from the skin and simply covered with an absorbent dressing, e.g. following abscess drainage. Fluids drain under gravity. Alternatively, they may be connected to a vacuum container. If the wound is not airtight, or if there is persistent accumulation of fluid, the drains may be placed on continuous low pressure suction.

'Shortening a drain' means withdrawing it bit by bit to allow the cavity to seal up gradually, while still allowing fluids to drain. This is rarely necessary following head and neck surgery, as most drains are usually quite small. It may be of use, however, following incision and drainage of an extensive abscess, e.g. Ludwig's angina, to prevent further collection of pus.

⑦ Scars

All **wounds extending deeper than the epidermis heal with scarring**. The aim is to minimize this to cosmetically and functionally acceptable levels. In uninjured skin, collagen synthesis and breakdown is balanced. However, during healing there is a marked rise in collagen production. This reaches a maximum at around one month, then falls slowly to pre-injury levels. Early on the scar is red, hard, and sometimes itches. Temptation to try and improve the scar before maturation must be resisted. However, improvements in its appearance can be achieved by regular wound massage with a moisturising cream, which encourages breakdown of collagen. It takes about 9–12 months for a scar to mature, during which significant improvements in appearance can be achieved. The wound eventually becomes less vascular, softens, and flattens. Scarring is due to an excess of collagen in the proximity of the wound.

Factors that promote poor scars:
- healing by secondary intention;
- healing of wounds under tension;
- continuing tension on a maturing scar;
- poor vascularity, e.g. diabetes,irradiation;
- dead tissue, e.g. crushed;
- linear wounds running perpendicular to crease lines or linear lines.

Hypertrophic scars and keloids

In some cases scar tissue continues to thicken. A hypertrophic scar remains confined to the wound closure and may soften and flatten after several years. A keloid, however, continues to overgrow and may involve previously undamaged tissue. They can become very bulky. The difference between the two is one of extent rather than structure. Keloids occur more commonly among blacks than whites and are often seen after burns. In the early stages, massage with a moisturiser maintains the suppleness of a scar. Regular intra-lesional steroid injection over 3–4 months may be useful for rapidly growing keloids. Alternatively, steroids may be applied topically (Helan tape). Sustained pressure on the scar (some silicone dressings) has been shown to improve flattening and softening. However, this must be continuous and maintained for 6 months to be of any use. Face masks have been designed and are of most use in burns patients. Surgical excision may be necessary for very large keloids, however, there is a high incidence of recurrence. Radiotherapy was used in the past but is no longer used because of the risk of radiation-induced cancer.

Management of established scars

This depends on the particular characteristics of the scar.
- Shortened scars—scars contract during maturation, and may distort adjacent structures, particularly around the mouth, base of nose, and eyes. Lengthening of the scar may be carried out by rearrangement using a technique of 'Z-plasty'.
- Shelf scars—semi-circular scars contract unequally along each side and the inner part often bulges over the outer (pin-cushioning). This is difficult to correct, but may be improved by increasing its length using multiple Z-plasties.
- Widened or stretched scars—tension across the wound or repeated movement can lead to this. These can be excised and resutured. Supporting the wound with adhesive tape (e.g. steristrips or subcuticular suture) during the first month will minimize recurrence.
- Tattooing—this occurs following inadequate removal of grit, etc., at the time of primary closure. Dermabrasion or excision and primary closure is the best way of removing tattooed tissue.
- Badly aligned scars—scars running in natural skin creases are less noticable than those running across them. Some may therefore be realigned using a Z-plasty changing the direction of the scar by 90 degrees.
- Uneven scars—these can be improved by multiple interdigitating flaps ('W' plasty, 'geometric broken line closure') following excision of the scar. By creating irregularities in the new scar, this breaks up the straight line appearance.

⚠ Paediatric facial trauma

General considerations

Paediatric facial injuries commonly occur following falls, bicycle accidents, road traffic accidents, and sporting accidents. Emergency admission to hospital can be a very stressful, frightening, and anxiety-provoking experience for the child and family. The injured child will be unprepared for what is about to happen and will need constant explanations. If possible, the parents should be allowed to stay with their child during all investigations and treatments. They too will require support and information.

During an emergency admission, children are often in pain while being subjected to a strange and unfamiliar surrounding. They need a calm, relaxed, and unhurried admission process. Children are compliant if they are comfortable and pain-free, if they understand what is happening to them, and if they have their parents in attendance with them. Most paediatric emergency admissions are not life-threatening and time can therefore be spent explaining and preparing the child and parent for their surgery and hospital stay.

Unfortunately there is a tendency with emergency admissions to perform procedures and treatments quickly, and sometimes the child's needs can be overlooked. Any emergency admission is made worse by any need for surgery. Remember, this may be the first time the child has been admitted to hospital, let alone have to undergo a surgical procedure. All explanations given to the child must be age-appropriate, allowing them to understand the treatment they will receive. Children need to participate in their care in order to maintain a sense of control and an understanding of all events.

Parental participation should be welcomed, the child/parent relationship is unique and can help the child cope with the special tests, procedures, and surgery they may need to undergo. Parents know their children better than anyone and if they are supported and kept informed of their child's condition, this will benefit the child.

Facial lacerations

Childhood accidents resulting in abrasions, scratches, cuts, and bruises are generally normal events in a child's lifetime. **However, do not forget the possibility that injuries may be non-accidental.**

Facial lacerations need to be assessed thoroughly. Facial lacerations can bleed profusely and this adds to what already is a stressful and anxious time. For some children, assessment and management may require a short general anaesthetic, in others it may be possible to use local anaesthetic. This avoids general anaesthesia, but must only be undertaken with the full consent and co-operation of the child and parent.

Initial treatment should be directed towards controlling blood loss and cleaning up the wound. It should be irrigated gently with normal saline and a non-adhesive dressing applied. Analgesia or sedation (if no contra-indications) may be given prior to this if necessary. Consider also:

- X-ray for any foreign bodies;
- was the child was knocked out;
- the child's tetanus status.

If there are no complicating factors, the child should be taken to theatre as soon as possible. Children should only be fasted for the minimum of time required for a safe general anaesthetic. Protocols vary slightly between units but this is approximately 4 h for food and 2 h for clear fluids. The child and parents should be warned of the possibility of post-operative bruising and swelling, and reassured that this will settle quickly.

Post-operatively, suture lines can be left exposed to the air or supported by steristrips. With traumatized wounds, some surgeons prescribe an antibiotic course, especially if the wound was dirty. The child's stay in hospital should be short and they can be considered for discharge when fit. At home the suture line will require daily cleaning with normal saline and the parents can be taught this prior to discharge. Crust formation on the wound can prevent optimum healing, resulting in a larger scar.

Sutures are generally removed 4–5 days following surgery. Depending on the number of sutures and the area of injury, the child may need to return to the ward or wound care clinic, or attend the family's GP practice for removal. If the wound has a large number of fine sutures and is in an awkward place, then an experienced nurse will need to remove them. Some children may require a light oral sedation prior to suture removal. Following removal, the repaired laceration can be supported with steristrips.

The parents should be advised to keep the steristrips in place until they fall off. After 2–3 months they should be encouraged to massage the scar with a moisturising cream to prevent thickening and shrinkage of wounds.

Facial fractures
Do not forget the possibility that injuries may be non-accidental.

Children's bones are elastic, i.e. they tend to bend or buckle rather than fracture. Therefore, any fracture in a child is a marker of a serious injury and the underlying soft tissues should be considered injured also (e.g. rib fractures and lung contusion).

Children who have sustained facial fractures require immediate assessment of their injuries. A full examination should be performed, as other injuries are often associated. Facial fractures are often associated with a head injury and the neurological status must be investigated and treated accordingly. Facial fractures can also involve the orbit—assess visual acuity. Depending on the age, use a Snellon chart or pictures for younger children.

Clinically there may be pain or tenderness, swelling, bruising, and non-occlusion of their jaw and teeth. Some fractures will be stable and require no further treatment, others may require surgical reduction once the facial swelling has reduced. If possible, nurse upright to reduce the facial swelling. Consider intravenous fluids if the child has difficulty taking fluids orally—**they can rapidly become dehydrated**.

Post-operatively the child should be nursed in an upright position, as soon as anaesthetic recovery allows. This will help to reduce facial swelling. Ice packs can also be used to reduce swelling, if tolerated. Fluids and a soft diet can be introduced, as tolerated, and any intravenous fluids discontinued. The child should start oral hygiene as soon as possible and must understand the importance of doing so. Mouthwashes should be used regularly, especially following diet, and the child should be encouraged to continue normal teeth-brushing using a soft toothbrush.

Paediatric maxillofacial trauma—non-accidental injury

Any child presenting with an injury to the head and neck that does not appear consistent with the history warrants further investigation. Injuries such as facial fractures, torn frenulum, bites, puncture wounds, and ocular trauma should arouse suspicion. Where there is suspicion of abuse, advice should be sought from a more experienced individual such as a paediatrician or child protection advisor.

Diagnosis can be difficult at times but a number of clues exist:

- there may be a **delay** in seeking medical attention;
- the **history given is vague** and lacking in detail, the account may **vary with every telling**, and the accounts may differ from person to person;
- the explanation and account of the accident is **not consistent with the injury** observed;
- **parent shows inappropriate reaction** to severity of injury;
- the **parent's behaviour** gives cause for concern: obvious signs of irritability, and hostility, seldom touches or speaks to the child;
- the child appears fearful, withdrawn, sad, and avoids physical contact with parents;
- when there is disclosure of an abusive act.

The eye

⑦ Basic anatomy and physiology

The eye is a highly specialized organ with an average axial length of 24 mm and a volume of 6.5 ml. Except for its anterior aspect, it is protected by the bony orbit. The orbit is otherwise filled with orbital fat, which together with a suspensory ligament, suspends the eye in the cavity. Six muscles (four recti and two oblique) are attached to the eye and move it to the nine positions of gaze.

The eyeball (globe)

The eyeball itself consists of three coats that surround the contents of the eye (aqueous humor, lens, and the vitreous body). The three coats are:

- Tough fibrous outer layer. This layer is transparent anteriorly (**cornea**) and opaque in the larger posterior portion (**sclera**). They meet to form a small depression around the cornea (**limbus**).
- Pigmented and vascular middle layer. The **uveal** tissue is continuous and forms the choroid posteriorly and the ciliary body and iris anteriorly.
- Neural inner layer. **Retina** is the inner most layer and gives rise to the nerve fibres that leave through the optic disc to form the optic nerve and convey visual stimuli to the brain.

The ocular contents need to be transparent for light to get through to the retina. The **lens** is a specialized structure situated behind the iris and can be stimulated by the ciliary body to change its shape and focus objects on the retina. It divides the eye into a large posterior and a small anterior segment. The anterior segment is further divided into a small posterior and a bigger anterior chamber by the iris and is filled with aqueous. The vitreous gel fills the posterior segment.

Eyelids

These protect the eyes from the environment, injury, and light, and also maintain the cornea by spreading the tears evenly over its surface. They are composed of an outer skin layer, a middle layer of muscle and connective tissue, and an inner layer of conjunctiva. The skin is thin and loosely attached to the underlying tissues. This allows significant amount of fluid to gather underneath it, and hence the characteristic swollen and bruised eye. The meibomian glands line the edge of the lids. These produce oil that helps lubricates the eye. The lashes protect the eyes from the elements and debris.

The **orbicularis oculi muscle** closes the lids and goes into spasm for protection when the eye is painful. The conjunctiva is the mucous membrane of the eye covering the inside of the eyelids. It is continuous at the fornix with the conjunctiva covering the eyeball up to the cornea. The conjunctival sac is, therefore, only open anteriorly and it is impossible to lose a contact lens around the back of the eye (a common worry among patients).

Lacrimal system

The lacrimal gland is situated supero-temporally in the anterior orbit. The tears are spread on the surface of the eye by blinking and then pumped into the lacrimal drainage system. This forces the tears into the puncta at the inner corners of the upper and lower eyelids. The puncti are the openings for the tubes (canaliculi) leading to the lacrimal sac in the medial canthal area. The tears then go down the naso-lacrimal duct into the nose. Any disruption in this system gives rise to watery eyes, a condition many patients find very frustrating.

Tear film

The tear film serves several purposes: it keeps the eye moist, nourishes the front of the eye, creates a smooth surface for light to pass through the eye and provides protection from injury and infection. It is comprised of three layers: oil, water, and mucous. The mucous layer helps the film adhere to the eye. The outer oil layer, produced by the meibomian glands, reduces evaporation. The watery component is produced by the lacrimal glands.

Conjunctiva

This is the thin, transparent mucos membrane that covers the outer surface of the eyeball from the corneal limbus to the inside of the eyelids. It contains accessory tear glands and mucous secreting goblet cells that moisten and lubricate the eye.

Sclera (the 'white of the eye')

This is a tough, opaque tissue that forms the eye's protective outer coat. In children, the sclera is thinner and more translucent, allowing the under-lying tissues to show giving it a bluish cast. As we age, the sclera tends to become more yellow.

Cornea

The cornea is a dome-shaped, transparent window through which light passes. It is responsible for approximately two-thirds of the eye's focusing power. It is normally clear and has a shiny surface. It is avascular and is maintained by the aqueous and tear film.

The cornea is extremely sensitive—there are more nerve endings in the cornea than anywhere else in the body. There are five layers: epithelium, Bowman's membrane, stroma, Descemet's membrane, and the endothelium. The epithelium is a layer of cells that covers the cornea and quickly regenerates when the cornea is injured. However, deep injuries may lead to scarring and growth of blood vessels, and result in an opaque area.

Iris and pupil

The iris is a muscular diaphragm with a central aperture called the pupil. Fine muscles enable it to dilate and constrict the pupil, and thus control the amount of light that enters the eye. The iris is flat and separates the anterior chamber from the posterior chamber.

The pupil constricts in response to bright light and also when looking near. If a bright light is shone in one eye, the afferent pathway leads to the stimulation of bilateral parasympathetic nuclei in the midbrain. Both pupils then constrict via the efferent fibres in the third nerve. Therefore, there is a direct and consensual response of the pupils to light. However, the near gaze response follows a different path within the midbrain and can be spared when the light reflex is affected and vice versa. Any disruption of the afferent and efferent pathways or damage to the iris muscles will affect pupillary function.

Ciliary body

Part of the uveal tract, it lies between the iris and choroids, and is important in supporting the lens and changing its shape (accommodation). It also produces the aqueous humour that fills the front of the eye.

Choroid

A posterior portion of the uveal tract, the choroid lies between the sclera and the retina. It is composed of layers of blood vessels that nourish the back of the eye. Anteriorly it connects with the ciliary body and posteriorly it attaches to edges of the optic nerve.

Aqueous humor

This watery fluid is constantly produced by the ciliary body to nourish the lens and cornea, as well as maintaining the intra-ocular pressure. The aqueous circulates in front of the lens, through the pupil, and out of the eye via the drainage angle.

Drainage angle

The eye's drainage system is made up of several structures: the priphery of the iris, the ciliary body, the trabecular meshwork, and the canal of Schlemm. Aqueous is made in the ciliary body behind the iris and passes through the pupil into the anterior chamber. From there, fluid passes into the angle structures, where it drains from the eye. The aqueous eventually flows into the adjacent blood vessels.

If the drainage angle slowly blocks, the pressure in the eye rises without causing symptoms or pain, eventually leading to glaucoma. In acute-angle closure glaucoma, the peripheral iris quickly blocks the angle and the rapid rise in pressure causes the clinical picture and pain characteristic of the condition.

Lens and accommodation

The crystalline lens is just behind the iris and is composed of an inner nucleus surrounded by a softer cortex. The lens is encased in a capsule, suspended from the ciliary body by tiny 'wires' called zonules. Its purpose is to focus light onto the retina. One-third of the eye's focusing power is supplied by the lens, which can increase its refractive power to allow objects nearing the eye to stay in focus. This process is called **accommodation** and is possible because the young lens can change its shape. With age, the nucleus gradually hardens, diminishing its ability to accommodate (**presbyopia**) and reading glasses are required.

Refraction

For the eye to see clearly, (Fig. 9.1), the light needs to be brought into focus on the retina (refraction). In **emmetropia** (normal sightedness), the light rays are brought into focus on the retina. In **short- and long-sightedness** the light is focused in front or behind the retina, respectively. In all refractive errors, the unfocused light that falls on the retina creates a circle of confusion and therefore vision is blurred. If a lens is used to move the focus of the eye onto the retina, vision improves. **Astigmatism** is when a point focus of light cannot be created on the retina. This occurs because the optical system of individual focuses the light differently on its

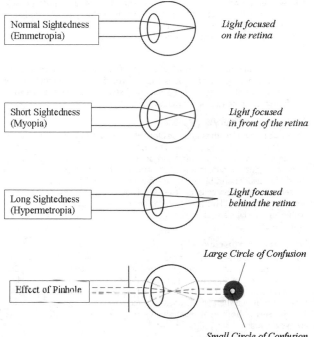

Fig. 9.1 Ray diagrams showing the path of light in normal, myopic, and hypermetropic eyes and the pinhole principle.

horizontal or vertical axis. Special cylindrical lenses are needed to correct this error.

Vitreous humor
This is a clear gel that occupies the posterior chamber of the eye (between the lens and the retina). It comprises about 80% of the volume of the globe. Light is transmitted through the vitreous to the retina.

Retina
This is a multi-layered photoreceptor tissue that lines the back of the eye, converting light into electrical impulses that are recognised by the brain as visual stimuli. There are two types of photoreceptors in the retina: rods and cones. Cones are contained in the macula and are responsible for

detailed central vision and colour perception. They are most densely packed within the fovea and function best in bright light. The rods are spread throughout the peripheral retina and function best in dim light. They are responsible for peripheral and night vision.

Macula

This is a small but highly sensitive part of the retina responsible for detailed vision (e.g. reading). It is located roughly in the centre of the retina, just lateral to the optic nerve, and between the vascular arcades. The **fovea** is the centre of the macula.

Optic disc and nerve

The optic nerve transmits impulses from the retina to the brain and forms the optic disc as it leaves the eye. The optic disc rim is pink and represents the retinal nerve fibres viewed head on as they dip into the disc. The cup is the area not containing any fibres and is pale. The margin of the disc should be distinct and blood vessels occupy a central position. There are no sensory receptor cells on the disc itself and hence everyone has a normal 'blind spot'. This is not normally noticeable because the vision of both eyes overlaps and the brain 'completes the picture' with information from the other eye.

Extra-ocular muscles

There are six muscles that surround the eye and control its movements. The four recti muscles control movements from left to right and up and down. The two oblique muscles rotate the eyes inward and outward, as well as assisting the recti in their function. All muscles need to work together to move the eye. As one contracts, the opposing muscle relaxes. The muscles of both eyes must also work in unison so that the eyes are always aligned.

⑦ History taking

A good history is vital to assessing a patient with an ophthalmic complaint.
**The two main symptoms to ask about are pain and visual disturb-
ances**.

Eye discomfort can be described in two ways:
- a **gritty/foreign body sensation** tends to indicate an ocular surface
  problem such as a foreign body;
- an **aching sensation** is more suggestive of a deeper aetiology such as
  uveitis, raised pressure, and scleritis;
- a combination of these symptoms can exist.

Visual disturbances mainly fall into three categories:
- **reduced visual acuity** can be anything from blurring to total loss of
  vision;
- **unusual visual experiences** can take the form of floaters (shapes
  floating across the vision), flashing lights (can be quick like lightening or
  prolonged shimmering), shadows (permanent shadow obscuring part of
  the visual field), and distortion (objects wavy or bent instead of
  straight);
- **diplopia** (double vision) may be described as objects being side by side
  (horizontal), one above the other (vertical) or tilted in relation to one
  another (torsional).

Try to ascertain the onset, duration and associated features of the
presenting complaint. In a setting of trauma, specific questions will be
relevant to the eyes. Was the injury of low (grinding) or high velocity
(hammering, drilling)? Was the patient wearing eye protection? Sharp and
blunt injuries cause a different pattern of injury and the size of the
offending object will determine if the bony orbital rim took the main brunt
of injury instead of the eyeball. The presence of chemical or organic
matter can cause severe sight-threatening complications requiring immediate treatment.

Previous ocular history

This is of utmost importance. Does the refractive error (needing glasses)
and amblyopia (lazy eye/poor vision since childhood) explain the reduced
vision or is the trauma responsible? Pre-existing ocular conditions, such as
a squint, may be responsible for the abnormal eye movements and not a
blow-out fracture. Previous ocular surgery can make the eye more susceptible to trauma. Patients do not always volunteer such information or feel it
is not relevant.

General medical history

This will indicate risk factors for many ophthalmic emergencies
(arteriosclerosis and retinal artery occlusion, diabetes and vitreous haemorrhage). Drug history, allergies, social and family history will all guide
diagnosis and management strategy.

⑦ Basic eye examination

Following trauma, a systemic examination of the patient, with careful attention to the ABCs, must take precedence. When stable, it is important to make the patient as comfortable as possible in order to allow adequate ophthalmic examination. Eye pain can result in eyelid spasm, making examination near impossible. **Usually a drop of a local anaesthetic agent (amethocaine, benoxinate) can relieve surface pain (corneal abrasion, foreign body) and relax the lids. The room lights can be turned down to reduce photophobia**. Also, a calm and confident approach by the doctor can relieve the anxiety of patients with eye disease. Occasionally systemic analgesia or local anaesthetic infiltration to the branches of the facial nerve supplying the orbicularis oculi muscle is required. An examination under sedation or general anaesthetic can be performed as a last resort in children or if the patient is going to surgery for other reasons.

Visual acuity

This is the measurement of how well a person sees. It is the most vital element of examination, and sadly a frequently neglected one. This must be performed using a **back-illuminated Snellen chart at a distance of 6 m with the patient wearing their spectacle correction for distant vision**. Each eye is tested separately and results recorded as a fraction. The numerator is 6 (i.e. test performed at 6 m) and the denominator corresponds to the line on the chart they could read. If the patient only manages to read the top line (60 line), the vision is recorded as 6/60. This simply means that the patient was tested at 6 m but could only read the line a normal person should have managed to read at 60 m.

If the patient does not have their glasses or has not been tested for them, then a **pinhole** can be used to try and obtain the best possible vision (Fig. 9.1). A pinhole works by eliminating the peripheral rays of light entering the eye and hence creating a smaller circle of confusion on the retina. If this improves the visual acuity, the reduced vision was due to a refractive error rather than a disease process. But a pinhole has a limited effect if the glasses' prescription is high. If a vision chart is not available, or the patient is immobile, then any documentation of vision is better than none. Mini Snellen charts can be used with the patient wearing their reading glasses. Alternatively, comments on improvised tests, such as 'able to read small newspaper print or only able to count fingers at one meter', should be documented.

Colour vision

This should be tested with an Ishihara book. The patient is asked to read numbers on test pages and scored according to how many they got right. Colour-vision defects are common in men and affect one in eight males. The commonest problem involves confusing reds and greens. Loss of colour perception is one of the early signs of optic nerve compression after trauma.

Visual fields

The patient's field of vision can be assessed by using your own visual field as a normal control (assuming it is normal). Sit opposite the patient and use your left hand to cover your left eye and ask the patient to mirror you (right hand over right eye). Ask the patient to look at your open eye all the time. You then move a white hatpin (held half-way between you and the patient) in from the periphery until the patient reports seeing it. If this corresponds to your own field of vision then the patient has a normal field. Repeat this in all quadrants of vision and in the fellow eye. A red hatpin can be used to plot the central field of vision and the blind spot.

Pupils

Assessment of the pupil is vital in assessing optic nerve and retinal function, as they form the afferent pathway in the pupillary reflex. The patient must look in the distance when performing the light test to avoid stimulation of the near response. Also it is vital to have a torch bright enough to stimulate a response. This is the commonest cause for failure in pupil assessment.

An afferent pupillary defect (APD) is recorded if a bright light in one eye fails to constrict either pupil (i.e. no message reaching the midbrain). If one of the pupils constricts, then it is likely that a pupil defect (sphincter muscle tear or dilating drop in the eye) or efferent pathway defect is responsible for the abnormality.

An important test of the afferent pathway is the 'swinging light test' or **Relative Afferent Pupillary Defect (RAPD) test**. An APD may be subtle and the pupil may react sluggishly but nevertheless react. The test therefore compares the two eyes to pick up the defect. The light is shone in the normal eye (both pupils briskly constrict), then the light is moved over to the other eye with a delay of 1s. During this delay, both pupils should start to dilate, and when the light shines in the eye, they should briskly constrict again. But if there is a subtle afferent defect, the pupil first continues to dilate before constricting again in a sluggish manner.

Eye movements

The patient is asked to look straight then follow a target to the other eight positions of gaze and report if they see double at any stage. Any report of diplopia indicates asymmetrical eye movement. You must still observe for restricted range of movement, as **patients may not necessarily appreciate diplopia**, especially if they have poor vision in one eye.

Eyelids

The lower eyelid normally sits at the level of the inferior limbus and the upper lid 1–2mm below the upper limbus. The eyelids should be examined for any lacerations, noting their position, length, and depth. Care must be taken to exclude underlying globe damage, retained foreign body, and penetrating orbital and brain injuries. **When opening a swollen eyelid you must not press on the eye, as this can cause or exacerbate globe injury**. The direction of applied force should be up and down towards the orbital rims. **Medial canthal injuries can involve the lacrimal drainage system**.

Upper-lid injuries may affect the levator muscle; its function should be noted by asking the patient to look down then up whilst pressing on the eyebrow to neutralize occipito-frontalis muscle function. The range of movement is noted in millimeters (normal >15mm). Lid closure also needs to be assessed, to ensure adequate closure is possible to protect the cornea from exposure.

Slit-lamp examination

Examination with a slit lamp provides a superior view of the ocular contents. It provides a magnified and 3D view of the eye in sections. However, there are different manufacturer designs and it can take a lot of practice to learn how to use it. Each emergency department needs to liaise with the ophthalmologist in their hospital to arrange tutorials on their particular slit lamp, as this is beyond the remit of this chapter. Even without the slit lamp, a considerable amount of information can be obtained using a good ophthalmoscope.

Conjunctiva

Subconjunctival haemorrhage is seen as fresh layer of blood beneath the conjunctiva. It is distinct from injected conjunctiva, which has a pink colour, and the dilated vessels can be easily seen. If blood is reported in the tear film after trauma in the absence of a lid laceration, then at least a conjunctival laceration must have occurred to account for the blood. You must examine for and **exclude globe damage**.

Cornea

The normal cornea is **always clear**. In the elderly, a peripheral rim of white deposit known as arcus senilis can be seen but it does not affect vision. Generally speaking a cloudy cornea indicates corneal oedema and a white area is either scarring or active infiltration. Foreign bodies and prolapsed tissue are usually dark in colour but can be any colour and consistency.

Intra-ocular pressure

The pressure inside the eye is usually between 12–21 mmHg. Formal measurement requires equipment and skill not commonly available to the non-ophthalmologist. Subjectively, however, high pressure can be assessed using ones fingers to diagnose glaucoma. Ask the patient to close their eye and look down. Using your two index fingers, press through the upper eyelid to feel if the eyeball is hard. Your own eye can act as a normal control. **In post-operative patients and if globe rupture or a penetrating injury is suspected, the intra-ocular pressure should not be assessed, as pressure on the eyeball can open up the wound or further expulse ocular contents**.

Anterior chamber

The normal anterior chamber should be deep and contain aqueous humor making it an optically empty space. Blood and inflammatory debris can settle and form a fluid level called **hyphema** and **hypopyon**, respectively.

Iris

Iris is a muscular structure with a central aperture (pupil). The pupil should be round and reactive to light. Any irregularity in its shape is abnormal. A defect in the iris periphery is called a **dialysis** and indicates significant trauma avulsing the iris root from the ciliary body.

Lens

The lens is normally behind the iris and can be viewed through the pupil. It is usually clear. Any opacity in the lens is known as a **cataract**. Incidence of cataract increases with age and most patients over sixty have a degree of cataract. Any displacement of the lens or disruption of its capsule is easily recognizable especially if the pupil is dilated.

Fundoscopy

The direct ophthalmoscope can be used to examine the vitreous and fundus. Sit opposite the patient at the same eye level. Ask the patient to look straight ahead, look through the ophthalmoscope to obtain the red reflex, whilst you are approximately 30 degrees off their visual axis. Then follow the red reflex in as you move towards the patient until you get the fundal view. Following the red reflex stops you from 'losing' the eye. This way you are likely to get the view of the disc with little effort. If you do not see the disc, just follow the branching of the vessels in towards the disc (remember that the vessels branch away from the disc).

A **poor red reflex** indicates opacity in the media (cataract and vitreous haemorrhage). However, it must be noted that pigmented fundi tend to have a significantly duller red reflex. Once on the disc assess its margin (distinct or blurred), rim colour (pale or hyperaemic), cup (full or empty), and blood vessels (congested, pulsating, or attenuated). Papilloedema is suspected if the margin is blurred, colour hyperaemic, cup is full, and vessels congested. The rest of the fundus is examined by rotating the ophthalmoscope to view different quadrants and macula.

Dilating the pupils using tropicamide 1% or cyclopentylate 1% can make examination of the fundus much easier. Pupils should not be dilated if the patient is likely to need neuro-observations. ALSO patients who are very longsighted (their glasses magnify images), have shallow anterior chambers and those with a history of angle closure glaucoma should not be dilated as this can precipitate a rise in intra-ocular pressure.

ⓘ Quick reference list

The following lists are by no means exhaustive but provide a list of common and important diagnosis for reference.

Red eyes

- **Blepharitis and dry eyes**—gritty eyes and itchy lids, usually no discharge, inflamed lid margin.
- **Subconjunctival haemorrhage**—layer of fresh blood rather than injected vessels, usually in one sector.
- **Foreign body**—gritty sensation, watery and usually a clear history of FB.
- **In-turning lashes**—local irritation and redness, usually visible and easily removed.
- **Abrasion**—gritty sensation, usually a clear trauma history, and watery discharge.
- **Conjunctivitis**—gritty and discharge is watery (viral), purulent (bacterial), muco-purulent (chlamydia).
- **Acute angle closure glaucoma**—pain, nausea, and vomiting, cloudy cornea, fixed semi-dilated pupil, and raised intra-ocular pressure.
- **Contact lens problems**—gritty, watery or discharge if infected, usually over-wear or poor compliance with cleaning, corneal opacity if ulcerated.
- **Corneal ulcer**—painful and photophobic, purulent discharge, opacity on the cornea, reduced vision.
- **Uveitis**—painful and photophobic, watery, mostly injected around cornea, vision can be reduced.
- **Scleritis**—sectoral injection, dull ache to boring pain, vision can be reduced, pain on eye movement.
- **Episcleritis**—sectoral injection, dull discomfort, vision normal, no pain on eye movement.
- **Carotid cavernous fistula**—dilated and arterialized vessels, if direct fistula proptosis, ophthalmoplegia and chemosis, raised intra-ocular pressure, usually a history of trauma.
- **Thyroid eye disease**—generalized mild injection and discomfort, proptosis, any thyroid state possible.
- **Orbital cellulitis**—painful proptosis with ophthalmoplegia, fever and generally unwell, possibly vision, colour vision, and pupils are affected, swollen optic disc.

Examination and signs in trauma

- **Observation**—lid bruising and oedema, lacerations, bony deformity, proptosis, severity of other injuries.
- **Visual acuity—reduced vision**.
- **Colour vision**—loss of colour perception.
- **Visual fields**—restricted field.
- **Pupils**—afferent pupilary defect, irregular shape, or iris dialysis.
- **Eye movements**—asymmetrical or restricted movement, any nerve palsy (III, IV, VI).
- **Lid and orbital rim**—peri-orbital swelling and bruising, lacerations, emphesema, step in orbital rim.
- **Conjunctiva and sclera**—injection, haemorrhage, lacerations, prolapsing tissue.

- **Cornea**—any cloudiness or opacity, lacerations with prolapsed tissue.
- **Intra-ocular pressure**—high in blunt trauma, low in penetrating injuries and ruptured globe.
- **Anterior chamber**—presence of hyphaema (blood), hypopyon (pus), flat chamber.
- **Lens**—dislocation, cataract formation, or rupture of capsule.
- **Vitreous**—loss of red reflex if haemorrhage.
- **Retina**—detachment, tears, haemorrhages, vascular occlusion.
- **Optic disc**—haemorrhages, papilloedema.

Painful loss of vision

- Acute angle closure glaucoma.
- Chemical burns
- Corneal ulcers.
- Uveitis: especially posterior and intermediate.
- Scleritis: especially posterior.
- Herpes zoster ophthalmicus.
- Temporal arteritis.
- Orbital cellulitis.
- Blunt and penetrating ocular trauma.
- Retrobulbar haemorrhage.
- Optic neuritis.

Painless loss of vision

- Retinal artery occlusion: central or branch.
- Amaurosis fugax: transient ischaemic attack involving the optic nerve.
- Retinal vein occlusion: central or branch.
- Age-related macular degeneration: loss of central vision.
- Retinal detachment.
- Vitreous haemorrhage.
- Cataract: although not acute may be noticed acutely by the patient when one eye covered.
- Advanced glaucoma: although not acute may be noticed acutely by the patient when one eye covered.
- Occipital cortex strokes: one half of vision lost (homonymous hemianopia).

Painful eye

- All the causes listed under painful loss of vision.
- Corneal abrasion.
- Foreign bodies.
- Conjunctivitis.
- Contact lens related hypoxia, malposition, drying, debris, and infections.
- Blepharitis: itchy and crusty eyelids irritating the eye, uncomfortable not painful.
- Dry eyes: can be severe but usually uncomfortable rather than painful.

Proptosis

- Thyroid eye disease.
- Orbital cellulitis.
- Retrobulbar haemorrhage.
- Neoplastic lesion in the orbit.
- Orbital inflammatory disease.
- High myopia (short-sightedness).
- Congenital.

☠ Vision-threatening injuries

- Penetrating globe injuries.
- Blunt injury and ruptured globe.
- Loss of eyelids.
- Retro bulbar haemorrhage.
- Traumatic optic neuropathy.
- Chemical injuries.

Ocular injuries occur commonly in maxillofacial trauma, especially with injuries to the upper face and forehead. These range from simple corneal abrasions to penetrating globe injuries and optic nerve compression. It is worth remembering that the brain is not far behind or above the orbit, and is separated from it by some of the thinnest bones in the body. **Brain and eye injuries should be excluded in all high-velocity and penetrating orbital trauma**. The force required to damage the globe can leave the surrounding tissues relatively unscaved. Unless specific attention is paid to the eye, such injuries can be missed. The eye can receive the full impact of small high-velocity missiles (explosions, glass, metal-on-metal impact) at the time of accident. Ruptured globes and perforations with retained intra-ocular foreign body, need to be borne in mind. **All ocular injuries listed above require urgent ophthalmic referral**. Visual loss becomes a significant concern once the acute stage of trauma has passed, because it both impedes rehabilitation and dramatically reduces the quality of life.

☢ Penetrating ocular trauma

Full-thickness penetration into the eye wall (cornea or sclera) can occur with a sharp object. There may be a retained intra-ocular foreign body. Work place accidents and interpersonal violence are the commonest causes of injury.

There is variable loss of vision, which may be accompanied by pain and bleeding, depending on size, location, and extent of injury. Associated lid laceration, bruising, and subconjunctival haemorrhage may be observed. The entry site is usually obvious and the eye looks collapsed. Uveal tissue, retina, and the vitreous gel may be prolapsing out of the eye. The lens may be damaged and cataractous. A hyphaema and vitreous haemorrhage are usually present. The intra-ocular pressure is low and aqueous fluid may be seen leaking from the wound when a fluorescein drop is instilled. In cases of small high-velocity objects (metal and glass chips) the eye may appear intact and a small entry wound overlooked. The **history is therefore important** in alerting the doctor to the possibility of an intra-ocular foreign body (IOFB). An IOFB may be visible if the view of the fundus is clear.

Care must be taken not to apply pressure to the eye during examination, as this can further expulse ocular contents. The possibility of penetrating orbital and brain injury should be borne in mind.

If intra-ocular blood or lid oedema prevent examination, an ultrasound or CT scan can detect intra-ocular foreign bodies, retinal detachment, and globe integrity.

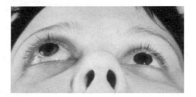

Fig. 9.2 Proptosis and ophthalmoplegia.

Management

Analgesia and anti-emetics should be administered, as required. A hard plastic shield should be taped over the eye to stop eye-rubbing, especially in children. Tetanus status must be checked. Primary surgical repair of the globe by an experienced ophthalmologist should be performed as soon as possible. Usually the foreign body is removed at the same time. The use of oral ciprofloxacin is thought to reduce the risk of endophthalmitis. Prognosis is variable and can be very good. A good initial visual acuity carries a better prognosis. Large defects and posterior involvement are poor prognostic indicators. Corneal scarring, glaucoma, cataract, and retinal detachment are the main complications leading to poor vision.

:☺: Blunt ocular trauma

Blunt trauma can result in intra-ocular damage with an intact eyeball or cause a ruptured globe (same as seen when an orange is dropped from a height; the force may only cause bruising of the fruit or cause rupture of its skin). Antero-posterior compression of the eye during trauma expands the eye at the equator. This is the mechanism of tearing of structures within the eye leading to the clinical picture. The force of trauma may not appear to be severe but an object small enough to fit within the bony orbital rim will transmit all its energy to the eyeball. Globe rupture will be discussed in the following chapter.

In blunt trauma, visual acuity is usually reduced without an afferent pupillary defect. The patient may report floaters and that the vision has improved since the incident. This is because the intra-ocular blood has settled at the bottom of the eye with the patient in an upright posture. Associated lid laceration, bruising, and subconjuctival haemorrhage may be present. Iris sphincter muscle tears, iris dialysis, hyphaema, and a displaced lens may be observed. The intra-ocular pressure is usually high due to blood blocking the trabecular meshwork in the drainage angle. Posterior segment complications of trauma are vitreous haemorrhage, choroidal ruptures, retinal commotio, and tears leading to a retinal detachment. An ultrasound scan can detect globe rupture, retinal tears, and detachment, if the view of the fundus is poor.

If the eye is soft in the setting of blunt trauma, a globe rupture must be excluded.

Management

The aim of management is to control the inflammation, pain, and intra-ocular pressure, while the eye settles. Steroid, cycloplegic, and anti-hypertensive drops need to be initiated by the ophthalmologist, as required. Careful follow-up to look for complications of retinal detachment, glaucoma, cataract, and retinal membrane formation is required. Prognosis is generally good and depends on whether any of the above complications arise. Choroidal rupture and retinal detachment involving the macula carry the worst prognosis.

☺ Ruptured globe

Ruptured globe is defined as the loss of integrity of the eyeball following blunt trauma. The bony orbit offers protection to the eye but is deficient anteriorly. This is even more relevant in individuals with prominent eyes, as they are more susceptible to blunt trauma. Interpersonal violence and falls are the commonest causes of globe rupture. There is a history of significant blunt ocular trauma, usually with an object small enough to fit within the bony orbital rim, e.g. knuckles, squash ball. or the edge of table. Previous ocular surgical history is important. as the scar is a potential site of rupture.

Patients present with severe and sudden loss of vision with pain. Visual acuity is usually down to perception of light with afferent pupillary defect. Associated lid laceration and bruising may be observed. A subconjunctival haemorrhage is invariably present. Uveal tissue, retina, and the vitreous gel may be prolapsing out of the eye. The eye is collapsed, and if the rupture is posterior, the anterior chamber looks very deep. The lens may be displaced and a hyphaema is usually present. The intra-ocular pressure is very low and the eye movements are reduced.

If severe lid bruising and oedema is present, it will be difficult to examine the eye. Care must be taken not to press on the eye in an attempt to open the lids, as this will further expulse ocular contents. If severe lid oedema prevents examination and a rupture is suspected, then an ultrasound or CT scan can detect globe integrity.

Management

Analgesia and anti-emetics should be administered, as globe injuries can be painful and vomiting is common. Uncontrolled vomiting can further expulse ocular contents. A hard plastic shield should be taped over the eye to stop eye-rubbing, especially in children. Tetanus status must be checked. Primary surgical repair of the globe by an experienced ophthalmologist should be performed as soon as possible. Many advocate use of oral ciprofloxacin to prevent endophthalmitis. Prognosis is generally poor and depends on the site and extent of rupture. Posteriorly positioned and large defects carry the worst prognosis.

☺ Eyelid lacerations

In eyelid lacerations, **assessment and management of the underlying ocular damage is more important than that of the eyelid**. Visual acuity, fields, colour vision, ocular movement, pupillary defect, and the fundus should be examined. Conjunctival, corneal, and scleral lacerations, hyphaema, lens dislocation, and globe rupture must all be excluded. The position, length, and depth of eyelid lacerations should then

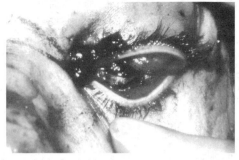

Fig. 9.3 Ruptured globe flow kick by a horse.

be documented under local anaesthesia, if required. **Upper-lid injuries may affect the levator muscle** and its function should be noted. Full neurological examination is required if penetrating brain injury is suspected or in the presence of altered consciousness.

Failure to detect damage to underlying structures is the main source of error when evaluating lid lacerations. Penetrating globe, orbital, and cranial injuries must be excluded in all penetrating lid lacerations. Small lid laceration may conceal a large retained foreign body. Globe rupture and blow-out orbital fractures are likely with blunt injuries.

Plain orbital X-rays may reveal fractures and retained foreign bodies but CT scan is the investigation of choice if the history suggests a significant risk of the above.

Any associated injury must be treated accordingly and the tetanus status checked. Especially in the unconscious patient, **eyelid lacerations can compromise the cornea**, which dries very quickly and loss of vision can ensue. Until the defect is repaired, eyelid remnants should be pulled over to provide corneal cover (a traction suture may be required for this). Plenty of chloramphenical or artificial-tears ointment should be administered and the whole area covered with a wet gauze swab.

Simple lacerations can be explored and cleaned under local anaesthesia and closed in layers as with any laceration. **Care must be taken to ensure suture ends do not rub the cornea and cause abrasions.** Many shallow cuts appose with no sutures; they scab over and heal extremely well, as the lid is very vascular. Complex lacerations (including any involving the lid margin, lateral and medial canthal regions, medial-third of the lids, and levator muscle) must be referred to an ophthalmologist for repair. These lacerations can disrupt the lacrimal drainage system and functional integrity of the lid and require detailed understanding of the functional and cosmetic anatomy of the region. As the lid is very vascular, even necrotic-looking tissue can survive and thus no tissue should be excised. Adequate cosmetic and functional results can be achieved but it may require further operations. Unsightly scars, watering, exposure of the cornea, and loss of vision are complication of lid lacerations.

:☺: Retrobulbar haemorrhage

Retrobulbar haemorrhage results from bleeding and associated oedema behind the orbital septum. It is effectively **a form of compartment syndrome**. Blood can collect within or outside the cone formed by the recti muscles, the former being more severe. As the pressure rises, it rapidly compromises the orbital and retinal vessels, with a concomitant increase in the intra-ocular tension. Left unchecked, blindness and ophthalmoplegia can result. These changes are irreversible in a few hours. Classically, the onset of symptoms is within a few hours of injury, but there are documented cases occurring after several days. Key symptoms are:

- severe pain;
- progressive loss of vision;
- proptosis;
- ophthalmoplegia;
- development of a fixed dilated pupil.

The combination of **pain, proptosis, and loss of vision** are the cardinal diagnostic features. However, the unconscious or agitated patient may not complain of pain, nor may it be possible to assess the visual acuity. A **tense proptosis** with resistance to retropulsion of the eye and a dilated pupil with an afferent defect may be the only clues to the presence of a retrobulbar haemorrhage. Again, it is essential to maintain a high index of suspicion and frequently review the patient. CT scanning will demonstrate severe proptosis with stretching of the optic nerve and a tented posterior sclera as the eye is forced anteriorly. Very often the diagnosis of retrobulbar haemorrhage is clinical, as treatment needs to be instituted as soon as possible.

Management is essentially surgical, although medical measures may be used while preparing the patient for theatre. The aim of treatment is to decompress the orbit. **A lateral canthotomy with lateral canthal tendon division may be performed as a temporary measure**. Lignocaine1% with adrenaline (1 in 200 000) is injected into the lateral canthal area of the affected eye and the lateral canthus is incised to the orbital rim and the identified canthal tendon cut. The lower eyelid is then pulled forward and its lateral attachment to the orbital rim divided. This allows the globe to translate forward, so partially relieving the pressure by increasing the retro bulbar volume. If necessary, the same procedure can also be applied to the upper eyelid, laterally. This is usually a temporary measure to buy time, while preparing for surgery. Formal decompression is carried out under a general anaesthetic. The orbital and intra-conal space is entered allowing the blood and oedema to escape via a drain left *in situ*. Various approaches are possible, the infra-orbital approach is the most commonly used. In addition, high-dose intravenous steroids, acetazolamide (250–500 mg) and mannitol (1 g/kg) are often utilized before and after surgery until the globe pressure is seen to be falling.

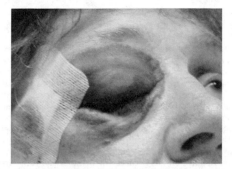

Fig. 9.4 Retrobulbar haemorrhage.

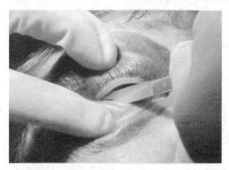

Fig. 9.5 Lateral canthotomy.

Traumatic optic neuropathy

Traumatic optic neuropathy occurs when there is disruption around the optic canal resulting in either compression of the optic nerve, shearing forces to the nerve as it passes through the canal, or haematoma formation within the nerve itself. Untreated it can render the patient blind and the diagnosis needs to be made early to allow the best chance of visual recovery. The signs that suggest an optic nerve injury include: **decreased visual acuity, decreased colour vision, poorly reactive pupil, and an afferent papillary defect with a relatively normal ocular examination**. This is an ophthalmic emergency and should be referred accordingly.

Treatment of optic nerve compression is controversial and again may be either medical or surgical. The options include: observation, IV corticosteroids, and optic nerve decompression. Medical treatment aims to reduce the oedema and inflammation that contributes to nerve damage. Time is of the essence; best results are obtained if steroids are given within 8h of the injury. The surgical option is carried out via either a craniotomy approach or lateral facial approach.

✴ Chemical injury

Chemicals that have a pH different to that of the eye (pH = 7.4) can cause a burn. Domestic and industrial accidents and assault are the commonest causes. **Alkalis cause more damage than acids, as they breakdown lipid membranes and penetrate deeper. Many household cleaning detergents contain sodium hydroxide**. Damage is caused by ischaemia and necrosis of the ocular surface with loss of epithelial stem and goblet cells. Loss of vision results from severe dry eyes and scarring. More severe cases result in cataract, glaucoma and uveitis as well.

Patients present with severe pain, blepharospasm, watering, and variable reduction in vision. Try to obtain the pH of the offending chemical and establish the baseline pH of both eyes. **All eyes must be given local anaesthetic drops, pH assessed, and irrigation with copious amounts of saline (litres) started immediately. This must continue until the pH is normal before anything else is done (it is not unusual to need more than 5 l)**. Note vision, epithelial defects, corneal clarity, cataract, and residual particulate matter. Immediate referral to ophthalmology is then made, once the pH has come back to normal. Further management with intensive antibiotics, steroids, potassium ascorbate, cycloplegia, and vitamin C usually requires admission.

The prognosis can be extremely poor. This depends on the pH of offending chemical and the extent of initial damage. **Hence the first-aid treatment received on site and in casualty is vitally important if the patient is to have a good prognosis**.

✴ Abrasion

This is an area where the corneal epithelium is deficient. The patient complains of pain, watering, and has a foreign-body sensation. They have difficulty keeping the eye open. Usually there is a history of trauma or contact lens wear. The eyelids may be in spasm and the conjunctiva is injected. With topical anaesthesia, the vision is normal. The area of abrasion stains with fluorescein.

Chloramphenical drop or ointment should be prescribed four times daily for 5 days. Although an eye-pad is not essential, it helps keep the eye closed and patients tend to feel more comfortable. It can be kept on for 1 day. The abrasion heals rapidly and the patient should be a lot more comfortable in 2 days. No contact lens should be worn for 2 weeks and after the patient has seen his/her own optician. If the patient is very distressed, cycloplegic drops given stat and oral analgesia will provide some relief until abrasion heals.

Refer only if a secondary corneal ulcer or a **recurrent erosion syndrome** develops. The latter develops if the epithelium does not adhere properly to the underlying Bowman's membrane. It therefore is likely to be scraped off by the upper eyelid first thing in the morning when the patient opens their eyes or in response to minor trauma and eye-rubbing. The problem may manifest itself months after the original trauma and at first presents with minor foreign-body sensation in the morning, which resolves completely in a few hours. Treat the acute abrasion as above. Long-term use of lubricating eye ointments, bandage contact lens, and occasionally surface treatment by needle puncture or laser may be required.

Ensure that there is no opacity of the cornea (which indicates a secondary infection of the underlying stroma) and there are no foreign bodies.

☼ Arc eye

This is a specific condition caused by ultraviolet injury from welding, tanning lamps, and high-altitude snow. Ultraviolet light injury causes oedema and sloughing of the corneal epithelium leading to punctate erosions or abrasions. Patients complain of pain, tearing, blepharospasm, photophobia, and blurred vision several hours after exposure. Treatment is as with an abrasion.

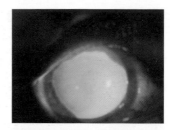

Plate 3: Large corneal abrasion stained with fluorescein (under cobalt blue light).

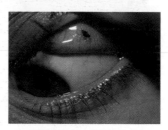

Plate 4: Subtarsal Foreign Body.

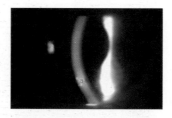

Plate 5: Corneal Foreign Body.

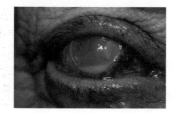

Plate 6: Corneal Ulcer with Hypopyon.

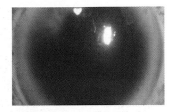

Plate 7: Hyphaema. Note some blood is in suspension and obscuring the view of iris and pupil.

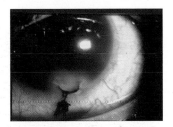

Plate 8: Penetrating eye injury. Note jagged corneal laceration with shreds of iris prolapsing.

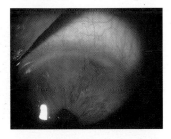

Plate 9: Irido-dialysis following blunt trauma.

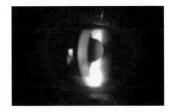

Plate 10: Hypopyon and keratic precipitates in Uveitis.

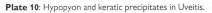

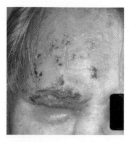

Plate 11: Herpes Zoster Ophthalmicus. (Courtesy of Mr. B Burton.)

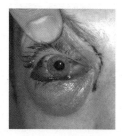

Plate 12: Orbital Cellulitis. Note swollen, proptosed eye with chemosis.

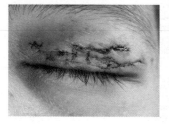

Plate 13: Three jagged lacerations to the upper lid. Always exclude penetrating injury.

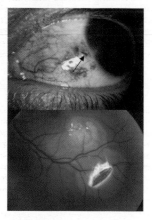

Plate 14: Intra-ocular Foreign Body. The small entry wound is easily missed (arrowed).

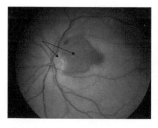

Plate 15: Central Retinal Artery Occlusion. Note the Cilio-retinal artery which has preserved part of the macula (arrowed). Retina is otherwise pale.

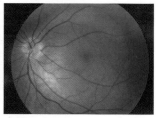

Plate 16: Swollen optic disc. Note the blurred margins and absence of disc cup.

ⓘ Foreign bodies

Surface foreign bodies (FB) are found on the cornea, conjunctiva, or under the lids. Slow velocity (grinding, welding, and wind borne) foreign bodies do not have the force to penetrate the eye and only embed themselves superficially in the epithelium. There is a FB sensation or grittiness in the eye, watering, and variable photophobia. A clear history of FB may not always be present or precede symptoms by hours. On examination the vision is normal, unless the FB is on the visual axis. The eye is injected and may be in spasm until anaesthetic drops are instilled. **Everting the lids is essential**. FBs can sometimes be seen more readily if fluorescein drops are instilled. Surface FBs should be directly visible and do not require radiological investigation. Instill local anaesthetic drops. A moistened cotton bud is effective for removing most conjunctival and subtarsal FBs. However, a green needle used with a slit-lamp is often needed for corneal FBs. Prescribe chloramphenical ointment four times a day for 5 days and padding for the first day. Referral is not required unless a rust ring remains on the cornea or an infected corneal ulcer has developed under the FB.

Intra-ocular FBs that have penetrated the eye as a result of high-velocity injuries, are discussed under penetrating injuries.

ⓘ Sore and itchy eyes

Sore and uncomfortable eyes are a common presentation to the doctor. In many cases, the eyes do not look red and the patient does not look in pain. However, the irritation can be considered severe enough to interfere with comfortable daily life. The aetiology of this clinical picture is varied and large overlap exists. But in general, the eye has **tear film insufficiency (dry eyes), blepharitis, or both**. As a rule, these problems are more prevalent with increasing age and co-exist. The problems can be exacerbated by tiredness, wind, air conditioning, central heating, and contact lenses. **Take care to exclude foreign bodies and in-turning lashes in any patient with a sore eye**.

⑦ Tear film insufficiency

The tear film consists of three layers: mucous, water, and oil. Lack of any portion or imbalance of their various proportions can make the tear film unstable. The mucous layer allows the watery portion to adhere to the epithelial surfaces, and the oil layer reduces evaporation and gives a degree of surface tension to the tears to stop its break up. The aqueous portion of the tear film is deficient in most patients but few have true Sjögren's syndrome. Deficient goblet cell activity and meibomian gland disease can disturb mucous and oil layer production.

Clinically, complaints of sore, dry eyes with intermittent blurring (tear break-up or mucous strands) are commonplace. Paradoxically, intermittent watering is reported in milder cases due to reflex hyper-lacrimation. The eye may be injected and papillary conjunctival reaction seen when lids everted. Fine punctate erosions on the corneal epithelium are seen with fluorescein staining under slit-lamp examination and larger abrasions can develop. In severe cases, the vision is reduced and fine strands of mucous are seen attached to damaged epithelium.

Management

Simple measures

Avoid sitting near air-conditioning, wear side-guards on glasses when outside to minimize evaporation, or reduce contact lens wear to a few hours.

Tear replacement

Many are commercially available in drop, gel, or ointment form. In general, ointments provide longer-lasting comfort but blur the vision, as they are more viscous and are reserved for night-time use or severe cases. Drops do not blur but drain away quicker. **Drops may need to be administered up to every half hour. In these instants, and if contact lenses are being worn, preservative-free drops should be used**.

Tear preservation

The lacrimal drainage system can be blocked using plugs or surgery to stop tear drainage in moderate to severe cases.

Tear modification

Mucous strands (excess production) can be reduced with acetylcysteine.

Tear stimulation

Oral pilocarpine can be used in severe cases to stimulate tear production. However, side-effects from other cholinergic stimulation can limit its use (sweating and gastro-intestinal symptoms).

It is important for the patients to realize that their condition can be controlled but not necessarily cured and that long-term use of drops and their compliance is very important for the eye to be comfortable.

⑦ Blepharitis

Blepharitis is a common condition characterized by chronic inflammation of the eyelid margins. It can be classified into seborrhaeic or staphylococcal disease, but the aetiologies often overlap. Its prevalence increases with age and often co-exists with tear film insufficiency. It is associated with eczema and rosacea in some patients.

Clinically, the patient complains of sore, red, and itchy eyelids and eyes. Crusting of the eyelids and recurrent conjunctivitis, hordeolums, and chalazions may be reported. The eyelids are thickened and red with crusting around eyelashes or oily clumps on the lid margin. The eyes may be injected and a papillary conjunctival reaction seen on everting the lids. Corneal ulcers can develop in some patients as a hypersensitivity reaction to bacterial by products.

Management

Aim of treatment is to reduce the bacterial load on the eyelids and to ensure meibomian secretions flow freely and not solidify or irritate the lid margin.

Lid hygiene is the cleaning of the lids with warm compresses to achieve:
* liquification of the oily meibomian secretions and clearing them off the lid margin to allow flow;
* reduce the bacterial load on the lid margin.

Using baby shampoo or bicarbonate of soda dissolved in the water can aid this process. Cleaning should be done twice daily followed by administration of antibiotic ointment (fucidic acid) to the lid margin if staphylococcal disease is predominant. After the eye has settled, maintenance cleaning once a day will control the situation.

Oral antibiotics—in severe cases, a regimen of doxycycline over 4 months can help. The mode of action is thought to be by alteration of meibomian secretion. This is best started by an ophthalmologist to assess its efficacy.

It is vital for the patients to realize that their condition can be controlled but not cured. Long-term compliance with lid hygiene and the use of artificial tear drops to treat any associated tear film insufficiency is very important for the eye to be comfortable. It is common for patients to be non-compliant with long-term lid hygiene.

? Contact lens related problems

Contact lenses are widely used to correct refractive errors and provide a good functional and cosmetic alternative to glasses. For this reason they are often worn more than their prescribed limit. Also, due to expense and inconvenience, they are not looked after, replaced, and cleaned properly by all patients. The combination of the above factors can lead to problems with sight-threatening complications.

Contact lenses can be hard, gas permeable, or soft. The latter can be flexed between fingers and generally speaking is more comfortable than the others. With better technology, many soft lenses are daily disposable and are therefore thrown away after each use. Hence they are less likely to get infected or build up lipo-protein deposits that reduce oxygen permeability, comfort, and clarity. On the other hand, extended-wear lenses (left *in situ* for weeks) and lenses designed for yearly disposal are more likely to cause problems.

Over-wear is by far the commonest cause of problems. This leads to hypoxia and damage to the epithelium of the cornea. Epithelial microcyst formation, abrasions, blood vessel growth, and increased risk of microbial keratitis are complications of over-wear.

Contact lens history taking

- What type of lens is worn?
- How old is the lens? How old is the lens case and solutions? Look at how dirty the case is!
- What cleaning regime is used? All-in-one solutions are not as good as hydrogen peroxide cleaning (2-step).
- Do they ever clean the lens in water, swim with lenses?
- How many hours and continuous days are lenses worn? Least break in wear = more problems.
- Pre-existing eye diseases: dry eyes, blepharitis, and corneal scarring increase infection risk.

Abrasions

Usually caused by over-wear and hypoxic damage to the epithelium, which then swells and easily sloughs off when the lens is removed or mishandled.

Contact lens intolerance

The patient complains of increased discomfort and redness leading to reduced wear time. The commonest reason is dry eyes. Contact lenses require a minimum level of tears to hydrate them (soft) or form a tear meniscus under them (hard and gas permeable). Artificial tear drops (preservative free) may alleviate the problem but if the eye is too dry, then lenses cannot be worn. Other reasons for intolerance are build-up of deposits on lens, lens solution allergy (usually to the preservative in them), and giant papillary conjunctivitis. In the latter, large papillae are seen under the upper lids. It represents an allergic response to lens deposits or mechanical irritation from rubbing against the lens.

Lost contact lens

Many patients fear that a lens has become 'lost' around the back of their eye. This is impossible, as the conjunctival sac is closed at the fornices and it is more likely that the lens has fallen out without the patient realizing or it has lodged somewhere under the eyelid. Everting the eyelids will reveal any lost lens or a clean glass rod can be carefully swept under the lid to find the lens.

Infections

Conjunctivitis and microbial keratitis need to be treated promptly by an ophthalmologist, as serious complications can arise. These are described in the relevant chapter and the patient must be told to not wear their lens or use the lens case and solutions again or in the fellow eye.

Management

General advice on contact lens care, cleaning, and avoiding over-wear must be emphasized to minimize all of the above problems. Dry eyes can be managed with artificial tears suitable for the type of lens being worn or the lens type can be change to suit the eye better. These and cases of intolerance can be dealt with by the patient's optician. **Patients must be told to stop lens wear when the eyes are inflamed**. Abrasions can be treated in the usual manner with chloramphenical QDS for 5 days, if there is no infection. No lens should be worn for at least 2 weeks after the eye has settled and after the patient has seen their optician for a check-up to assess suitability to continue wear. **All infections should be referred to an ophthalmologist**.

☼ Herpes zoster ophthalmicus (HZO)

HZO is shingles affecting the ophthalmic division of the trigeminal nerve. Re-activation of the herpes zoster virus in the nerve ganglion leads to shingles. The elderly are usually affected by shingles and any young person should be suspected as being immuno-compromised.

Patient presents with a **painful vesicular rash in the dermatome supplied by the nerve**. The rash is over the upper eyelid, forehead, scalp, and on the side of the nose. There may be a prodrome of fever, malaise, tingling, and pain up to a week before the rash. The vesicles soon ulcerate and crust over. Marked swelling of the lower eyelid and face is frequently encountered as oedema spreads in tissue planes. Eye examination may be difficult due to severe lid oedema. Reduced vision, conjunctivitis, corneal epithelial defects, and opacity, as well as raised intra-ocular pressure and uveitis, can occur. Rarely, scleritis and optic neuritis is present.

People who have not had chicken pox can catch the infection from a patient with shingles in the vesicular and ulcerating stages.

If the side of the nose is involved in shingles (Hutchinson's sign), there is a high risk of intra-ocular complications.

If shingles affects the young or more than one dermatome, the patient should be investigated for immune deficiency (e.g. HIV).

Management with acyclovir 800 mg five times daily for 1 week needs to be initiated as soon as possible. Immunodeficient patients need admission for intravenous treatment. Adequate analgesia must be prescribed. Ocular inflammation requires topical steroid drops and the intra-ocular pressure must be closely observed and treated. Skin scarring and chronic pain can result from shingles. Usually the prognosis for vision is good but intra-ocular involvement can lead to anaesthetic cornea, scarring, and iris atrophy.

:☼: Orbital cellulitis

This is severe infection posterior to the orbital septum. Commonest source of infection is from infected peri-orbital sinuses or spread of pre-septal cellulitis posteriorly. Tooth abscesses and organisms introduced by trauma are less common causes.

Patients are often unwell with a **high fever and a painful, swollen eye**. There is a quick onset of rapidly worsening symptoms often with a history of sinus disease, peri-orbital infection, or injury. There is marked **proptosis, chemosis, and lid oedema**, which is red, hot, and tender to touch. Visual acuity and colour vision are reduced, together with an RAPD, if there is optic nerve compromise. Eye movements are reduced and painful. Fundoscopy may show swollen optic nerve head and artery or vein occlusions.

The main differential diagnosis is pre-septal cellulites, which is less severe and represents an infection anterior to the septum. It generally follows on from an infected lid cyst. If the conjunctiva is injected, even without other signs of posterior involvement, you must assume orbital cellulites until proven otherwise. In children, a rhabdomyosarcoma can mimic orbital cellulitis.

Orbital cellulitis can lead to meningitis, brain abscess, cavernous sinus thrombosis, septic shock, and death. It is vital for it to be diagnosed and managed promptly.

Commonly associated pathogens are *Staphlococcus aureus, Streptococcus pneumoniae* and *pyogenes* and (in children) *Hamophilus influenzae*. Full blood count, biochemistry, and blood cultures should be performed. CT of orbit and brain is necessary. Patient should be admitted. High-dose broad-spectrum intravenous antibiotics that cover both anaerobic and aerobic organisms should be administered after blood cultures are taken. Metronidazole and ceftazidime are one such combination. Surgical drainage of orbital, sinus, tooth, and brain abscesses is planned, as required, after scanning. Prognosis is good if treated early. Optic neuropathy and vascular occlusions carry poor visual prognosis. Cavernous sinus thrombosis has poor prognosis for life.

ⓘ Conjunctivitis

Conjunctival inflammation has many causes including bacterial, viral, or chlamydial infections, and allergic disease. Bacterial and viral infections usually start in one eye and then spread to the second eye, which is generally less severely affected. There may be a preceding upper respiratory tract infection or contact with an affected individual. Gram-positive cocci and adenoviruses are the commonest pathogens. Chlamydial infections are usually unilateral and a sexually transmitted disease is likely even if asymptomatic, therefore sexual risk factors need to be assessed. Allergic conjunctivitis affects atopic individuals and a history of eczema, asthma, and hayfever is usually present. It tends to be seasonal and grass pollen is a major trigger. **Neonatal conjunctivitis** is a notifiable disease and is caused by organisms infecting the eye during vaginal delivery. Herpetic, gonococcal and chlamydial infections are common causative organisms and need to be treated in the baby and parents. Respiratory and systemic infection can be life threatening for the baby and paediatric opinion must be sought.

Presentations of conjunctivitis
- Bacterial—purulent discharge, red eyes, and grittiness.
- Viral—watery discharge, red eyes, and grittiness.
- Chlamydial—muco-purulent discharge, gritty red eye.
- Allergic—watery, red, and gritty eyes, which may be associated with allergic rhinitis.

In infective conjunctivitis the eye is red and uncomfortable, with variable lid swelling. Vision should be normal when anaesthetic drops are given and the discharge is washed away. Chemosis (conjunctival oedema) is common. Bacteria cause a papillary conjunctival reaction and viruses and chlamydia a follicular reaction. Pre-auricular lymph nodes may also be palpable in the latter two types. Unless chlamydia is strongly suspected, no eye swabs are required. Otherwise genito-urinary medical referral, as well as eye swabs, are needed. In allergic disease, large papillae can be seen under the eyelids or large follicles around the limbus (vernal allergic conjunctivitis in Afro-Caribbean children).

Reduced vision and corneal opacities require further ophthalmological assessment. Gonococcal conjunctivitis rapidly leads to corneal ulceration and perforation, and must be considered in all with an active sexually transmitted infection.

Management
Bacterial
Respond well to a broad spectrum antibiotic such as chloramphenical drops four times daily for 1 week.

Viral
No specific treatment is proven to be effective. Cold eye compresses and artificial teardrops give some symptomatic relief.

Chlamydial

Needs systemic treatment by GU specialists after swabs are taken. Doxycycline 100mg twice daily for 1 week or azithromycin 1g once are effective treatments. Tetracycline eye ointment may be required if severe.

All patients must be told not to share a towel and pillow with others, and to observe strict hand hygiene to avoid spreading their infection. The prognosis is generally very good. Viral infections can take up to 6 weeks to settle. Specialist assessment and treatment with steroids may be required if vision is affected due to corneal scarring.

Allergic

Many patients will be taking over-the-counter medication for their allergy already but may not necessarily be using them correctly. Systemic antihistamines, steroid-containing nasal sprays, and lubricating eye-drops can all relieve symptoms. Antihistamine eye drops (levocobastine, emedastine) are also useful. Mast cell stabilizers (sodium cromoglycate) need to be used regularly for 4 weeks to have a significant effect. If a patient is very badly affected despite trying the above options, referral for topical steroids as a stabilizing treatment should be considered. **Long-term steroids by any route can lead to cataract and glaucoma, therefore intra-ocular pressures should be monitored**.

⊙ Corneal ulcer

This is an infective or inflammatory disease of the cornea with loss of the epithelium and stromal involvement. Usually a degree of trauma has lead to a breach of the epithelium and allowed organisms to invade the corneal stroma. Bacteria, fungi, protozoa, and viruses can be the offending organisms. Also, hypersensitivity reactions to eyelid bacteria can cause a milder peripheral inflammatory ulcer (marginal keratitis).

Patients present with a painful, pussy, watery red eye with variable loss of vision. There is a short history of increasing symptoms, usually in a contact lens wearer, following trauma or foreign body. Poor contact lens hygiene, cleaning with tap water, and over-wear are risk factors for corneal ulcer. Vision is reduced and there is intense photophobia. Lid swelling and conjunctival injection and oedema are noted. An opaque lesion on the cornea, which stains with fluorescein is invariably present, and a fluid level of pus (hypopyon) may be seen in the anterior chamber. Management is with intensive topical anti-microbial treatment (up to half-hourly as an in-patient) guided by the clinical picture and microbiology. Atropine 1% will stop iris adhesions and relieve pain. Ciprofloxacin 750 mg twice daily has good ocular penetration and is used in severe bacterial keratitis. Systemic antiviral and antifungals can be used as appropriate.

Immediate referral to ophthalmology is required for corneal scraping (microscopy and culture) before treatment is commenced. Any opacity on the cornea, in a painful red eye, should be considered an ulcer until proven otherwise.

A **dendritic ulcer** is a specific condition caused by the herpes simplex virus. An active cold sore history may be present but is not required for diagnosis. The eye is watery and photophobic. A dendrite has a linear branching shape, which stains well with fluorescein. Refer to ophthalmology for treatment with acyclovir 3% ointment five times daily with out-patient follow-up. Herpetic disease can be recurrent and involve central cornea as a disciform keratitis.

Acanthamoeba keratitis is a protozoal infection of the cornea. It is a rare but severe complication of contact lens wear caused by washing and storing lenses in water or swimming and bathing with contact lenses in the eye. The infection is extremely difficult to diagnose and treat. Therefore the disease is usually tackled late and runs a long course with severe inflammation.

Corneal ulcers can be devastating to vision as a result of scarring, irregular astigmatism, and, rarely, endophthalmitis or perforation following corneal melting. Central ulcers caused by fungi and protozoa have the worst prognosis.

☼ Uveitis

This is inflammation of the uveal tract (the pigmented layer) of the eye. If only the iris is involved, it is called iritis or anterior uveitis. Involvement of the ciliary body and choroid are termed intermediate and posterior uveitis, respectively. Pan-uveitis involves the entire uveal tract. Although most cases are unilateral, both eyes can be affected. Uveitis can be associated with systemic inflammatory diseases, such as sarcoidosis, systemic lupus erythematosis, and various arthritides. Endophthalmitis is when an infection is responsible for the uveitis.

Patients usually have a dull ache over the eye and may have reduced vision and floaters. Photophobia can be severe. Ciliary (around the cornea) or generalized conjunctival injection is present. On slit-lamp examination, inflammatory cells can be seen in the anterior chamber, which can stick to the corneal endothelium (keratic precipitates) or form a hypopyon. The pupils may be irregular and immobile if the iris adheres to the lens (posterior synaechae). Vitritis and yellow retinal infiltrates may be present on fundoscopy in posterior uveitis.

Refer as soon as possible to ophthalmology. Investigation is not required initially if the patient is otherwise well. Steroids (topical, local injections, and systemically, depending on severity) and cycloplegics must be started under ophthalmology supervision. Generally the prognosis is very good but uveitis can be chronic and recurrent. Posterior uveitis in association with systemic disease carries a poorer prognosis.

☼ Scleritis and episcleritis

This is an inflammation of the scleral or episcleral coat of the eye. There may be an association with systemic and connective tissue diseases, such as rheumatoid arthritis and SLE. Onset is generally over a few days. Usually there is unilateral aching in the eye associated with a sectoral injection of the eye. Scleritis is much more severe and can cause reduced vision, chemosis, proptosis, and pain on eye movement. Episcleritis should not affect any eye functions.

Check for lid oedema, chemosis, nodules, reduced vision, proptosis, pupillary defects, and eye-movement restriction. Exudative retinal detachment, disc oedema, and vascular occlusions can occur with scleritis. There may be evidence of secondary uveitis and keratitis (corneal inflammation). A drop of phenylephrine 2.5% will constrict episcleral but not scleral vessels and can help to distinguish between the two. Ultrasound B-scan may be required to show scleral thickening in posterior scleritis.

Management

Episcleritis is generally self-limiting in up to 4 weeks and can be managed conservatively if mild. Episcleritis and mild scleritis respond well to non-steroidal anti-inflammatory drugs (e.g. brufen 400 mg three times daily for 4 weeks). Moderate to severe scleritis usually requires systemic and topical steroids under ophthalmology supervision. The prognosis is very good for episcleritis and depends on system associations for scleritis.

Refer as soon as possible for scleritis. Although this is not required for episcleritis, refer in severe or non-resolving cases and when diagnosis is in doubt. Local irritation from lashes and foreign bodies need to be excluded if there is sectoral injection of the eye with a gritty sensation.

:☀: Glaucoma

Glaucomas are a group of eye diseases with the common features of optic nerve head damage and visual field loss usually associated with an abnormally elevated intra-ocular pressure (IOP), although a significant number of patients can have normal eye pressures (12–21 mmHg). **A high IOP left untreated will ultimately lead to loss of vision**. Glaucoma is a common condition with an estimated prevalence in the over 40s of 1%, and is usually asymptomatic. The intra-ocular pressure is normally maintained by a controlled balance between formation of aqueous within the eye and its subsequent drainage via a complex trabecular network of tissues at the 'drainage angle'.

A pathological increase in IOP usually occurs as a result of obstruction to the outflow of the aqueous. Obstruction can occur if the periphery of the iris becomes displaced forwards so that it covers the drainage angle of the anterior chamber. This results in angle closure and affects patients whose angle is very narrow. This will result in **closed angle** glaucoma. In **open angle** glaucoma, however, pathological changes occur within the microstructure of the drainage system and so obstruct the outflow of aqueous. In these cases the angle is not closed but remains 'open'.

Acute angle closure glaucoma (AACG)

AACG occurs when rapid closure of the drainage angle leads to an acute rise in the intra-ocular pressure. Patients with narrow drainage angles are predisposed to closure of the angle when the pupil dilates. This bunches the peripheral iris over the angle and blocks it. The increasing size of the lens in the ageing eye pushes the iris forward, which further narrows the angle and hence the condition mainly affects the elderly. Also long-sighted patients are at risk, as they have smaller eyes and therefore narrower angles.

Patients present with a short history of increasing eye pain. This becomes very severe, with nausea, vomiting, reduced vision, and haloes seen around lights. The cornea becomes cloudy and the pupil unreactive and mid-dilated. The eye becomes hard to palpation. Both eyes have shallow anterior chambers. There may have been previous milder attacks, which resolved spontaneously and started at night when the pupil naturally dilates.

Refer immediately to ophthalmology, as the pressure in the eye must be reduced urgently. Intravenous acetazolamide 500 mg stat, topical apraclonidine 1% three times daily, timolol 0.25% twice daily are given to reduce the pressure, if there are no systemic contra-indications. Dexamethasone 0.1% four times daily is used to control inflammation. Pilocarpine 1% is given to the opposite eye to prevent acute closure until laser peripheral iridotomies can be performed to prevent an attack of angle closer. In resistant cases, administration of IV mannitol or oral glycerine can reduce the IOP by increasing the hypertonicity of the blood and hence osmotic forces draw fluid out of the eye. Caution must be observed in patients with heart failure. If the pressures are controlled quickly the prognosis is good.

Some patients are wrongly treated as an acute abdomen in casualty due to severe nausea and vomiting.

Open angle glaucoma

Open angle glaucoma is the commonest form of glaucoma and is an insidious, slowly progressive disease, which occurs bilaterally with no symptoms until considerable visual impairment has occurred. Early diagnosis is therefore imperative and may be achieved by regular eye examination of the over 50s and those with a known family history. Patients may notice nothing until much of their peripheral vision is lost, however the clinician or optician can detect three signs of glaucoma:

(1) cupping of the optic disc;
(2) raised intra-ocular pressure;
(3) visual field losses detected using automated perimetry.

Treatment can be both medical and surgical, the medical treatments aim to increase the outflow and/or suppress the secretion of aqueous. Surgical treatment aims to create an alternative outflow for the aqueous or partially destroy ciliary body to reduce inflow.

Secondary glaucoma

In secondary glaucoma the raised IOP is secondary to a recognized local cause such as iritis, injury, rubeosis (iris neovascularization due to diabetes or central retinal vein occlusion), and inappropriate use of steroid eyedrops. Treatment involves controlling the underlying factors and then medical or surgical treatment of glaucoma, as appropriate. Secondary glaucomas generally have a poorer prognosis.

Congenital glaucoma

Congenital glaucoma may present at birth or in the ensuing months and years. The condition is caused by the abnormal development of the drainage angle, which results in raised IOP, which in turn causes the immature eye to enlarge. This is referred to as buphthalmos, which literally means 'ox eye'. Other indicators of disease are a family history, cloudy cornea, large corneas (horizontal diameter > 12 mm) watery eyes, and photophobia. Treatment is almost invariably surgical. **Urgent ophthalmic referral is required**.

☼ Retinal artery occlusion

An occlusion of the central retinal artery or any of its branches can result from an embolus or thrombosis. Less common causes are temporal arteritis and collagen vascular diseases. There is sudden unilateral painless loss of vision, which may be severe and total (central retinal artery, CRAO) or partial with sectoral field defect (branch retinal artery, BRAO). The patient may have a history of ischaemic heart disease, diabetes, stroke, amaurosis fugax (sudden loss of vision which resolved within 24h), and smoking. The following features are noticed on examination:

- CRAO: visual acuity counting fingers to light perception, RAPD, narrow arteries, white oedematous retina with a cherry-red spot at the macula. If the patient has a **cilio-retinal artery** (separate artery from choroidal circulation to the macula in 20% of the population), central vision is spared in CRAO. The patient may have 6/6 vision with restricted fields.
- BRAO: variably reduced vision (depending on how much macula is affected), pupils usually normal, sectoral whitening of retina and arterial attenuation.

Refer immediately to ophthalmology. Get an ESR and CRP urgently to exclude temporal arteritis. A full cardiovascular work up can be done routinely including fasting glucose, cholesterol, triglyceride, ECG, and carotid dopplers.

Management aim is to try and dislodge the embolus by reducing the eye pressure within 24h of occlusion. The simplest method is ocular massage but intravenous acetazolamide 500mg stat or paracentesis (fluid drainage from the anterior chamber) are more effective, although the latter can cause severe complications. The above measures generally have a poor success rate. Usually the occlusion is not reversible and the visual loss is permanent.

Temporal arteritis must be excluded in all patients over 50 years.

:⚙: **Retinal vein occlusion**

An occlusion may involve the central retinal vein or any of its branches. The retinal vein and artery share a common sheath. The artery can therefore compress the vein as they cross leading to stasis and occlusion. The condition generally affects the elderly.

Patients present with unilateral, painless loss of vision developing over a few hours. There may be a history of hypertension, diabetes, glaucoma, hormone replacement treatment, or hyper-coagulability state. The vision is variably reduced and there may be an RAPD, visual field defect, and a raised intra-ocular pressure. On funduscopy, a swollen disc, congested and dilated veins, retinal haemorrhages, and cottonwool spots are seen in the area supplied by the occluded vein. Full blood count and hyper-coagulability state should be investigated, as indicated. A fluorescein angiogram may be performed under ophthalmology care.

No acute treatment is shown to reverse a vein occlusion. Control of vascular risk factors, hypertention, intra-ocular pressure, and hyper-coagulability states aim to protect the second eye. Patients require long-term ophthalmology follow-up to screen for treatable complications such as neo-vascularization, macular oedema, and glaucoma. The prognosis depends on the degree and extent of ischaemic damage and ensuing complications. Poor initial vision and an RAPD carry the worst prognosis. Up to 5% of patients can have the second eye affected.

A vein occlusion should be suspected in asymmetrical diabetic retinopathy.

① Third nerve palsy

Third nerve palsy results from the complete or partial palsy of the oculomotor nerve. The third nerve arises in the midbrain, passing through the subarachnoid space and over the edge of the tentorium cerebelli. It then passes near to the vessels in the circle of Willis before entering the cavernous sinus and finally the orbit. It innervates the levator muscle of the upper eyelid, superior, medial and inferior recti, and inferior oblique muscles, as well as the parasympathetic supply for pupillary constriction and accommodation.

Third nerve palsy can be broadly divided into having a surgical or a medical aetiology. Surgical causes include **increasing intra-cranial pressure, tumours, and aneurysms around the circle of Willis** leading to compression of the nerve. Medical causes include **diabetes and hypertension** leading to ischaemic damage of the nerve.

Patients may present with **double vision** if the **ptosis** (drooping eyelid) is not blocking the visual axis. Surgical causes may have a history of trauma or progressive involvement of the pupil and muscles of extra-ocular movement. In medical palsies, risk factors for vascular disease (hypertension, diabetes, obesity, smoking, increasing age, and other vascular disease) exist. Headache can be a feature of both causes and should not be considered diagnostic. There may be partial or total ptosis, which can stop the patient's appreciation of double vision if it occludes the visual axis. The eye is turned to a down and out position and cannot elevate or adduct. The pupil may be dilated and unreactive. **Medical third nerve palsies usually do not involve the pupil. If the pupil is involved, or becomes involved later, a surgical cause should be considered**. Examine the fundus for papilloedema. **Associated cranial nerve palsies and other neurological deficits should be excluded**.

Refer urgently for CT or MRI scanning if a surgical cause for the palsy is suspected. Trauma patients need regular neurological monitoring for development of a fixed dilated pupil. Neurosurgery to evacuate a haematoma or to clip an aneurysm may be indicated. All patients need to have expert orthoptic evaluation of their eye movements and full work-up to manage vascular risk factors. Diabetes and hypertension should be controlled. **Troublesome double vision can be relieved by patching of one eye or by using prisms to align the visual axis**. Recovery from a third nerve palsy is variable and can take months. Squint surgery if required usually has limited success.

ⓘ Fourth nerve palsy

Forth nerve palsy is palsy of the trochlear nerve. The forth nerve nucleus is in the caudal midbrain. The slender nerve leaves midbrain posteriorly and decussates to wrap around the brainstem on its long path to supply the contralateral superior oblique muscle. This muscle intorts and depresses the eyes as its main functions. A palsy generally makes reading and going down stairs difficult.

Trauma accounts for up to 40% of forth nerve palsies. **Decompensation of congenital palsies and ischaemia are other common causes**.

Patients present with vertical double vision and torsion, if the palsy is of adult origin. There may be a history of significant head trauma. In congenital cases, a long-standing **abnormal head posture** may be observed on reviewing the family albums. Vascular risk factors are present in ischaemic cases.

The affected eye is hypertropic (deviated up), especially if the head is tilted to the side of the palsy (Bielschowsky test). Patients may be adopting an abnormal head posture to compensate for the defect (chin down and head turned and tilted to the opposite side). **Associated cranial nerve palsies and other neurological deficits should be looked for. Bilateral palsies may be more difficult to detect and are commoner with trauma**.

Orthoptic and ophthalmologic assessment is necessary, rarely is imaging is required if atypical presentation. Prisms can be prescribed to help symptoms. Patients generally manage well with head posture, prisms, and occasionally surgery.

① Sixth nerve palsy

Sixth nerve palsy is the complete or partial palsy of the abducens nerve. The sixth nerve nucleus is in the pons and its course takes it around the facial nerve nucleus to leave the brainstem anteriorly. It travels up the base of skull and over the petrous bone towards the cavernous sinus and the orbit. It supplies the lateral rectus muscle and abducts the eye.

Isolated sixth nerve palsies are **usually ischaemic** in origin. **Basal skull fractures** can damage the nerve directly. Also **space-occupying lesions** can displace the brainstem down and stretch the nerve over the edge of petrous bone.

Patients present with horizontal double-vision, especially when looking to the side of the lesion. There may be a history of general vascular disease, trauma, or headaches, depending on cause. The affected eye will not abduct and is convergent (turning in) when looking straight. Vision should be normal and optic disc assessment is mandatory to exclude papilloedema. **Associated cranial nerve palsies and other neurological deficits should be looked for. Bilateral palsy is indicative of trauma or space occupying lesions**.

Imaging is required if intra-cranial pathology is suspected. Medical work-up should be done for ischaemic causes. Acutely, patching of the eye or prisms can give symptomatic relief from double vision. Any underlying pathology should be treated. There is variable recovery of function over few months. Ischaemic palsies have the best prognosis for full recovery.

Chapter 10

The ear

⑦ Applied anatomy

Structurally there are three parts:

- **External ear:** pinna, external auditory meatus (EAM), and tympanum. The skin on the outer part of the EAM contains hair follicles and wax-producing glands. These are absent on the inner part. The ear is a self-cleansing organ. Cotton buds should not be used—all they do is impact wax within the canal.
- **Middle ear:** this is an air-containing space allowing sound transfer to the cochlea. It contains the three ossicles, two muscles, and part of the facial nerve. Equalization of pressures occurs via the Eustachian tube. The mastoid air cells communicate with the middle ear and both are closely related to the brain, jugular bulb, and labyrinth. Infections, therefore, are potentially very serious.
- **Inner ear:** this comprises the cochlea, vestibule, and semicircular canals. The 'membranous' part is surrounded by fluid, which communicates with the CSF. The cochlea contains the organ of hearing. The vestibule and semicircular canals are involved in balance.

The ear is innervated by the V, IX, and X cranial nerves, and by the posterior roots of C2 and C3 (see Referred pain).
Useful points in the history include:
- **hearing loss**—onset and progression;
- **pain;**
- **discharge;**
- **tinnitus;**
- **imbalance;**
- **noise exposure;**
- **nasal obstruction/discharge;**
- **drugs (ototoxic);**
- **family history.**

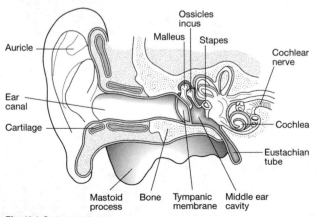

Fig. 10.1 Basic ear anatomy.

Remember that naso-pharyngeal pathology can result in secondary ear involvement—always look at the throat and nasopharynx.

Complications of ear infections include:

- mastoiditis;
- facial palsy;
- labyrinthitis;
- meningitis;
- brain abscesses;
- thrombosis of the dural venous sinuses.

① Otalgia ('earache')

This is a common symptom usually due to local disease. It may, however, be referred. **If the ear looks normal check distant sites.**

Local causes

- **Acute otitis externa**. Local infection may follow injuries or may be seen in patients with eczema of the ear or who swim a lot. Streptococci, staphylococci, pseudomonas, and fungi are the main organisms. Gentle tugging on the pinna is painful. A short course of antibiotic/steroid drops or dressing may be required.
- **Furuncles (infected hair follicles)**—drain and prescribe antibiotics.
- **Acute and 'malignant' otitis externa**—refer to ENT.
- **Perichondritis**—the pinna is swollen and tender due to infection of the cartilage.
- **Barotrauma.**
- **Herpes zoster.**
- **Tumours.**

Referred pain

Due to its varied innervation, pain can arise secondarily from diseases of the following:

- **tonsillitis and upper respiratory tract disease;**
- **Eustachian tube dysfunction;**
- **dental pathology;**
- **disorders of the TMJ;**
- **parotid disease;**
- **the oropharynx;**
- **the larynx and pharynx;**
- **cervical spondylosis;**
- **malignancy of any of the above, but particularly the tongue base.**

Never forget tumours of the upper aerodigestive tract as possible causes of earache in adults.

① Otorrhoea

Discharge from the ear may arise from several causes. The commonest is due to middle-ear infections. The nature of the discharge may give a clue to its cause:

- **watery**—CSF or eczema;
- **mucoid**—chronic suppurative otitis media;
- **purulent**—furunculosis or local abscess;
- **bloody**—trauma/acute otitis media/malignancy;
- **foul-smelling**—cholesteatoma.

ⓘ Mastoiditis

Mastoiditis is a potentially very serious complication of aggressive or untreated acute otitis media. Here, infection passes to the mastoid air cells causing further suppuration and bone necrosis. Remember that an infection that can track to the mastoids might also travel elsewhere—**always consider other possible complications** of acute otitis media with your diagnosis:

- intra-cranial (meningitis, brain abscess, extra and sub-dural abscess, lateral sinus thrombosis);
- extra-cranial (labyrinthitis, facial nerve paralysis, mastoiditis).

Presentation

Patients complain of a **persistent and throbbing pain with increasing deafness**. Discharge (otorrhoea) is present, which is usually creamy and may be profuse. Clinical signs include:

- systemic upset: unwell/pyrexia/tachycardia;
- tenderness over the mastoid prominence often with a post-auricular swelling that pushes the pinna forwards;
- otoscopy may show bulging of the roof or posterior wall of the external auditory canal; the tympanic membrane is usually red, perforated, and discharging.

Investigation

- **Full blood count:** will show a raised white cell count (neutrophils).
- **Mastoid X-rays:** will show opacity of the air cells.
- **CT scans** will give far more information but are rarely indicated.

Treatment

Patients often need **admission** for intravenous antibiotics, fluid resuscitation, and control of pyrexia and analgesia. If the causative organism is unknown, then broad-spectrum antibiotics are given, e.g. amoxycillin and metronidazole. In the absence of a rapid or complete response to antibiotics, or if a subperiosteal abscess is present, surgery may be indicated. A cortical mastoidectomy is performed. Here the mastoid air cells are opened to remove any necrotic debris, whilst leaving the middle ear intact.

℗ Otitis media

Inflammation of the middle ear (otitis media) is a common condition, usually occurring bilaterally, which may be either acute or chronic. Acute otitis media frequently occurs in children following an upper respiratory tract infection and may be viral or bacterial in origin. *Streptococcus pneumoniae* and *Haemophilus influenzae* are common bacterial pathogens.

Acute otitis media (AOM)

The pathological sequence of events in AOM begins with inflammation, oedema, and exudates of the mucous membrane of the middle ear. This obstructs the Eustachian tube preventing further drainage. Pressure builds up, and exudate and pus causes the eardrum to bulge. Unrelieved, necrosis of the tympanic membrane results in perforation. The middle ear can then drain and the infection may partially resolve.

Presentation

Patients are often systemically unwell. They complain of a throbbing earache (otalgia), which progresses in intensity until perforation of the drum relieves some of the pressure. Conductive deafness is present, possibly with tinnitus. The tympanic membrane ranges in appearance from the loss of the light reflex, to red and bulging, culminating in perforation with discharge (otorrhoea).

Deafness in children is a treatable cause of developmental delay—early detection and appropriate investigation and treatment is therefore imperative.

Management

- **Antibiotics**. Penicillins are often the first line of treatment, but culture and sensitivities should be carried out. If the signs and symptoms do not resolve, consider altering the choice of antibiotic and further assessment for infection elsewhere (mastoid, nasopharynx, sinuses).
- **Analgesics/antipyretics**.
- **Decongestants.**
- If a patient persists with a bulging tympanic membrane despite adequate antibiotic therapy, **myringotomy** under general anaesthetic allows the ear to drain.

Otitis media with effusion (OME) 'glue ear'

This condition is said to affect 30–40 % of children at some stage in their development and presents with deafness and a mild otalgia, occasionally associated with tinnitus. OME is due to a build-up of fluid in the middle ear. Although many cases will resolve spontaneously, antibiotics may be necessary if there is the suspicion of underlying infection.

If pain or hearing loss persists for over 10 weeks, surgery should be considered:

- **Myringotomy and grommet insertion**. Under GA, a small incision is made in the tympanic membrane and a plastic grommet (drainage tube) is then inserted. The grommet will self-extrude after an average period of 6 months—repeated insertions may be necessary if the effusion persists.
- **Adenoidectomy**. May be beneficial in the long-term.

⑦ Deafness

Many forms and causes of deafness exist, but a simple classification may be:

- **sensori-neural:** nerve impulses are prevented from being transmitted to the brain by a defect of either the auditory nerve (CN VIII) itself or the functioning of the cochlea;
- **conductive** sound is prevented from reaching the cochlea apparatus by some form of mechanical obstruction in the outer or middle ear;
- **mixed deafness:** a combination of sensori-neural and conductive deafness in the same ear.

Assessment

- A simple **clinical** assessment of a patient's degree of deafness may be made by an examiner repeating certain words at different intensities and at different distances to each ear in turn. By convention this is recorded as, for example, WV @ 200 cm (whispered voice at 200 cm).
- **Tuning-fork tests:**
  - **Rinne's test**—a 512 Hz tuning-fork is struck and held close to the ear; it is then placed firmly on the ipsilateral mastoid process and the patient is asked to say whether the tuning fork is heard better by bone conduction (BC, i.e. when on the mastoid) or air conduction (AC):
    - AC > BC Rinne +ve (middle/outer ear functioning normally);
    - BC >AC Rinne –ve (defective middle/outer ear).
  - **Weber's test**—a struck tuning fork is held on the vertex of the patient's head and they are then asked to say whether the sound is heard centrally or more to one ear than the other:
    - conductive deafness—sound heard in deafer ear;
    - sensori-neural deafness—sound heard in better hearing ear.
- **Audiometry** specialist tests carried out in soundproofed rooms using precision equipment. Test may be Subjective (pure tone audiograms, speech audiometry), which require patient response, or Objective (impedance audiometry, evoked response audiometry).

Causes

Deafness in children is a treatable cause of developmental delay—early detection and appropriate investigation and treatment is therefore imperative.

Otitis media

Otitis media with effusion ('glue ear') is the commonest cause of deafness in children with reported figures of 60% of cases going undetected in the first year. Commonly presenting with hearing loss and otalgia, there is a higher incidence in children with Down's syndrome or cleft palate. Treatment in the short term involves antibiotics and decongestants, progressing to surgery if symptoms persist (myringotomy and grommets).

The main causes of deafness in the adult population are **wax impaction** and ageing (over 60s)—**presbyacusis**. Presbyacusis is a progressive loss of hair cells in the cochlea with age.

Otosclerosis

This is the formation of new bone occurring within the inner ear resulting in relative immobility of the auditory ossicles (fixation of the footplate of the stapes), and hence a conductive deafness.

Polypharmacy

Generally drugs that are renal toxic are commonly ototoxic, e.g. cytotoxics, systemic aminoglycosides.

Otitis media with effusion is rare in adults and so further investigation must be undertaken to exclude a neoplastic growth. Progressive unilateral sensori-neural deafness must raise the suspicion of an **acoustic neuroma** (a rare but treatable tumour of the vestibular element of the VIIIth cranial nerve) and appropriate investigation should be undertaken to exclude this diagnosis.

Table 10.1 There are many causes of deafness

	Sensorineural	Conductive
Congential	**Hereditary** **Infection** CMV/Toxoplasmosis/Rubella/Syphilis	**Atresia** Middle ear Agenesis
Acquired	**Degenerative:** Age/Noise induced (industrial) **Infective** Herps/Mumps/Meningitis **Trauma** Head injury **Neoplastic** Metastases/Acoustic neuroma **Ototoxic** Drug induced **Metabolic** Diabetes/Hypothyroidism **Other** Meniere's/Multiple Sclerosis	**External ear** **Wax/Foreign body** Otitis Externa Trauma **Middle ear** Otitis Media (acute/chronic) Barotrauma Tympanic membrane injuries Middle ear tumours Otosclerosis

① Dizzyness/'vertigo'

Disorders of the middle and inner ear can result in loss of balance.
Otological causes include:
- **Impacted wax.**
- **Acute otitis media.**
- **Otitis media with effusion.**
- **Chronic suppurative otitis media.**
- **Trauma** (temporal bone fracture)—check for facial palsy.
- **Labyrinthitis**—this is a localized and often self-limiting viral infection
  resulting in rapid and profound dizzyness. If prolonged consider
  herpes zoster infection. Usually hearing is unaffected.
- **Ménière's disease (endolymphatic hydrops)**—this typically affects
  young to middle-aged adults and occurs as clusters of severe
  imbalance. Symptoms include vertigo, fluctuating hearing loss, tinnitus,
  and a 'fullness' in the ear. Management includes betahistine and
  diuretics, avoidance of caffeine, salt, and cessation of smoking.
  Surgery may be required in chronic cases.
- **Otosclerosis.**
- **Otosclerotic drugs.**
- **Syphilis.**

⑦ Tinnitus

Noises in the ear can affect up to one in five of the population, especially
after noise exposure. Noises can also arise from the TMJ, Eustachian tube,
and carotid artery. **When unilateral and accompanied by hearing
loss, further investigations are required**. Causes include:
- **wax;**
- **insects;**
- **otosclerosis;**
- **glue ear;**
- **noise-induced;**
- **presbyacusis;**
- **Ménière's disease;**
- **trauma;**
- **ototoxic drugs;**
- **labyrinthitis;**
- **acoustic neuroma;**
- **AV malformations;**
- **TMJ disorders;**
- **glomus jugulare;**
- **carotid body tumours.**

Chapter 11

The mouth, lips, and teeth

ⓘ Bleeding from the mouth

Oozing following injuries and surgery to the mouth is common and **usually seems much worse than it actually is**. A lot of the 'blood' is blood mixed with saliva, which the patient may not be able to swallow.

Most cases need only simple reassurance and getting the patient to bite firmly on a clean handkerchief or gauze swab over the wound for at least 20 min. In the vast majority of cases bleeding settles and no further action is required other than care of the airway, if necessary using gentle suction. If bleeding persists, rinse the mouth out to clear any clots and look for the bleeding site. This can be dealt with by further suturing or packing the wound with 'surgicel'. Other measures include antifibrinolytic agents, such as tranexamic acid. Patients rarely need to go back to theatre.

If all else fails, patients need to be admitted for bed rest and investigated for bleeding disorders or liver disease.

Occasionally persistent bleeding following minor injuries is the presenting sign of an underlying clotting disorder such as haemophilia. The bleeding is managed initially as above and blood is taken for clotting studies. Clotting disorders should be managed following consultation with a haematologist. Known haemophiliacs often require admission for minor surgery and may be given factor replacement, tranexamic acid, and DDAVP at the time of surgery.

Bleeding sockets following dental extractions are rarely life-threatening. However, in the presence of significant co-morbid disease (for example, in the elderly with poor CV reserve), a bleeding socket may compromise the patient's well-being. Decide whether it is sufficient to simply deal with the local problem, or whether it is necessary to investigate further for systemic cause and effects of bleeding.

Classification

- **Primary** haemorrhage—a direct consequence of the surgical procedure.
- **Reactionary/delayed** haemorrhage—usually occurring after several hours, where the vasoconstrictor in the LA is wearing off.
- **Iatrogenic**—interference with fingers/clot disruption (rinsing too early).
- **Secondary** haemorrhage—after 48 h post-surgery, due to disturbed wound healing following infection.

Co-morbid factors

- Local infection.
- Bleeding diatheses.
- Drugs, e.g. warfarin, aspirin.
- Co-morbidity, e.g. liver disease.

Co-morbid factors need to be managed as soon as they are recognized. This may simply involve the use of antibiotics for local infection. When surgery is required, any possible risk of bleeding should be specifically questioned for **prior** to surgery, e.g. previous history of bleeding problems or the use of drugs such as warfarin.

Management

Good technique should prevent primary haemorrhage. However, persistent bleeding may be troublesome and require further action. **Pressure** is usually sufficient to arrest capillary ooze. A sterile warm swab must be applied directly over the surgical site. This will encourage clot formation. **Exploration under local anaesthetic** involves removal of sutures, clots, and debris to identify the bleeding site. **Arterial bleeds arising from the gums** are dealt with by cautery or ligation of larger vessels. **Bone bleeds** may need the application of sterile bone wax to arrest haemorrhage.

Once the socket has been irrigated and cleaned, the site may be packed with a resorbable haemostatic dressing (e.g. surgicel) to promote clot formation. The socket should then be over sewn to keep the dressing *in situ* and to provide local pressure.

In the absence of co-morbid disease, it is exceptionally rare that patients need to be admitted for resuscitation and observation. However, it is probably prudent to check the haematological status of patients (FBC, clotting screen, LFTs), if they present with more than simple oozing.

⑦ Bleeding gums (non-traumatic)

Bleeding from the gums is a common symptom and is almost always due to local inflammation caused by inadequate tooth-brushing—'gingivitis'. However, gingival bleeding **may be a marker of an underlying systemic disease** and recognition of this is important for early diagnosis and management. Certain medical conditions and drugs are known to affect the gingivae. Where oral hygiene is very good consider these.

Causes

Consider the following:

- infection—gingivitis, peri-odontitis, dental;
- drug-related;
- anticoagulants (warfarin, heparin);
- trauma;
- chemical irritants (asprin);
- self-inflicted (toothbrush abrasion, incorrect flossing technique);
- ill-fitting new dentures;
- vitamin deficiencies—notably C and K;
- pregnancy—hormonal changes;
- liver disease;
- idiopathic thrombocytopenic purpura (ITP);
- leukaemia.

Often the cause of bleeding gums is obvious and easily treated. Treatment of infection involves removing the cause—either plaque in the case of gingivitis, or appropriate treatment of dental infection (root canal therapy, extraction). The patient's dentist can advise on oral hygiene and arrange for the patient to see a hygienist. In vitamin deficiencies (serologically proven) supplements can be prescribed along with dietary advice.

Pregnancy

The hormonal changes that are associated with pregnancy will reverse after delivery, but during the pregnancy excellent oral hygiene must be maintained. Local gingival bleeding may also be associated with a pregnancy epulis. This may need to be surgically removed if troublesome, although they usually regress after delivery.

Drugs

Drug-related gingival bleeding must be managed in close association with the physician who prescribed the medication. Simply stopping any drug thought to be the cause of bleeding may have effects that are potentially far worse to the patient. The degree of urgency to alter a prescription is directly related to the severity of gingival bleeding and also to the presence of bleeding from other sites, e.g. nasal mucosa and GI tract. In the case of some drugs, immediate reversal is possible, e.g. warfarin, whereas for others supportive measures are all that is possible.

Idiopathic thrombocytopenic purpura (ITP)

ITP, thought to be an autoimmune disorder, is probably the most common cause of thrombocytopenia. Close liaison with a haematologist is essential for safe management. Regional local anaesthetic blocks may be contra-indicated if the platelet count is below $30 \times 10^9/l$, The vast majority of cases will be adequately managed by the administration of cortico-steroids. For major surgical cases, platelet transfusions and/or the use of immunoglobulins may be necessary.

Leukaemia

Leukaemias are potentially life-threatening conditions representing malignant proliferation of white blood cells. In acute leukaemias (generally seen in younger patients), primitive blast cells are released, whereas in chronic leukaemias (generally effecting older patients) the leukaemic cells retain most of their normal morphology. It is not uncommon for leukaemias, especially the acute types, to present with oral signs and symptoms:

- bleeding gums—a hyperplastic gingivitis (red, spongy, fragile gums), which bleed spontaneously;
- infection—the gingivae are highly susceptible to infection; secondary acute ulcerative gingivitis may be seen;
- localized masses of leukaemic infiltrates;
- candida/HSV.

⑦ Dry socket

This is localized inflammation of the cortical bone surrounding a socket following extraction, most commonly the lower wisdom teeth. Typically, the patient complains of severe dull throbbing pain, around 4–5 days later and often has a bad taste in the mouth. Pain is often exquisite, with inflammation, exposed bone, and halitosis. Predisposing factors include:

- mandibular extraction;
- difficult extraction;
- pre-existing infection;
- poor blood supply (e.g. Paget's disease, following radiotherapy);
- smoking—nicotene is a vasoconstrictor;
- systemic disorders, e.g. diabetes;
- oral contraceptive.

The socket is irrigated with warm saline. It is then dressed with an antiseptic pack, e.g. Aavogyl. This contains iodoform (antiseptic), eugonal (sedative), and seaweed (for bulk)—this is resorbed as healing occurs. Antibiotics may be necessary.

:⊙: The acutely swollen mouth

:⊙: Sublingual swelling

See also Ludwig's angina.

Swelling here is potentially very serious because of the threat to the airway. The tissues are delicate and can easily distend, pushing the tongue up and back. Usually infections are also associated with swelling in one or both submandibular spaces, in the neck. They are almost always due to dental infections. When significant swelling is present, urgent decompression is required, even if there is no obvious pus—the decompression also allows oedema to leak out and reduce tension.

① Palatal swelling

Infections arise most commonly from the lateral incisors and palatal roots of multi-rooted teeth. The differential diagnosis includes mucous extravasation cysts, pleomorphic adenomas, muco-epidermoid carcinomas, lymphomas, angina bullosa haemorrhagica, and carcinomas arising in the maxillary sinus.

:⊙: Peritonsillar abscess

See also: The acutely swollen neck.

⑦ Fascial tissue spaces

Sublingual space

The roof of the sublingual space is the tongue and floor of the mouth. Its floor is formed by the mylohyoid muscle. It contains the sublingual glands and the deep lobes of the submandibular glands. It communicates posteriorly with the submandibular spaces.

Palatal space

This is a potential space between the mucoperiosteum and hard palate. Pus tracks into this space most commonly from lateral incisors, as the apices of the roots are often closer to the palate than to the buccal plate of the maxilla. Infection from palatal roots of multi rooted teeth can also pass into the palate.

Parapharangeal space

This potential space extends from the base of the skull to the root of the neck and therefore communicates with the mediastinum. Its anterior boundry is the pharangeal wall, and its posterior boundary the carotid sheath and prevertebral fascia. Laterally and superiorly it is bounded by the deep aspect of the medial pterygoid and is known as the deep pterygoid space, which communicates with the floor of the mouth. **Dental infections here can potentially track down the neck and result in mediastinitis**.

Paratonsillar space

This is between the pillars of the fauces medially and the superior pharyngeal constrictor laterally. It contains the palatine tonsil. It communicates with the deep pterygoid space and hence the parapharangeal space.

⑦ Oral hygiene

Over 300 different species of organisms have been identified in the human mouth. These include:
- *Streptococcus*
- *Lactobacillus*
- *Fusobacterium*
- *Borrelia vincenti*
- *Actinobacillus*
- *Porphyromonas*
- *Actinomyces*
- *Candida*
- *Spirochaetes*

.... to name a few!

Colonization begins soon birth and persists for the remainder of life. Even after meticulous cleaning by a hygienist, bacteria are found on the gums within a few hours (up to 1 million per mm^3 after just 1 h). Dental plaque is a firmly adherent layer of mucopolysaccharides, proteins, and bacteria, which rapidly forms on teeth and is difficult to completely remove. It is this plaque that is responsible for tooth decay, gum disease, tartar, and wound infections. Some organisms are responsible for specific diseases, e.g. candida (oral thrush), fusobacteria (acute necrotizing gingivostomatitis), and actinomyces (actinomycosis).

Yet despite all these potential pathogens constantly present in the mouth, wound infection is remarkably rare or, if it occurs, usually mild. This is believed to be due in part to the antibacterial action of saliva and the presence of 'growth factors' that aid healing. This does not mean that we can be complacent about sterile technique or aftercare; those infections that become established can be extremely difficult to treat, especially if bone is involved.

The mouth is under constant threat of infection from the environment and therefore must be capable of fighting infection. Most people can care for their own mouths, but there are a number of patients who need assistance with oral care. In a healthy person, removing food debris is a normal oral function, but this is diminished in patients with ulcers and infections in the mouth. In health, saliva is produced in large amounts daily and acts as a mouthwash, maintaining a clean environment. It is also antibacterial and controls the pH of the mouth.

Following injuries or surgery, oral hygiene is more difficult due to pain, swelling, and so on. The patient should be encouraged in maintaining a clean mouth with the use of mouthwashes (corsodyl, hot salt water). These should be used regularly especially after meals. Gentle cleaning with a brush should be encouraged, as most patients are afraid that the wounds will fall apart if they use one. *Frequent* cleaning is the key to success, rather than occasional scrubbing. In most cases, a small-headed multi-tufted child-size toothbrush with a fluoride toothpaste is appropriate.

① Mucosal infections

① Viral

Vesiculo-ulcerative infections

Vesiculo-ulcerative lesions secondary to infections are mostly viral. There are many infective causes of oral ulceration; however, **not all mouth ulcers are due to infections**.

Herpes

The herpes viruses are a large family of viruses. Seven types affect humans and six of the seven affect the head and neck. These include:

- herpes simplex virus type I causes oral, peri-oral, and occasionally genital infections;
- varicella zoster virus causes chickenpox and herpes zoster;
- Epstein–Barr virus has been linked to infectious mononucleosis, Burkitt's lymphoma, naso-pharangeal carcinoma, and oral 'hairy' leukoplakia;
- cytomegalovirus is associated with salivary gland disease and systemic infections of immunocompromised patients.

Herpes simplex virus (HSV) infections

This is a common cause of vesicular eruptions on mucosa and skin. In healthy individuals it is usually self-limiting. Two forms occur: the primary (systemic) herpes and secondary (localized) herpes. Spread is by Physical contact.

Primary HSV

Most cases occur in children who present with mild primary herpetic gingivostomatitis. There is a vesicular eruption of perioral skin or oral mucosa, accompanied by fever, malaise, and lymphadenopathy. The lesions heal without scarring.

Secondary or recurrent HSV (cold sores)

Prodromal symptoms of pain, burning, and tingling precede eruption of multiple small vesicles. These may develop after a period of 'stress', such as a recent illness. Generally they heal without scarring, but can get secondarily infected. The lesions are contagious.

Immunodeficient patients may present with repeated attacks of secondary herpes and a predisposition to bacterial and fungal infections. The infection can become systemic, and fatal.

Herpetic whitlow

This refers to secondary HSV infection of the fingers and was seen classically on clinicians hands, especially dentists, prior to the advent of rubber gloves.

Treatment of HSV

This is usually unnecessary other than analgesia, fluids, and rest. Prompt topical application of 5% acyclovir ointment reduces the duration of infection. Immunosuppressed patients may need systemic treatment.

Varicella zoster (VZ) infections

Varicella (chickenpox)

This is primary infection with the VZ virus. Usually its occurs in childhood. A rash involving the head, neck, and most of the body erupts, and there is fever and general malaise. The rash develops into a general vesicular eruption, which turns into pustules and ulcerates. It is usually self-limiting. Rarely (and mostly among the very young or the immunosupressed), varicella can be severe, progressing to encephalitis, pneumonitis, and death. **Infection during pregnancy leads to fetal abnormalities**.

Herpes zoster (shingles)

This is an acute herpetic infection in any dermatome, commonly the Vth cranial nerve. It is the secondary manifestation of VZ. This usually affects older age groups. It specifically affects a sensory dermatome. Thus on the face it can erupt in the distribution of any of the branches of the trigeminal nerve, or cervical plexus. It is very painful and debilitating with severe complications if it affects the ophthalmic branch. **It has a very high incidence in the immunosupressed**.

Clinical features

- Burning, tingling pain in the skin. Pain may precede or follow eruptions and last from one to several weeks.
- Spontaneous permanent remission is common, although patient may progress to chronic (post-herpetic) neuralgia.
- **Post-herpetic neuralgia** is chronic pain and skin changes following acute herpes zoster. There may be burning, tearing sensations or itching and crawling dysaesthesias in skin.

In the acute phase, stellate ganglion blocks using local anaesthetic such as bupivacaine, may help for severe pain. Transcutaneous Nerve Stimulation (TENS), capsaicin cream, and tricyclic anti-depressants are also useful.

Ramsay Hunt syndrome

This is VZ involvement of the facial and auditory nerves. Facial paralysis is accompanied by vesicles in the ipsilateral external ear, tinnitus, deafness and vertigo.

Treatment is supportive. If immunocompromised, **acyclovir or vidarabine** can be given systemically.

Hand, foot, and mouth

This is caused by coxsackie virus. It affects children with mild systemic effects. The primary complaint is a sore mouth as a result of vesicles that rupture to become ulcers. These occur anywhere in the mouth. Multiple maculopapular lesions on the feet and hands help confirm the diagnosis. Treatment is supportive.

Herpangina

Caused by a coxsackie virus. Also affects children. Occurs endemically. They present with malaise, fever, sore throat, and dysphagia. A vesicular eruption is seen on the soft palate, pillars of fauces and tonsils. Treatment is supportive.

See also: Infections presenting as verrucal lesions.

⑦ Bacterial

Syphilis

This is caused by the spirochete *Treponema pallidum*. Until the use of penicillin this was an infection that was rampant for centuries. In the West it is not commonly seen any more. **Transmission is by sexual contact, by tranfusion, and transplacentally**. Its clinical stages are primary, secondary, and tertiary.

The infectious lesion of the primary stage is known as a **primary chancre** and forms at the site of innoculation. This is usually a painless ulcer with rolled margins. With oral sex the chancre can form in the mouth and lips, but otherwise is most commonly found on the genitals. There is often painless lymphadenopathy. The chancre heals spontaneously after several weeks.

Secondary syphilis follows with general malaise and mucocutaneous lesions, which are **highly infectious**. They present as elevated verrucal plaques known as condylomata lata. These inflammatory lesions can affect any organ system.

After a latent period, one-third of patients will go on to develop **tertiary syphilis**, with lesions affecting many organ systems. These lesions are known as gummas. They have a predilection for neural and cardiovascular tissue. Intra-orally they present on the palate. Generalized glossitis with mucosal atrophy in tertiary syphilis may have a predisposition for squamous cell carcinoma.

Diagnosis involves serological tests (VDRL), immunologic staining of biopsied tissue, and darkfield microscopy of scrapings. **Treatment** is with penicillin.

The differential diagnosis of a chancre must include squamous cell carcinoma, traumatic ulcers, tuberculosis, and histoplasmosis.

Gonorrhea

This is caused by *Neisseria gonorrheae*, a diplococcus. It is spread by direct sexual contact. In the mouth, they may be seen as non-specific ulcers following oral sex. **Treatment** is with penicillin.

Tuberculosis

This is caused by *Mycobacterium tuberculosis*. A resurgence has taken place in the developed world because of drug resistance, migration, and immunosupression. Spread is by droplet or direct inoculation. Clinically it can appear in any mucosal surface. The typical lesion is a non-healing, chronic, and painful ulcer.

Treatment includes isoniazid, rifampicin, streptomycin, and ethambutol. Refer to public health authority for contact screening. Prevention by good socio-economic standards is the long-term solution.

Actinomycosis

Caused by *Actinomyces israeli*, an anaerobic Gram-positive bacterium. It is a commensal in the mouth. Previous infections, surgery, and trauma predispose to an infection by actinomyces. **Treatment** is by long term, high dose penicillin, and debridement.

Acute necrotizing ulcerative gingivostomatitis (ANUG)

This is also known as 'trench mouth' because of the pungent anaerobic smell. It is caused by anaerobic bacterial invasion of the oral tissues. There is usually some **predisposing condition, such as malnutrition or immunosupression**. ANUG affects specifically the interdental gingival papillae, destroying them. If untreated, it will continue to necrose adjacent tissues. Cancrum oris (noma) is like ANUG, but is more aggressive, attacking other mucosal surfaces. It can result in substantial tissue loss of the face. **Treatment** is debridement of the necrotic tissue, penicillin, or metronidazole.

① Fungal infections

These may present with ulcers. With the exception of candida, these are relatively rare infections and their presence should prompt **enquiry into oversees travel and immunodeficiency**.

Deep fungal diseases are characterized by primary pulmonary involvement. However, oral manifestations include histoplasmosis, coccidioidomycosis, and cryptococcosis. These present as ulcers. Oral infection follows direct implantation. **Treatment** is by systemic antifungals.

See also Infections presenting as white and red lesions.

⑦ Candida

Candida are fungal organisms normally seen as part of the commensal flora in up to 90% of the population. However, infection may be a marker of immunosuppression. Consider:

- immune suppression—drugs/infection (HIV);
- trauma;
- neoplasia;
- malnutrition;
- diabetes.

If the host's resistance to candida is low, a more diffuse lesion or widespread systemic infection may be seen.

Various clinical presentations exist.

Pseudomembranous candidiasis ('thrush')

Presents clinically as white plaques, which can be wiped away often leaving an inflamed mucosa behind. The 'pseudomembrane' is a meshwork of candidal hyphae penetrating superficially into the mucosa, with aggregates of fibrin and cellular debris. **Treatment:**

- identification of any predisposing cause;
- antifungal agents (nystatin, amphotericin, imidazoles, e.g. miconazole).

Acute erythematous candidiasis

This resembles thrush but without the overlying pseudomembrane. Clinically, the mucosa is red and often painful. Classically it is seen in patients with immune suppression (e.g. HIV infection) or patients on long-term antibiotic or steroid therapy. **Treatment:** topical antifungals.

Chronic erythematous candidiasis (denture-induced)

This is a secondary infection of traumatised mucosa following prolonged denture wearing. There is a red, angry mucosa, localized to the fitting

surface of the prosthesis, commonly affecting the upper arch only.
Treatment is directed at the causative factors:

- infection—antifungals as lozenges or cream applied to the denture
  fitting surface;
- trauma—removal of the cause and provision of appropriately
  constructed dentures with tissue conditioners, as necessary.

Chronic hyperplastic candidiasis (candidal leukoplakia)

Mucosal hyperplasia, with histological features of atypia, can be associated
with local candidal infection. Debate continues as to whether this
represents a progression of a tenacious candidal infection or a secondary
infection of a mucosal lesion. Some feel these lesions may have premalign-
ant potential and so excision.

⑦ White patches in the mouth

White patches of the oral mucosa covers a myriad of conditions. Some lesions may be instantly recognizable, e.g. the reticular 'lace-like' white striations of lichen planus. Often an obvious cause may be apparent, e.g. frictional keratosis from a poorly finished dental restoration. For less obvious lesions consider:

- a family history of similar conditions;
- associated dermatological conditions;
- associated ocular conditions;
- infections;
- possible causative agents, e.g. tobacco smoking.

White patches of the oral mucosa may be considered in four broad groups:

- **leukoplakias (functional/ idiopathic);**
- **familial;**
- **inflammatory;**
- **dermatological conditions.**

Leukoplakias (functional/idiopathic)

The term 'leukoplakia' literally means 'white plaque'. It is often used to describe any white patch associated with a physical/chemical irritation (e.g. tobacco smoke). It is also used to describe lesions of undetermined origins. Leukoplakias as a whole have a **reported 10–15% incidence of malignant change**. Of all conditions *speckled* leukoplakia is considered the most sinister.

Histopathological diagnosis should be sought for any non-healing/ suspicious lesion. The more common findings are as follows.

Neoplastic change associated with leukoplakia

Oral cancer may manifest itself as a new white patch or may occur within a long-standing lesion (dysplasia → carcinoma *in situ* → invasive squamous cell carcinoma). The process may show a variable time-scale. Certain features should be considered as sinister:

- firm/fixed;
- induration;
- ulceration (non-healing);
- painless;
- friable/bleeding.

Cancers are often plaque-like in appearance with white raised/everted/rolled edges surrounding an area of central ulceration. Common sites are the 'sump' areas of the mouth: the vestibule, floor of mouth, and the lateral posterior tongue.

Trauma-induced leukoplakias (frictional keratoses)

These lesions are akin to calluses one may see on feet due to ill-fitting shoes. Likewise in the mouth the causative agents are often poorly fitting dentures or poorly finished restorations: the location and outline of the white patch often corresponds well to the cause. Removal of the cause usually results in resolution of the lesion: persistent lesions should be biopsied.

Tobacco-associated leukoplakias

Commonly seen as areas of homogenous leukoplakia in the buccal mucosa, these are white patches caused by chronic chemical irritation of tobacco substrates. The mucosa is seen to have undergone hyperkeratosis as a protective measure against the assault. 'Smoker's keratosis' is a particular condition affecting the palate, where the mucosa is greyish-white with red spots (which represent the openings of minor salivary glands). There is an association between these leukoplakias and malignant change—all suspicious lesions should undergo biopsy for histological diagnosis.

Idiopathic leukoplakia
- **Verrucous leukoplakia** (verrucous hyperplasia)—thick white patches of papillary or warty appearance that generally affect the alveolar mucosa or vestibule. Reports have shown the presence of HPV (human papilloma virus) to be a common finding. May mimic verrucous carcinoma and so biopsy may be necessary.
- **Speckled leukoplakia**—presents as an area of velvety red mucosa with multiple white plaques; commonly seen in the floor of mouth and lateral tongue. Considered to be 'pre-malignant'.

Familial white patches
Various conditions show a genetic preponderance. These are very rarely associated with malignant change, but may be present with other systemic conditions.
- **White sponge naevus**. Bilateral, diffuse white lesions of the buccal mucosa, occasionally also affecting the tongue. The lesions may be so dense as to show corrugated folds. No treatment necessary/biopsy will confirm a diagnosis.
- **Leukoedema**. Considered by many as a variation of normal as oppose to a pathological process. Appears as a grey/white film ('mother-of-pearl') bilaterally in the buccal mucosa. The white appearance is reduced when the mucosa is stretched.

Inflammatory white patches
- **Candidiasis**. White plaques that can be easily wiped away leaving an erythematous mucosa—may be associated with the immune compromised patient.
- **Koplik's spots**—multiple white spots covering the buccal mucosa; seen in children in the prodromal stages of measles infection.
- **Hairy leukoplakia**—a marker of HIV infection. Vertical, parallel, hair-like white lesions are seen on the lateral aspects of the tongue. May be superimposed with candidal infection; however, the Epstein–Barr virus (EBV) has been implicated as the causative agent.
- **Chemical burn**—agents such as aspirin (saliacylic acid) may produce a mucosal burn with subsequent epithelial inflammation. Initially the overlying necrotic tissue will be a white plaque that will eventually slough away.

Dermatological conditions
Lichen planus—classically reticular, 'lace-like' striations are seen in the buccal mucosa. Of unknown aetiology, although various drugs (e.g. thiazides) and the mercury in amalgam restorations have been implicated. Multifocal or plaque-like white lesions, with local erythema may also be seen. Pre-malignant changes have been reported in the *erosive* forms of this common condition.

⑦ Red patches in the mouth

Red lesions of the oral cavity generally represent an inflammatory process—the 'redness' being a reflection of the increased local vascularity. There are, however, a number of other conditions that can result in red patches.

Local red patches

- **Burns**—chemical burns can cause white patches. Less severe chemical or thermal burn may produce inflammation only, seen as a red patch. The white slough produced by superficial necrosis is not present.
- **Functional**—red patches may represent mucosal irritation, e.g. ill-fitting dentures.
- **Chronic erythematous candidiasis** may present as red mucosa beneath the fitting surface of a denture.
- **Port wine stain** (macular haemangioma)—developmental in origin; tend to be localized to the neurovascular divisions of the trigeminal nerve (V).
- **Erythroplakia**—the red equivalent of leukoplakia, this term simply means 'red patch'. May also be used to describe red patches with multifocal white patches (speckled or leukoerythroplakia): **these lesions are prime suspects for malignant change**.

Diffuse red patches

Many conditions may present as diffuse or multifocal red patches; those commonly encountered include:

- **Geographic tongue**—irregular patches due to loss of the filliform papillae on the dorsum/lateral tongue surface. Variable progression with recurrent episodes at different sites. May be associated with discomfort (glossodynia).
- **Vitamin deficiencies**—commonly seen in the elderly and alcoholics. B vitamins and folic acid deficiency may be associated with atrophic glossitis, an important marker for pernicious anaemia.
- **Candidiasis**.
- **Bullous/erosive disease**—such as herpetic lesions, varicella zoster, impetigo, pemphygoid and pemphygus, and erosive lichen planus. A common feature of these lesions is diffuse erythematous change of the oral mucosa accompanying the localized disease lesions.
- **Dysplastic field change**—just as local erythroplakias may be seen, so may widespread multifocal red lesions, which have the same features as focal erythroplakias.
- **Radiation mucositis**—commonly seen in patients post-irradiation for head and neck malignancy. Super-infection may occur often with candida.

⑦ Pigmented lesions

Pigmented lesions of the skin and oral mucosa, other than red lesions, are generally **blue, brown, or black**. They may result from accumulations of intrinsic pigments (e.g. melanin, haemoglobulin) or extrinsic pigments (e.g. heavy metal particles), which are either locally or systemically absorbed. A further group of lesions that blanch on pressure represent vascular anomalies.

Focal pigmentation

- **Amalgam tattoo**—dental amalgam traumatically implanted into the mucosa, either at the time of restoration placement, or as debris at time of extraction, produce a bluish/black pigmented lesion with irregular borders that does not blanch when pressed.
- **Mucoceles**—haemorrhagic mucoceles may appear as focal bluish/red lesions following trauma; they are most frequently seen on the buccal mucosa or lips.
- **Vascular—haemangiomas** are common hamatomatous lesions seen in childhood, generally affecting the lips, tongue, and cheeks. Typically they are flat and blanch on pressure, although some may be nodular as a result of calcification or thrombosis. **Varicosities** or **'venous lakes'** are seen in the more elderly population and commonly affect the sublingual veins or the lips.
- **Melanocytic naevus**—skin naevi ('moles') are very common, particularly in the skin of the head and neck. On the other hand, oral naevi are rare. They generally arise in childhood and reach a given size, after which growth stops. Various groups are described: compound, junctional, intramucosal, blue naevus.

Diffuse and multifocal pigmentation

Racial pigmentation

Diffuse macular multifocal pigmentation is commonly seen in certain racial groups. Generally occurring in darker skinned people, the patches are dark brown and may occur at any site in the oral mucosa, although the gingiva is the most commonly affected site.

Peutz–Jegher's syndrome

A genetically inherited (autosomal dominant) condition characterized by polyp formation in the small intestine and multifocal macular melanin pigmentation in peri-oral locations. The bowel polyps are not thought to be pre-malignant although cases of malignant change have been reported and hence diagnosis of this condition may be of great importance to the patient. Pigmentation in and around the mouth usually affects the lips and buccal mucosa and resembles 'freckles'. The extremities may also show focal areas of pigmentation.

Kaposi's sarcoma

This is a rare type of malignant angiosarcoma that is usually mucocutaneous in its presentation. It is a marker disease of the acquired immune deficiency syndrome (AIDS) in HIV positive patients. Lesions of the oral mucous membranes frequently affect the palate and present as bluish/black or red macules, which may darken over time and ulcerate, at which stage they become painful.

Malignant melanoma

Neoplastic proliferation of melanocytes may give rise to malignant melanoma. Oral melanomas are rare; when present over 70% are reported in the posterior maxillae and hard palate. They present as dark brown/black irregular lesions often with an uneven surface. Prognosis is related to depth of invasion. Survival rates overall for skin and oral melanomas are exceptionally poor: less than 5% live in excess of 5 years.

⑦ Ulcers

Ulcers are a common problem in the mouth—they may be localized or part of a wider systemic disease. A careful history is therefore necessary. Consider involvement of the eyes, genitalia, joints, and skin. **Vesicular lesions may present as ulcers** if traumatized. Examination of all mucous membranes should be carried out for the possibility of other lesions.

Recurrent/generalized ulceration

Recurrent aphthous stomatitis

This term encompasses several groups of oral ulcers that frequently recur over time. They often present with prodromal burning and tingling of the mucosa. Many aetiological factors have been suggested, including: familial tendency, microbial infections, allergens, haematological disorders, hormonal disruption, and stress.

Minor aphthous ulceration

These present as crops of ulcers measuring less than 10 mm on the lips, cheek, and tongue. Usually less then ten in number, they are round and flat, often with an erythematous margin. Generally self-limiting they resolve within 7–10 days.

Major aphthous ulceration

These ulcers often larger than 10 mm may also be seen on the palate and pharyngeal wall. Major aphthae are generally painful and may have similar appearances to oral carcinoma—a crater like ulcer with rolled margins. However, they resolve usually within 2–3 weeks.

Acute necrotizing ulcerative gingitvits

This presents as multifocal necrotic ulcers primarily on the inter-dental papillae. Patients present with pain and halitosis. Anaerobic fusiform and spirochaete bacteria are the causative agents and antibiotic therapy is required (augmentin/metronidazole), followed by meticulous oral hygiene. It is thought that stress plays an important role as an exacerbating factor in this condition, and may be seen in students around exam time!

Focal ulceration

Traumatic

The most common cause of oral ulceration. There is usually a clear history from the patient, e.g. cheek biting, or an obvious local cause, e.g. a sharp dental restoration. Removal of the cause should lead to a quick resolution of the lesion.

Primary syphilitic chancre

Presents as a firm painless lesion with central ulceration, most frequently occurring on the lips or tongue. This is a sexually transmitted condition (causative organism *Treponema pallidum*) with the chancre occurring 3–6 weeks after sexual contact.

Squamous cell carcinoma (SCC)
Any oral ulcer persisting for over 3 weeks without an apparent cause should be considered a carcinoma until proven otherwise. Cigarette smoking, tobacco, or betel chewing and alcohol are known aetiological factors. The lesion may occur *de novo* or arise in established sites of leukoplakia or erythroplasia. Ulcers are often painless and growth rates vary. SCC of the oral cavity spreads to draining cervical lymph nodes in a predictable fashion before producing distant metastases, so early presentation and treatment is associated with a favourable outcome. Unfortunately, many of these lesions present late. Overall oral cancer has a relatively poor prognosis with 5-year survival rates for all stages of the disease reported at 45–50%.

:⚙: Blisters—vesicles and bullae

⑦ Vesicles

Vesicles are fluid-filled blisters generally less than 5 mm. Lesions over this size are termed bullae. The main vesicular diseases are primarily infections, commonly viral organisms. Some types may be harboured during dormant phases in sensory nerve nuclei.

Herpetic gingivostomatitis

Primary herpes virus infection (commonly type I) presents with multiple vesicular eruptions over the lips, gingivae, and buccal mucosa. The vesicles may rupture leaving an erythematous area or a white pseudomembranous erosion. Systemic upset with pyrexia is common. The conditon is contagious and usually runs it course in 10–14 days with uneventful healing. **Secondary herpes labialis** is recurrent infection of the lips by the same virus. Clusters of vesicles occur on the vermillion border. These may be painful and exudative, forming coalesced crusts. Systemic upset is not a feature. The virus is thought to lay dormant in ganglia and be reactivated by such factors as trauma, infection, sun exposure, and stress.

Varicella zoster

Primary VZ, 'chickenpox'. This is a dermal vesicular disease with an incubation of 2–3 weeks. Lesions generally start on the trunk and then become widespread—oral lesions predominantly affect the palatal mucosa. **Secondary VZ 'shingles'** affects adults and the elderly and is a reactivation of the virus. The virus remains dormant in sensory nerve ganglia and the pattern of eruption follows the sensory distribution. Prodromal neuralgia is followed by painful vesicular eruption persisting for 1 to 4 weeks. Post-herpetic neuralgia often follows.

① Bullae

Pemphigus vulgaris

This is an uncommon autoimmune skin disease characterized by bullae formation. Patients are often middle-aged females. The disorder is said to occur more commonly in Jews than other ethnic groups. Oral lesions may occur before skin lesions in up to 50 % of patients. The lesions present as painful, fragile blisters or diffuse gelatinous plaques that rupture easily leaving broad based areas of denuded skin with associated erythema. **Nikolsky's sign:** a bullous lesion may form after rubbing clear skin or mucosa. Control of the disease usually requires high dose, long term systemic steroids.

Benign mucous membrane pemphigoid

A bullous autoimmune dermatosis with a predilection for mucous membranes—the mouth and eyes being favoured sites. Often presenting in the late middle ages (50–60s), the disease is twice as common in females as males. It often runs a protracted course. The oral bullae of pemphygoid are thicker and so, unlike pemphigus, they form as tense blisters that remain intact for several days, but again rupture. Eye lesions may heal with scaring leaving symblepharon—fibrous bands between the sclera and the lids: entropian with blindness is also a major complication.

⚙ *Erythema multiforme*

This is a **potentially severe skin disorder**, which is thought to be precipitated by allergens (e.g. sulphonamide drugs) or as a post-viral immune reaction (e.g. post-herpetic). However, many cases arise spontaneously. The disease mainly occurs in young adults and is more common in males than females. Presenting lesions may be bullae, macules, or erosions. On skin the classic 'target' lesion is often seen—a circular wheal with circumferential halo. In the mouth, the lips are most commonly involved. Bullae develop and burst rapidly leaving raw painful erosions, resulting in difficulty eating and drinking. The condition usually runs its own course in 2–5 weeks but systemic antihistamines and antipyretics may be used—steroids may be needed in more severe cases.

Stevens–Johnson syndrome

This is a severe form of erythema multiforme: widespread involvement of skin and the oral, genital and ocular mucosae. Patients usually need to be admitted for IV fluids, antibiotics, and steroids. Fatalities have been reported.

⑦ *Angina bullosa haemorrhagica*

This is a benign condition characterized by the sudden appearance of a blood blister on the oral mucosa in the absence of an obvious cause. It affects mainly middle-aged and elderly people of either sex. No treatment is required.

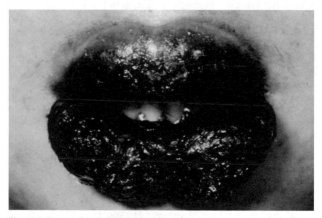

Fig. 11.1 Stevens–Johnson syndrome.

⑦ Dental emergencies

Emergencies affecting the teeth and supporting tissues.

Basic anatomy

An understanding of the form and function of the teeth, and their supporting tissues, is particularly relevant to the treatment of emergencies that affect the dental tissues. Developmentally, the pulp and periradicular tissues are one and the same. They remain intimately related throughout life at both a neural and vascular level through apical, lateral, and accessory canals.

It is useful to have the eruption, calcification, and apical closure dates at hand, particularly when treating the child and young adult. Be alert to the presence of congenital and development abnormalities that affect teeth, and the significant changes that occur to the internal anatomy of teeth during the process of development and ageing.

The basic tissues of the teeth and supporting structures can be described under the headings of enamel, dentine, pulp, cementum, periodontal ligament, and alveolar bone.

Enamel

This is the hardest and most impermeable of the tissues. It protects and supports teeth and, although 95% inorganic by weight, is permeable to certain ions and molecules and may demonstrate cracks and hypomineralized defects. Loss of enamel through caries, natural wear, and dissolution with acidic foods can lead to weakening of its structure and potential for the entry of micro-organisms.

Dentine

This has a tubular structure, which is bathed in tissue fluid from the pulp. It is 70% inorganic by weight. It is not as hard as enamel and is more resilient. The tubules in dentine have the diameter of a red blood corpuscle and their numbers range from 15 000/mm^2 at the enamel dentine junction to 65 000/mm^2 nearer the pulp. Dentine is highly permeable and its permeability increases with diameter and number of tubules. The tubular fluid occupies 20% of the dentine by volume.

Dental pulp

This consists of connective tissue within a pulp cavity surrounded by dentine. The pulp communicates with the periradicular tissues through the apical lateral and accessory canals, which allow the passage of inflammatory products to and from the periradicular tissues.

Cementum

Covers the surface of the roots and provides a point of attachment for the periodontal ligament. It is 40% mineralized by weight.

Periodontal ligament

This is dense fibrous tissue arranged in specific groups of collagen fibres providing support and attachment for the tooth in the alveolar socket.

Alveolar bone

Consists of outer cortical bone, beneath which is spongy bone consisting of trabeculae and bone marrow. It is easily resorbed under the influence of inflammatory changes.

Microbial plaque

This is the primary aetiological factor in both periodontal and endodontal disease. The plaque consists of bacterial colonies within a sticky matrix of proteins and bacterial products.

Calculus

Forms when supragingival and subgingival microbial plaque becomes mineralized. Saliva contains calcium phosphate that in susceptible people precipitates to form the hard deposit on teeth. Supragingival calculus is lighter in colour and forms near salivary duct openings. Subgingival calculus is darker in colour due to the inclusion of blood pigments. Calculus is not the direct cause of periodontal disease but it does encourage the formation of further plaque.

General principles

Dental emergencies arising from trauma to the teeth and supporting tissues are a common occurrence. Trauma can result in fractures of the crown and root and/or luxation or avulsion injuries. Such injuries may result in protracted treatment and it is most important that early diagnosis and management is undertaken correctly.

When examining the dental injuries ask yourself the following questions.

Do I understand the nature and extent of these injuries?

Examine the bony and soft tissue injuries first. Changes in contour, and displacement of teeth and alveolar processes should make you **suspect bony fractures**. Where soft tissue lacerations (e.g. lips) are present, the possibility of a **foreign body should be considered**. If fragments of teeth are suspected, get an X-ray of the soft tissues. **Establish the need for anti tetanus cover and consider antibiotics**.

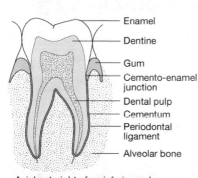

Enamel — Natural dental crown
Dentine
Gum
Cemento-enamel junction — Neck area
Dental pulp
Cementum
Periodontal ligament — Dental roots
Alveolar bone

Axial cut sight of an inferior molar

Fig. 11.2 Basic dental anatomy.

Are the damaged teeth salvageable?

Teeth that are damaged should be critically assessed. Loss of tooth substance and the presence of fractures make it important to decide whether the teeth are restorable. Vertical fractures involving the peri-odontal attachment have a poor prognosis. The future of the teeth should be assessed in the light of the patient's overall dental health status and treatment needs.

Has the blood supply to the teeth been damaged?

Damage to the vascular supply of the teeth is important where there is evidence of intrusion, extrusion, and lateral displacement. Loss of pulp vascularity leads to loss of the natural defence mechanisms in the pulp–dentine complex. Teeth are then less able to cope with bacterial insults and become vulnerable to **endodontic infection**. Vitality testing is a useful aid in establishing the state of the pulps of injured teeth. However, it gives an unreliable picture of the health of pulps for up to 12–24 weeks following trauma.

How contaminated is the tooth/teeth?

The degree of bacterial contamination of the involved teeth should be assessed. Crown fractures result in the loss of surface integrity and allow entry of micro-organisms. Early restoration of teeth to restore this integrity should be planned.

What is the degree of maturity of the injured teeth?

In teeth with immature roots with open apices, it is desirable to maintain the vitality of the pulps to help with root formation. Immature teeth with large pulp spaces may be difficult to root treat and restore.

Injuries range from chips off the enamel to crown/root fractures involving the pulp. The peri-odontal ligament and surrounding 'gum' support the teeth in their sockets and cushion the forces of mastication. These structures may be concussed (peri-odontal injury without loosening). Alternatively, intact teeth may be intruded (driven into the bone), displaced, or avulsed (pulled out the socket). Fractures of the teeth and/or supporting alveolar bone may or may not be associated.

Treatment

Treatment is required when there is:
- pain (pulp exposure);
- sensitivity to hot and cold (dentine exposure);
- recent avulsion;
- mobility (fracture or displacement);
- alveolar bone fracture;
- retention of part of the tooth;
- cosmetic deformity.

Principles of treatment include:
- pain relief;
- control of bleeding;
- dressing of exposed dentine or pulp;
- repositioning/replantation of the tooth. This is then splinted for a variable time depending on the nature of the injury;
- reduction and fixation of alveolar bone;
- cosmetic repair.

Dental caries

Dental caries is the most common cause of pulp and periradicular disease. This localized and progressive process destroys tooth tissue. The products of the metabolism of certain micro-organisms (i.e. organic acids and proteolytic enzymes) cause the destruction of enamel and dentine. Extensive invasion of dentine ultimately leads to bacterial infection of the pulp.

Host responses that tend to protect teeth from the insults of dental caries include:

- the buffering and bactericidal capacity of saliva;
- the physical barriers provided by enamel and cementum;
- the outflow of tubular fluid containing immunoglobulins;
- a decrease in permeability of dentine with the formation of peri-tubular dentine;
- intra-tubular calcification beneath carious lesions;
- the formation of tertiary dentine;
- inflammatory and immune reactions within the dental pulp.

Caries diagnosis

In the emergency situation, patients seek help as a result of the symptoms of dental caries. **Pain is usually at a fairly late stage in the carious process**. Cavities, discoloration of teeth, and symptoms ranging from reaction to hot and cold and intense pain may be evident.

Ideally identifying the presence of dental caries depends upon:

- a clean dry field;
- good magnified vision;
- appropriate bitewing radiographs;
- fibre-optic trans-illumination facilities.

Peri-odontal disease

In peri-odontal disease the root face becomes colonized by organisms from supragingival plaque. In susceptible patients, the chronic inflammation of the supporting tissues by the action of anaerobic micro-organisms leads to the apical migration of the attachment apparatus and bone loss. Peri-odontal disease may be site specific and localized.

Apart from when the peri-odontal tissues become acutely inflamed, peri-odontal disease tends not to give rise to emergencies.

Classification of dental pain

The sensory response of teeth is controlled by myelinated (Aδ) nerve fibres and unmyelinated (C) nerve fibres. Differences between the two fibres assist in the classification of dental pain.

Disturbances in the pulp dentine complex initially have their effects on the low threshold Aδ fibres, which produce a quick, sharp, pain. When inflammatory tissue damage occurs in the pulps of teeth, the high threshold C fibres become involved and produce spontaneous and lingering pain, which may become intense.

Pulpal states

- The *clinically normal pulp* is never spontaneously symptomatic. It reacts to thermal and electrical testing. Palpation and percussion does not elicit pain and the radiographic picture is normal.

- *Reversible pulpitis* suggests the presence of mild inflammation. The tooth reacts to thermal and electrical stimuli producing a short sharp pain for the period of stimulation. This is a typical Aδ nerve response. Radiographically, there is no evidence of pathology. Removal of the cause of inflammation (e.g. dental caries) leads to a resolution of the condition.
- *Irreversible pulpitis* describes an inflammation that results in the dull throbbing pain of 'toothache'. This C fibre pain may be difficult to localize and may be worse when lying down or bending down. Radiographic changes may be evident if the inflammation extends to the peri-odontal ligament.
- *Pulp necrosis* involves the complete or partial death of the pulpal tissue due to vascular impairment either from trauma or infection. The tooth does not normally respond to thermal and electrical testing. Where there is involvement of the peri-odontal ligament the tooth may respond to palpation or percussion.

'Toothache'

'Toothache' is the term used by the lay public to describe the continuous radiating pain experienced when the dental pulp of an offending tooth is irreversibly inflamed. The pain of toothache is often described as a constant throbbing pain. This pain is a C-fibre pain, for which the only definitive treatment is either extraction or endodontic therapy. It is often difficult to locate the tooth.

The ideal treatment is to remove the inflamed pulp and commence root-canal treatment. The use of 0.5–5.0% sodium hypochlorite solutions to irrigate the pulp space ensures good disinfection. Antibiotics need not be prescribed in the treatment of irreversible pulpitis. Pain can be controlled with peripherally acting analgesics. In severe cases a long-acting local anaesthetic (0.5% bupivacaine with 1:200 000 epinephrine) may be administered.

Dentinal hypersensitivity

This is the sharp, transient Aδ-type of pain generated by thermal, osmotic, chemical, and physical stimulation of exposed dentine. The pain is due to fluid movement within the dentinal tubules. It is seen in patients with gingival recession, loss of tooth tissue through abrasion, and in those patients where erosion of the teeth occurs because of an acid diet or vomiting. An essential aspect of care involves the sealing of the dentinal tubules with materials that bond to the dentine to limit fluid movement within the tubules.

Cracked-tooth syndrome

Patients with this condition complain of an acute pain on biting hard objects. The pain usually occurs on releasing the biting pressure, although patients are not always in a position to identify this themselves. The condition is again due to dentinal fluid movement affecting Aδ fibres. Treatment often involves the stabilization of the fracture and provision of restorations that give occlusal protection.

Acute peri-apical peri-odontitis

Acute inflammation of the peri-apical tissues may be the result of an extension of pulpal disease, direct trauma from high restorations, and chemical and physical irritation of these tissues during endodontic treatment. If the peri-odontitis is of occlusal origin, the pulp usually remains responsive to vitality testing. Teeth can be extremely painful and tender to touch. Radiographic changes may be minimal.

Emergency care for this condition depends upon the cause and involves:
- relieving the occlusion, where the inflammation is related to trauma or endodontic procedures;
- prescribing anti-inflammatory analgesics;
- removing micro-organisms and their toxins from the pulp space, where pulpal disease is the cause, by performing root-canal treatment.

Chronic peri-apical peri-odontitis

This is a chronic lesion produced in a tooth with a necrotic, infected pulp. The tooth may be totally symptomless or there may be mild symptoms. Radiographic changes are usually apparent and vary from widening of the peri-odontal ligament space to extensive peri-apical radiolucencies.

The lesions may be classified as:
- an apical granuloma—consisting of chronic inflammatory cells and granulomatous tissue;
- a chronic peri-apical abscess—often associated with a draining oral sinus;
- a dental cyst—characterized by a fluid-filled sac.

These conditions rarely present as emergencies but may become acutely inflamed and require emergency care.

Acute peri-apical abscess

This is a focus of purulent exudate containing leucocytes. It is generally a very painful condition. Teeth are non-vital, may be tender, and show signs of mobility. The condition is often accompanied with intra-oral and extra-oral swelling, and there may be lymph node enlargement, and affected patients may have a raised temperature.

Emergency treatment often involves:
- institution of dental and/or soft tissue drainage of pus;
- prescription of antibiotics where patients have toxic systemic effects (metronidazole 400 mg two to three times daily, may be better than penicillin);
- prescription of analgesics;
- commencement of root-canal treatment or extraction.

Where drainage is achieved through a tooth, the tooth should be left open to drain for no more than 24 h.

Acute peri-odontal conditions

The acute peri-odontal abscess arises when there is an acute exacerbation of infection within a peri-odontal pocket. Pain and intra-oral swelling, accompanied with swollen lymph nodes, makes the condition similar to the acute peri-apical abscess. Unlike teeth with acute peri-apical abscesses, teeth with peri-odontal abscesses respond to vitality testing.

Treatment involves prescription of antibiotics where there are toxic systemic effects, institution of drainage through the peri-odontal pocket, along with debridement of the pocket.

'Painful gums'

These are not a common occurrence. Where patients complain of pain and ulceration between the teeth and experience a characteristic taste and oral odour, **acute necrotizing gingivitis (ANG)** should be suspected. Fever, malaise, and swollen lymph glands may accompany the condition. The acute phase responds rapidly to metronidazole (200 mg three times daily).

Gingival pain preceded by a fever, malaise, and sore throat may indicate **acute herpetic gingivostomatitis**. The condition is self-limiting in 10–14 days. The use of various mouthwashes may provide symptomatic relief.

Acute pericoronal infection occurs most commonly during the normal eruption of impacted mandibular third molars. Pericoronal pocketing leads to plaque accumulation, inflammation, pain and trismus. Management includes:

- removing source of physical trauma where opposing teeth aggravate the inflammation;
- prescribing analgesics and antibiotics, where required;
- performing surgical pocket elimination to facilitate plaque control measures;
- surgical extraction of impacted teeth.

Foreign body reactions

These reactions can occur in peri-odontal tissues and are produced as a response to the presence of a foreign body. The lesions may be acute or chronic and are distinguished by the presence of multinucleate giant cells around the foreign object. The aetiological agent may be part of the patient's diet (e.g. fishbone) or a dental material that has been implanted accidentally into the tissues (e.g. a restorative material).

If the condition is acute, it should be managed with antibiotics and analgesics, and the offending agent should be removed to effect healing. The removal of the foreign object may involve surgery.

Post-endodontic pain

Patients may experience pain following canal preparation or following the obturation of the root canals. Incomplete cleaning, over-preparation, and over-medication may lead to acute periradicular peri-odontitis.

If there is any doubt about whether the canals have been completely cleaned, the tooth should be re-opened and the pulp space irrigated with sodium hypochlorite and dressed with calcium hydroxide. In all cases, the patient should be reassured and prescribed anti-inflammatory analgesics.

Pain occurring following obturation of root canals usually subsides within 48 h. Persistent pain is likely to be related to:

- traumatic peri-odontitis;
- inadequate cleaning of the root canals;
- extrusion of irritant material into the peri-odontal tissues;
- root fracture brought about by the obturation procedure.

Where treatment is required, it may involve reassurance, analgesics and antibiotics, endodontic retreatment, or surgical endodontics.

History taking—key questions

Taking a health history should be a matter of routine. Establishing a clear dental history requires an ability to listen to the patient's own account of the events that have led them to seek advice. Opening questions should be simple and not require just a 'Yes' or 'No' response. Examples include:

- 'What's the problem?'
- 'What can we do to help you?'

Time spent listening to patients is never wasted. Establish a clear history of the present complaint by asking:

- 'When did the problem start?'
- 'How long has it lasted?'
- 'Where's the pain?'
- 'What does it feel like?'
- 'What starts the pain?'
- 'When does it hurt most?'
- 'What provides relief?'

In essence, by simple questioning, it should be possible to establish the nature of the discomfort, its initiation, frequency, and duration. These key questions are likely to indicate whether the problem is of dental, peri-odontal, or unrelated origin.

Clinical examination

When taking a history, it is possible to observe skin colour, complexion, hands, and nails, to give some insight into the general health of the patient. Facial asymmetry, swelling, and lymph nodes should be noted along with their location, size, and consistency.

A brief general oral examination will indicate standard of oral hygiene, missing and worn teeth, peri-odontal condition, signs of inflammation, type and amount of dental treatment, and presence of untreated caries. Detailed examination of the area of main complaint should be made to note:

- colour, texture and architecture of hard and soft tissues;
- presence of swellings and sinuses;
- tenderness to palpation;
- vertical and horizontal mobility of teeth;
- tenderness to digital percussion of teeth;
- tenderness to biting on a wedge, e.g. wooden stick or golf tee;
- presence of fractures of the teeth using a fibre-optic light.

Peri-odontal indicators should be:
- gingival recession;
- bleeding on peri-odontal probing;
- pus on peri-odontal probing;
- furcation involvement.

Close examination of teeth may reveal:
- crazing and fracture lines;
- primary and recurrent caries;
- leaking restorations;
- exposed dentine and pulp;
- discoloration from pulp haemorrhage, microleakage, corrosion, and root-filling materials.

Radiographic examination

Valuable information is gained from radiographs. Peri-apical radiographic views should be taken using paralleling film/sensor holders. These films reveal:

- root form and root-canal anatomy;
- density of the alveolar bone;
- peri-odontal ligament continuity;
- lamina dura;
- coronal and root caries;
- peri-apical radiolucencies;
- pulp stones;
- state of restorations and root-canal treatment;
- horizontal and vertical root fractures.

Bitewing radiographs are particularly useful for the examination of approximal caries and pulp chamber anatomy. Occlusal radiographs may be used to view traumatized anterior teeth and large radiolucencies. Additional views taken with altered horizontal or vertical tube angles allow the application of parallax principles in the location of objects and the separation of superimposed images.

Special tests

Pulp testing

This is used to establish the responsiveness of the pulp. It does this by stimulating pulpal nerves. Methods employed include:

- electric pulp testing (EPT), where a positive response is usually due to the electric current stimulating Aδ nerve fibres;
- cold testing to stimulate Aδ nerve fibres with the use of ethyl chloride spray, ice sticks, and carbon dioxide snow;
- heat testing using hot gutta percha or hot water delivered from a syringe.

These tests usually produce an initial response that disappears with the removal of the stimulus, indicating the response of Aδ nerve fibres. A persistent dull ache following removal of the stimulus indicates C-fibre activity, indicative of irreversible pulpal inflammation.

When patients attend in pain, or pain can be precipitated, **local anaesthesia** may be used to identify the offending tooth. Intra-ligamental techniques are particularly useful in this situation.

Test cavity

Test cavity cutting (without a local analgesic) has been suggested as a means of identifying teeth with necrotic pulps. Other tests may include:

- excavation of caries to establish extent and possible exposure;
- removal of restorations to view remaining tooth substance;
- fitting occlusal diagnostic splints where occlusal problems are suspected.

Dental trauma

wn fractures

ures of the crowns may involve enamel only, enamel and dentine, or
el, dentine, and pulp. The teeth should be radiographed and tested
ality. Where the dentine is exposed, it should be coated with a liner
ealed with a bonded composite.

tures involving the pulps of teeth usually require pulp-capping,
pulpectomy, or root-canal treatment.

apping

indicated in small recent exposures and should be performed by:
ting the tooth with rubber dam;
oughly washing the exposure site with saline until haemostasis is
red;
ing the exposure with calcium hydroxide;
bring the crown with a bonded composite or glass ionomer.

pulpectomy or pulpotomy

procedures are performed in immature teeth with large exposures by:
nistering local anaesthetic;
ting the tooth with rubber dam;
oving a small portion of the pulp with a water-cooled diamond bur;
ing the pulp stump with saline until haemostasis is secured;
ring the pulp stump with calcium hydroxide;
re the integrity of the crown;
w at 6–12 weeks and at 6-monthly intervals thereafter to establish
ormation.

nal treatment

reserved for mature teeth with large exposures and immature
here, following partial pulpectomy, there is radiographic evidence
ption.

res involving the crown and root

nt here depends upon the site of the fracture and the mobility of
onal portion. Fractures with no displacement often require root-
atment to limit bacterial contamination. The long-term prognosis
cases depends upon the ability to seal both the fracture and the
ce with a bonded restoration, and provide adequate protection
esses which might displace the fracture.
e a mobile portion of tooth is present, it should be removed and
d to establish the extent of the fracture. Where restoration
asible, crown-lengthening procedures may be required to access
in of the fracture.

actures

ctures below the alveolar crest that are mobile may require
for up to 12 weeks to assist union of the fracture.
there is only little mobility, the tooth should be reviewed
and radiographically at 3, 6, and 12 months. Vitality testing is

①

Cro
Fract
enam
for v
and s
Fra
partia

Pulp
This is
- isol
- tho
  sec
- coa
- rest

Partia
These
- adm
- isola
- rem
- was
- cove
- resto
- revie
  root

Root-co
This is
teeth w
of reso

Fractu
Treatm
the cor
canal tre
in these
pulp sp
from str
Wher
examine
seems f
the mar

Root fr
Root fra
splinting
Wher
clinically

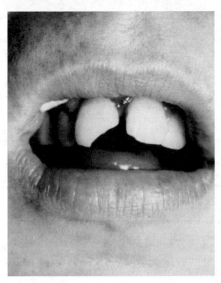

Fig. 11.3 Crown fracture—where is the missing fragment?

unreliable for up to 6 months. Where there is loss of vitality, it usually indicates that the pulp in the coronal portion has become necrotic.

In these cases, root treatment to the fracture line should be performed and the coronal pulp space dressed with calcium hydroxide to effect the formation of a hard tissue barrier against which a root filling may be compacted.

Traumatic peri-odontitis

This is painful inflammation around the apex of a tooth resulting from occlusal trauma. It may occur around both vital, non-vital, and endodontic-ally treated teeth. Radiographic examination may show very little, except for slight thickening of the peri-odontal ligament space. The tooth may be very sensitive to palpation and percussion. Management involves:

- electrical and thermal testing to establish the vitality of the tooth;
- paralleling peri-apical radiograph;
- occlusal adjustment to relieve the trauma;
- prescription of an anti-inflammatory analgesic to relieve the symptoms.

Luxated teeth

When there is evidence that the pulp of a previously luxated tooth has become necrotic, root-canal treatment should be performed.

The avulsed tooth

Immediate action is required when one or more adult teeth are knocked completely out of the mouth. If these teeth are put back into the socket, there is a good chance they will take. **The primary aim of treatment is to replant an avulsed adult tooth as soon as possible**. This does not apply to baby teeth, if one is knocked out it should not be pushed back into the socket because the developing adult tooth may be damaged. The chances of success depend on how long it has been out of the mouth, ideally encourage an adult at the scene of the accident to replant it. Unfortunately, many lay people (and a few doctors) are worried about pushing a tooth back into a socket and getting it the right way round. If unable to do this, store the tooth in an appropriate solution and refer as quickly as possible. The main reason why avulsed teeth do not re-attach is that the peri-odontal cells on the root dry out. **The tooth must be kept moist**. Milk is good storage medium. Provided that the tooth is kept moist in milk it can be replanted up to 24h later.

You therefore have two options when confronted by a patient with a tooth in his hand:

- replant the tooth back into its socket and refer the patient immediately to a dentist for splinting;
- make sure the tooth is safe (in milk or physiological saline) and arrange for immediate dental treatment.

Consider antibiotics and, if appropriate, a tetanus booster.

Avulsed teeth should be replanted as soon as possible after the injury and splinted for 7–10 days. Root-canal treatment should be performed after removal of the splint.

Splinting teeth

Rinse the tooth in clean water or milk, and place back into the socket from which it came. Ideally, this should be done by the patient or parent ASAP. Care should be taken to handle the tooth only by its crown and not by its root. If the parent or patient is unsure about re-implanting the tooth, it can be stored in milk or water. Alternatively, in *reliable calm* patients, the tooth may be gently held inside the mouth.

Many types of splint are available for stabilizing displaced and fractured teeth. These include:

- vacuum-formed polyvinyl splints;
- the use of etched enamel retained composite;.
- the use of polymethacrylate reinforced with wire or nylon.

A splint that allows *physiological movement* of the tooth during healing is less likely to produce ankylosis. Fixation for a period of 7–10 days is recommended. The exception to this rule is when there is avulsion or luxation of teeth accompanied with alveolar fracture. In this case, splinting may be required for 4–8 weeks. During this time, the patient should eat soft foods, avoid biting on the splinted teeth, and keep the mouth as clean as possible. In adults, the re-implanted tooth should have a root-canal treatment at around 1–4 weeks. In children (where the root has not completely formed) this may not be necessary. The tooth needs long-term follow-up as the pulp may still die resulting in pain, discoloration, or peri-odontal abscesses.

Consider antibiotics and tetanus in patients with accompanying significant soft tissue injuries.

Chapter 12

The salivary glands

⑦ Salivary gland diseases—general considerations

Saliva is produced by:
- **major salivary glands**—parotid, submandibular, and sublingual;
- **minor salivary glands**—these line the mouth, palate, and lips, and they can occasionally be found in the nose.

Common problems relating to these glands include:
- infections (mumps and other viruses, bacterial);
- swellings/lumps (obstruction/tumours);
- injuries (notably lacerations);
- dry mouth.

⑦ Tumours

Any of these glands can undergo malignant change. In the UK, the incidence of tumours of the salivary glands is approximately 3–4 per 100 000. Both benign and malignant tumours can occur at any age, although they are more commonly seen in the middle aged and elderly.

Patients may present with the following clinical features:
- swelling;
- pain;
- facial weakness (parotid gland);
- skin changes;
- poor hearing or earache;
- incidental finding.

Most parotid tumours present as a painless, localized swelling, which has been present for several months, although occasionally, it may have been present for many years. **Pain suggests infection or a rapidly growing malignant tumour**. **Other features suggestive of malignancy include facial nerve weakness, tethering of the lump, and rapid growth**. Investigations include CT scan or MRI scan. Fine needle aspirate cytology is often undertaken but its value is a source of hot debate.

Tumours of the submandibular gland constitute approximately 10% of salivary gland tumours. Around two-thirds of these are benign, the remainder being malignant.

Tumours of the minor salivary glands constitute about 10% of salivary tumours and usually occur in the palate and upper lip; 45% of these tumours are malignant. **A lump in the upper lip and hard palate should, therefore, always raise suspicions of a salivary gland neoplasm**, and will nearly always require a biopsy.

Not all swellings of the major salivary glands are due to salivary tumours. Tumours can also arise from associated blood vessels, nerves, fat, and lymphatic tissue. 'Tumour-like' conditions presenting as swellings include sarcoid, toxoplasmosis, and sialosis. The latter is a painless swelling, which may be associated with alcoholic cirrhosis, diabetes, acromegaly, or bulimia.

⑦ Calculi (stones) and strictures

Most calculi occur in the submandibular gland and duct, although they also commonly occur in the parotid gland. Calculi in the other salivary glands are rare. Strictures may arise from trauma, e.g. from cheek biting, dentures, following surgery, or a previous calculus. Both stones and strictures result in obstruction. Patients therefore usually complain of:

- recurrent or persistent swelling especially at meal times;
- pain on eating;
- symptoms relieved by discharge of saliva or pus from duct.

If saliva is allowed to stagnate in the gland, infection may develop. Long-term obstruction leads to permanent glandular destruction and a positive cycle of recurrent obstruction, infections, and further destruction.

Treatment

Depending on the type of obstruction, site, and presence of glandular destruction, this may include:

- dilation of stricture;
- removal of calculus;
- reconstruction of duct;
- repositioning of duct;
- excision of gland.

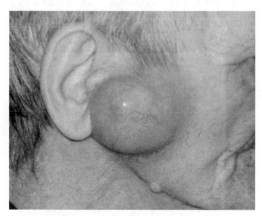

Fig. 12.1 Parotid tumour.

ⓘ Infections

Both the major and minor salivary glands can become infected. 'Ascending' infection, i.e. bacteria in saliva passing back along the ducts to the glands, commonly involves the parotid and submandibular glands. In such cases, predisposing conditions may be associated, e.g. dehydration, diabetes, or immunosupression. Fibrosis following radiotherapy or pre-existing obstruction from a calculus or stricture may also predispose to infection.

Common clinical features
These include:
- fever;
- pain;
- erythema;
- tender swelling;
- discharge of pus from the duct;
- dry mouth;
- dehydration.

If infection is not treated early, this may develop into chronic or recurrent infection. Progressive destruction occurs that aggravates the situation resulting in a non-functional gland.

Treatment
In the absence of an obvious abscess, which requires incision and drainage, this initially consists of antibiotics, rehydration, analgesia, and correction of any systemic conditions, e.g. diabetes. If an obstruction is found, e.g. stone, this needs to be removed to enable drainage. Gland massage, especially after meals, and 'lemon drops' to stimulate salivary flow, help to maintain a flushing effect and prevent stagnation of saliva. Abscesses need to be incised and drained on an urgent basis. If infection persists or continues to recur, excision of the gland may be necessary. This is best done when there is no active infection.

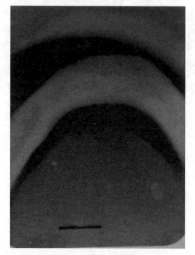

Fig. 12.2 Lower occlusal X-ray showing small stone in submandibular duct.

Infections of the parotid glands

Acute parotid sialadenitis

Mumps is the commonest cause of parotid swelling, even unilaterally. It has a peak incidence in childhood but can occur in adults. In teenagers, coxackie and echoviruses can also cause acute sialadenitis. Clinically there is pyrexia and malaise. Pain is the most striking symptom. There is diffuse swelling of the gland and often trismus. Treatment is supportive.

Acute suppurative parotid sialadenitis

This is the result of salivary stasis either from obstruction (calculus or stricture), glandular disease (Sjögren's, chronic sialadenitis), or a decrease in saliva production. Major predisposing factors are dehydration, the infirmed or elderly, and poor oral hygiene. It was more prevalent in the past, in old, debilitated, and dehydrated, hospitalized patients. The chief agent is *Staphylococcus aureus*. Treatment is rehydration of the patient, encouraging salivary flow (lemon drops), gland massage, and antibiotics. If an abscess occurs, it will need surgical draining.

Chronic recurrent sialadenitis

This is an incompletely understood entity. It is characterized by recurrent unilateral or bilateral diffuse swelling of the parotids in children and adults. Some go on to develop Sjögren's syndrome. The sialogram is useful, showing sialectasis. Treatment is conservative monitoring; troublesome glands may be removed.

HIV salivary gland disease

This clinically resembles Sjögren's syndrome in that it is bilateral diffuse enlargement of both glands. It has characteristic multicentric cystic appearance. Positive HIV serology will make the diagnosis.

Infections of the submandibular glands

Acute submandibular gland sialadenitis

The majority of infections are secondary to a calculus in the duct. Other causes include surgical scarring or strictures secondary to radiation. The whole of the gland swells up and there is malaise, pyrexia, and pain. Submandibular gland calculi are radio-opaque in 80% of cases, so a radiograph may aid in the diagnosis. Antibiotics are required. If the stone is easily felt in the mouth, it can be removed intra-orally. Alternatively, the whole gland can be excised electively. If the infection leads to a collection, then incision and drainage of the submandibular fascial space must be carried out as an emergency, and the gland removed electively later.

Chronic submandibular gland sialadenitis (Kuttner's tumour)

This results from repeated episodes of acute sialadenitis. The structure, parenchyma, and function of the gland are gradually destroyed. The gland ends up feeling very hard to palpation and may be mistaken for a tumour. Treatment is by surgical excision.

⑦ Salivary gland diseases—miscellaneous considerations

A variety of autoimmune and degenerative conditions can involve the salivary and lacrimal glands. Many of these do not require surgery, but occasionally surgery is carried out to establish a diagnosis, or remove painful/unsightly glands. Recurrent infection in a non-functioning gland is also an indication for removal. **Sjögren's disease carries a risk of lymphoma** and removal may be required to establish this. Biopsy of minor salivary glands can usually be done under local anaesthesia. More extensive excision of major salivary or lacrimal glands requires a general anaesthetic.

Patients may present with:
- xerostomia;
- swelling of the salivary gland or lacrimal gland;
- 'burning mouth';
- keratoconjunctivitis sicca;
- cosmetic deformity.

Cysts of the salivary glands

'Retention' or 'extravasation' cysts are commonly seen in the cheek and lower lip. They occur following trauma, usually a bite to the minor salivary glands resulting in scarring and obstruction. Every now and then they burst, discharging the saliva, only to re-occur at a later date. A ranula is a similar cyst arising from the sublingual gland. A sialocoele may arise in a major salivary gland following obstruction or previous surgery. Treatment usually involves excision of the cyst and associated gland.

Burns

:✿: Introduction

Burns are systemic injuries, which result in significant morbidity and mortality. They present a major challenge, not only during the resuscitation phase, but also with later reconstruction. With burns of the face, a **high index of suspicion for smoke inhalation is essential**. Not only may there be **carbon monoxide poisoning, but cyanide and other toxins** may have been inhaled. In addition, there may be **direct thermal injury** to the upper airway and lungs, resulting in **airway oedema**. This is especially the case if steam has been inhaled, which has a high latent heat of evaporation and has a very high mortality rate. **Burns involving the eyelids, nose, mouth, ear, and scalp cause significant functional and cosmetic problems**. These patients also need a great deal of psychosocial rehabilitation in later life.

Anatomy of skin

The skin consists of two main layers: epidermis (which is composed of stratified squamous epithelium) and dermis (composed of connective tissue). Associated with the skin are epidermal appendages, e.g. sweat glands, sebaceous glands, and hairs. It is via the cells in these app endages that the epidermis can regenerate following partial thickness burns.

There are four or five layers to the epidermis, depending on the thickness of skin. Beginning at the deepest part and moving towards the surface of the epidermis, these are: the stratum basale, stratum spinosum, stratum granulosum, stratum lucidum, and corneum. The stratum lucidium is not present in thin skin.

Functions of skin

- **Thermoregulation**. Skin is the largest organ in the body and provides a barrier to heat loss. Burn patients have difficulty maintaining their core body temperature. Every effort must be made to warm the patient and **prevent hypothermia**.
- Skin is a **barrier for evaporation. Burn patients loose large amounts of fluid**, which must be actively replaced during the resuscitation phase.
- **Immunological organ**. Skin provides a barrier to infection and burn patients are at **increased risk of sepsis**.
- **Neurosensory**. Superficial burns expose nerve endings resulting in pain. Deep burns destroy these nerves, leaving an insensate area.
- **Vitamin D metabolism**.

Types of burns

- Thermal burns; dry (flame).
- Thermal burns; wet (scald).
- Cold injury; frostbite.
- Chemical burns: acid and alkali burns.
- Electrical (contact) burns.
- Electro-thermal burns (arc flash burns).
- Friction burns.

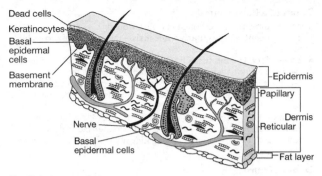

Dead cells
Keratinocytes
Basal epidermal cells
Basement membrane
Nerve
Basal epidermal cells

Epidermis
Papillary
Dermis
Reticular
Fat layer

Fig. 13.1 Anatomy of skin.

Causes of burns

Chip-pan fires, open unguarded flames, hot beverages, bath water, radiator contact burns, electrical burns, industrial burns, chemical burns, explosions, cement burns, hydrofluoric acid burns, fireworks, sunburn, and so on.

Mechanism of burns

Burns (with the exception of alkalis) coagulate tissue protein, causing necrosis of tissue. The main difference between thermal and chemical burns is the period of contact. **Chemical burns will continue to destroy tissue until the substance is neutralized or removed**. For thermal burns, the period of contact is often momentary. In addition to this, **some chemical agents cause systemic toxicity**, i.e. hydrofluoric acid by chelating calcium and magnesium ions. **Alkali burns tend to penetrate more deeply than acids** by causing saponification and liquefactive necrosis.

The mechanics of electrical burns are complex. Two mechanisms of cell damage predominate: current-generated heating with direct thermal burn, and denaturation of cell membrane lipids and proteins. The electrical current itself can punch large holes in the cell membrane (electroporation), which allows ions, metabolites, and even large molecules, such as DNA to escape.

Most fire-related deaths result not from the burn itself but from **inhalation of the toxic products of combustion**. This depends on the ignition source, concentration, and the solubility of the gases produced.

Zones of a burn wound

There are three zones described in a burn wound:

- **Zone of central coagulative necrosis**—this consists of non-viable tissue.
- **Zone of stasis**—this tissue is initially viable but has poor bloodflow. If the patient is not adequately resuscitated, the zone of stasis will become part of the zone of necrosis and the burn will deepen. One of the aims of burns management is to prevent this zone undergoing necrosis.
- **Zone of hyperaemia**—this is the outermost area of a burn and manifests an inflammatory response with increased blood flow. In burns >25% TBSA, the whole of the body will be included in the zone of hyperaemia.

Depth of burn

This depends on the **temperature** and **duration** of burn. It also depends on the **thickness of skin**, which varies with age, sex, and area of the body—the eyelids have the thinnest skin (0.5 mm) and the soles of the feet are the thickest (1.5 mm).

Initial assessments of burn depth may not be accurate as a superficial burn may progress to a deeper burn, due to infection or inadequate resuscitation. Historically, depth of burns have been classified as first, second, or third degree. This classification is often difficult to apply and has largely been superceded. When in doubt, it is always better to describe the burn to the receiving burn unit. The British Burn Association (BBA) recommends the following classification:

- **superficial (first degree);**
- **superficial dermal (second degree);**
- **deep dermal (second degree);**
- **full thickness (third degree)**.

Superficial: erythema only

This is akin to sunburn and should not be included in any of the assessments of burn area. It is very painful.

Superficial dermal

Characterized by **erythema and blistering**. The epidermis and most superficial dermis are involved only. These areas are very painful. They may be hypersensitive even to air currents. These burns heal without scarring in about a week.

Deep dermal

These extend deeper into the dermis; however, skin adnexal structures are undamaged, allowing spontaneous healing. They are **dry to touch** and may take up to 3 weeks to heal if uncomplicated by infection.

Full thickness

All the dermal elements are destroyed. The skin appears **translucent, mottled, or waxy white**. However, if there is significant leak of red blood cells from damaged vessels, it **may have a deep red appearance**. These areas are usually painless to pinprick. There may be involvement of underlying subcutaneous tissue, muscle, tendons, or bones. The classic finding is thrombosed vessels.

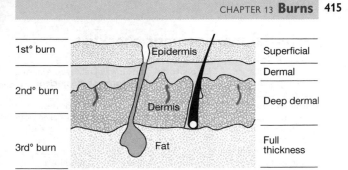

Fig. 13.2 Depth of burn.

Blisters

Blisters occur as the epidermis lifts from the dermis, due to damage of the dermo-epidermal junction. Plasma leaks from the damaged vessels and the osmotically active particles within the blister attract more fluid, resulting in enlargement over time. The fluid within a blister contains harmful inflammatory mediators. **There is much debate as to whether blisters should be burst or left intact, as a dressing**. If you are arranging transfer to a specialist burns unit, then it would be advisable to leave the blisters intact.

Escharotomy

This simply means opening the eschar, which is a thick layer of dead inexpansile skin. The eschar is **incised in areas that have circumferential full-thickness burns**, which may impede circulation or ventilation, as the underlying tissues swell. Burns of the neck, which require an escharotomy, are likely to be associated with severe inhalational injury and carry poor prognosis.

☼ Initial management checklist

Always follow local protocol, if available.

- Management as per **ATLS protocol**. The **airway** is always the initial priority. **Consider intubation or escharotomy of the neck or chest. Address airway, breathing, and circulation**.
- **Remove all clothing to stop the burning**. First-aid measures include irrigation or the application of cold water or saline-soaked cloth to decrease heat damage. Chemical burns require careful removal of the chemical-soaked clothing or chemical particles. Then dilute the chemical with copious irrigation (with water rather than trying to neutralize). Attempting to neutralize the chemical can produce an exothermic reaction with further burning.
- **Calculate the depth and area of burn**. Continue fluid resuscitation, as appropriate. The type of resuscitation should be discussed with the receiving burns unit as soon as possible.
- **Analgesia**.
- A **flow sheet**, outlining the patient's management should be initiated when the patient is admitted to the casualty department. This sheet should accompany the patient to the burns unit. A clinical photograph, if available, is a useful record of the event. The area and depth of burn should be recorded on an appropriate Lund and Browder chart.
- **Clingfilm is a useful temporary dressing**, which allows assessment of the burn with minimal distress to the patient. Clingfilm is sterile as it comes off the roll. **Avoid the application of flamazine** (silver sulphadiazine) for the first 48–72 h. Flamazine is a useful topical antimicrobial but it makes burns look deeper than they actually are. If you apply flamazine prior to transfer, you will be the only person to have seen the true extent of the burn and further assessment will be impossible. **Flamazine should not be applied to the face, as the silver can cause alteration in pigmentation**.
- A **urinary catheter** must be inserted for recording of hourly urinary output. Fluid resuscitation should be altered according to the hourly output.
- Large burns (>20%) can cause gastric ileus leading to nausea, abdominal distension, and vomiting. A **naso-gastric tube** must be placed for gastric decompression. This can be also useful for giving antacid and enteral feeding. Burns are hugely catabolic and a burn >50% total burn surface area (TBSA) increases the basal metabolic rate by approximately two times.

:⊙: Initial management

Always follow local protocol if available.

Consider the mechanism of injury—has there been an explosion, fall, assault, etc.? These patients need to be assessed according to the ATLS protocols.

Stop the burning process; protect yourself if chemical burns are suspected.

Airway

The larynx protects the subglottic airway from direct thermal injury; however, the supraglottic passage is quite vulnerable to heat exposure and may easily and **rapidly become obstructed as oedema develops**. In addition, the skin and soft tissues of neck itself may swell or contract with eschar, threatening the airway. Rapidly assess (and reassess) for airway involvement and signs of respiratory distress. The following problems exist:

(1) **direct thermal injury** causing upper airway edema and/ or obstruction;

(2) **inhalation of toxic fumes** from the products of combustion, leading to chemical tracheobronchitis, oedema, and pneumonia;

(3) **carbon monoxide poisoning**.

Consider intubation.

Inhalation injury
Suspect inhalation injury in:
- facial burns;
- singeing of eyebrows and nasal vibrissae;
- carbonaceous sputum;
- carbon deposits and swelling mouth and throat;
- history of confinement;
- confusion;
- explosion with burns to head and torso;
- carboxyhaemoglobin greater than 10%.

Symptoms of inhalation injury:
- lacrimation;
- severe brassy cough;
- hoarseness;
- shortness of breath;
- anxiety;
- wheezing.

The clinical manifestations of smoke-inhalation injury are subtle in the early stages and may not become obvious till 24h. The decision to intubate is clinical rather than findings of a chest X-ray or blood gas results. **A high index of suspicion must always been maintained and an anaesthetic opinion +/− fibre optic bronchoscopy is essential if there are any concerns. Disorientation, drowsiness, and coma indicate significant exposure to carbon monoxide (in the absence of other injuries).**

Breathing

Assume carbon monoxide (CO) exposure in any patient involved in a burn in a closed environment. CO levels of <20% may not be symptomatic. Manifestation of symptoms are headache and nausea (20–30%), confusion (30–40%), coma (40–60%), and death (>60%). Carbon monoxide shifts the oxygen dissociation curve markedly, due to its high affinity for haemoglobin (240 times, its half-life is 250 min). Patients suspected of exposure to CO should be administered **high-flow 100% oxygen** via a reservoir mask. CO levels from blood taken at the A&E may not represent the true level at the time of injury. A nomogram chart is available to extrapolate the value obtained and to calculate the original levels of CO.

Some patients may require endotracheal intubation and mechanical ventilation. **Arterial blood gases** should be determined as a base line prior to intubation.

Circulation

Burns in children >10% and >15% in adults require IV fluid resuscitation. As soon as the airway is under control, insert two large venflons, preferably in the antecubital fossae. Do not worry if you have to insert these into areas of burned skin, although it is preferable to use uninjured skin if possible. **Consider central lines in patients with cardiac problems** (not for access, but to assess fluid balance). Take blood for routine blood investigations, group and save. **Arterial blood gases** are necessary PO_2/PCO_2, carboxyhaemoglobin estimation and base excess.

There is no ideal formula for fluid resuscitation. There are several formulas around but they are all **guidelines**. In the UK most units use either the Muir and Barclay or Parkland regimens. The amount of fluid to be infused is calculated from the time of injury, **not** the time of arrival in the casualty. If the arrival of the patient is delayed, then you must 'catch up' the deficit. Erythema is ignored for estimation of total burn surface area (TBSA).

Parkland formula: 4 ml × weight (kg) × %TBSA = ml Hartmann's solution given in 24 h, half of this volume to be given during the first 8 h.

Muir and Barclay formula: weight (kg) × %TBSA/2 = ml colloid (i.e. albumin) given per unit time. The time periods are 4 h, 4 h, 4 h, 6 h, 6 h, and 12 h. In addition to the resuscitation fluid you must also give maintenance fluid at 1.5–2 ml/kg/h of dextrose.

The goal of the fluid resuscitation is to obtain a urine output in the range of 0.5–1 ml/kg/h adults, 1–1.5 ml/kg/h for children, and 1.5 ml/kg/h for infants. Urinary catheter must be inserted at admission to monitor the urinary output. In children, the help of a paediatrician may be required. Adjustments in the resuscitation fluid are made based on patient's response by changing the hourly infusion rates. A fluid bolus is recommended only in the presence of marked hypotension, not low urine output.

Halt the burning process

Remove all items of clothing to stop the burning. First-aid measures include irrigation or the application of cold water/saline-soaked cloth to decrease heat damage. This is often achieved at the scene and paramedics sometimes apply tea tree oil to the burn, which helps to reduce the heat as it evaporates.

Pain relief

As soon as the patient's state of shock and respiratory status has been assessed, relieving the pain and anxiety must be considered. Analgesics must be given intravenously since intramuscular absorption is unpredictable during the fluid-resuscitation period. Small, frequent, repeated doses of narcotics (morphine) are effective.

☼ Assessing the burn patient

History
It may not be easy to get a detailed history, if the patient is brought in unconscious or with airway compromise. However, the history of injury is extremely valuable, particularly:
- the time of injury (for fluid resuscitation);
- details of the environment (whether the patients was in a closed or open space);
- the mechanism of escape from the scene of fire may give some idea about the associated injury (did they jump from a window?);
- any pre existing illnesses (diabetes, hypertension, cardiopulmonary, and or renal problems);
- drug history;
- allergies;
- tetanus status.

Assessment of burn area
Record the patient's weight in kilograms. This is important for calculating fluid requirements and in assessing nutritional requirements later on.

Accurate assessment of the extent of burns is important in the calculation of fluid requirements. Be as accurate as possible, but remember that the volumes derived are only a guide and regular re-evaluation of fluid balance is essential. The 'rule of nines' (Wallace) is a useful guide to determine the approximate extent of burns. The adult body is divided into anatomical regions, which represent 9% or multiples of 9% of the total body surface. Hence head and neck = 9%, each upper limb = 9%, anterior torso = 18%, posterior torso = 18%, each lower limb = 18%, perineum = 1%. This is not applicable in children, as they have a larger surface area/body weight and the head accounts for more of this. Special charts are available for estimation of burn area at all ages (Lund and Browder). These are more accurate than the 'rule of nines' and should be available in every A&E department. They also help in graphic representation of the area and also depth of burns. **It is also useful to note that the surface area of the patient's palm, including the fingers, is approximately equal to 1% of their body area.** This is particularly useful when a patient has patchy areas of burn.

Special considerations
Chemical burns
These require careful removal of the chemical-soaked clothing or chemical powder. Then dilute the chemical with **copious irrigation** (with water rather than trying to neutralize). However, do be aware that **burns caused by sodium, potassium, or lithium will spontaneously ignite when exposed to water!** The burn should be covered with cooking oil to isolate the metal from water. Phenol actually penetrates more in dilute solution and should therefore not be irrigated. Oxalic and hydrofluoric acids will result in severe hypocalcaemia and hypomagnesaemia. They require treatment with topical and IM calcium gluconate. If in doubt, discuss with the burns unit or drug information centre.

Electrical burns

These cause more deep injury than superficial skin burns. They are arbitrarily divided into low (<1000 V) and high voltage (>1000 V). Direct current travels from a site of high potential to that of a lower potential, resulting in entrance and exit points. The greatest generation of heat occurs when electrical energy passes along a tissue of high resistance, such as bone. **Ventricular fibrillation** is a common cause of immediate death. These patients must be monitored for **compartment syndrome, haemochromogenuria, and cardiac dysrhythmias**. Muscle damage leading to rhabdomyolysis can lead to **renal failure**. They can also have associated fractures, corneal injury, and tympanic perforation.

All patients with facial burns should be suspected of having a corneal injury. Patients who are conscious at the time of burn often screw up their eyes, thereby protecting the eyelids and cornea. However, unconscious patients, such as epileptics, are often at risk of corneal damage due to the thin skin of the eyelids. The initial attending physician should not miss the opportunity of a careful ophthalmic examination using fluorescein dye, as eyelid swellings develop rapidly. If the patient has a corneal ulcer, then they should be referred for an ophthalmic opinion and given chloramphenicol eye ointment.

Ears

Full-thickness burns to the ear can result in perichondritis. After formal assessment, flamazine should be applied. The cartilage may need excision after 3–4 weeks.

Admission criteria

If there is any suspicion of inhalational injury, a fibre optic bronchoscopy should be performed. This may reveal deposits of carbonaceous particles and/or mucosal oedema. However, it is important to re-assess the patient, as mucosal oedema may not be present if the examination is performed soon after injury or the patient is inadequately resuscitated.

In the event of smoke inhalation, transfer to a burns unit is mandatory. Arrange for intubation beforehand. Exclude any other life-threatening injuries before transfer (? ruptured spleen, pneumothorax, etc.).

- Burn >10% TBSA in under 10 years or over 50 years of age.
- Burns >20% TBSA in other age groups.
- Burns involving face, hands, feet, genitalia, perineum, and joint areas.
- Full-thickness burns >5% any age group.
- Smoke inhalation injuries.
- Electric burns/lightening.
- Significant chemical burns.
- Burns associated with co-morbid medical conditions.
- Associated trauma.
- Non-accidental burn injuries (children).

DATE: WEIGHT:

Age: 7½ years to Adult

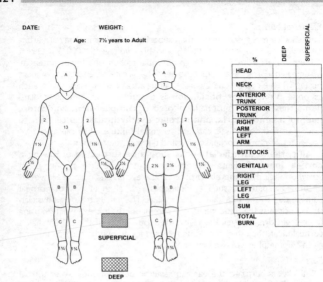

%	DEEP	SUPERFICIAL
HEAD		
NECK		
ANTERIOR TRUNK		
POSTERIOR TRUNK		
RIGHT ARM		
LEFT ARM		
BUTTOCKS		
GENITALIA		
RIGHT LEG		
LEFT LEG		
SUM		
TOTAL BURN		

SUPERFICIAL

DEEP

RELATIVE PERCENTAGES OF AREAS AFFECTED BY GROWTH

AREA	AGE 0	AGE 1	AGE 5	AGE10	AGE 15	ADULT
A = ½ OF HEAD	9½	8½	6½	5½	4½	3½
B = ½ OF ONE THIGH	2¾	3¼	4	4¼	4½	4¾
C = ½ OF ONE LEG	2½	2½	2¾	3	3¼	3½

Fig. 13.3 Lund and Browder burns chart (adult).

DATE: WEIGHT:

Age: Birth to 7½ years

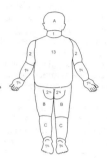

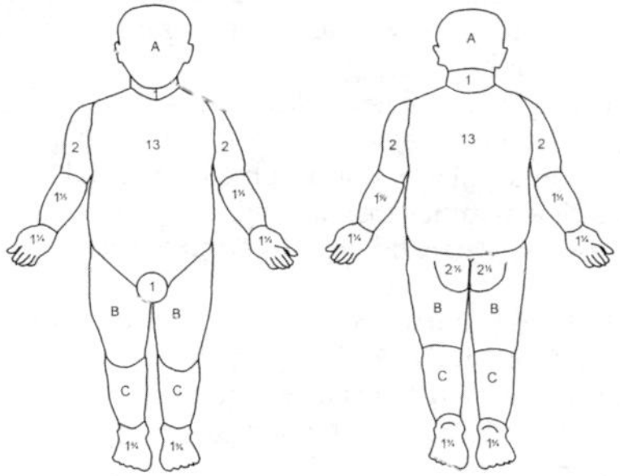

%	DEEP	SUPERFICIAL
HEAD		
NECK		
ANTERIOR TRUNK		
POSTERIOR TRUNK		
RIGHT ARM		
LEFT ARM		
BUTTOCKS		
GENITALIA		
RIGHT LEG		
LEFT LEG		
SUM		
TOTAL BURN		

[///] SUPERFICIAL   [XXX] DEEP

RELATIVE PERCENTAGES OF AREAS AFFECTED BY GROWTH

AREA	AGE 0	AGE 1	AGE 5	AGE10	AGE 15	ADULT
A = ½ OF HEAD	9½	8½	6½	5½	4½	3½
B = ½ OF ONE THIGH	2¾	3¼	4	4¼	4½	4¾
C = ½ OF ONE LEG	2½	2½	2¾	3	3¼	3½

Fig. 13.4 Lund and Browder burns chart (child).

☼ Stabilizing the burn patient

Before a patient is referred to the specialized burns unit they will need to be stabilized. It is important to communicate with the receiving unit, as regards the fluid-resuscitation protocol, as well as the management of the wound, specifically with regards to the dressing.

- **Airway**—history of burn injury in a confined space must arouse suspicion of airway injury. Clinical manifestation of smoke inhalation injury is subtle in the early stages and may not become obvious till 24 h. The decision to intubate is clinical rather than findings of X-ray chest, or blood gas results. The **airway must be stabilized prior to transfer**.
- **Breathing**—administer high-flow **100%** oxygen via a non-breathing mask. CO levels from blood taken at the A&E may not represent the true level at the time of injury. Some patients may require endotracheal intubation and mechanical ventilation. Arterial blood gases should be determined as a baseline prior to intubation.

Care of the burn wound

Cold saline soak or water for 15–20 min is helpful in reduction of, not only pain but also, local oedema. Burns wounds of the face are generally treated by exposure method. A bland dressing, such as jelonet or mepitel, may be applied to prevent exudation of fluid from burn areas. For superficial burn areas, liquid paraffin application is adequate. It is important to discuss with the receiving hospital regarding dressing materials, since various wound dressings have different advantages and disadvantages.

As a rule, antibiotics are not given in adults. However, in paediatric burns, most units recommend a 5-day course of flucloxacillin to prevent toxic shock syndrome.

⑦ Surgical management of burns

The surgical management of burns patients can be divided into immediate (escharotomy, tracheotomy), early/intermediate (excision and grafting), or late (post-burn reconstruction).

The first stage in grafting a burn wound is to excise the burn in a tangential fashion, until a viable bed is obtained. A split skin graft is then harvested from a donor site and secured to the wound with tissue glue, sutures, or staples. This is indicated for deep, partial, or full-thickness burns and should be performed at the earliest possible stage, once adequate resuscitation has been achieved. It is important to excise wounds if healing is likely to take longer than 21 days, in order to achieve the best functional and cosmetic results. **Facial burns tend to heal well as a result of their vascularity, and they can be managed conservatively in the initial stages**. For these burns split skin grafts are best left unmeshed and sutured in aesthetic units (e.g. forehead, side of nose, cheek).

Particularly in large burns (>50% TBSA), there may not be enough donor skin to cover the burn area, even if the grafts are meshed. Wound dressing alternatives include:

- Synthetic wound dressings—a variety of these are available, e.g. biobrane, which is composed from an outer layer of silicone and nylon, and an inner layer of collagen. It is applied in theatre with glue or staples, following debridement of the burn. Such dressings can also be used to cover donor sites. Unfortunately, they also provide an ideal culture medium.
- Cadaveric allograft—this is meshed 1:1.5 and laid over a meshed 3:1 autograft. Skin is highly immunogenic, but burn patients are immunosupressed and will not reject the allograft in the initial stages of their recovery. It helps to reduce fluid and electrolyte losses and reduce wound infection. Once the allograft is rejected, it will peel off to leave the autograft underneath.
- Xenograft—porcine skin. This is used as above.
- Integra—this is a dermal matrix derived from shark proteoglycan and bovine collagen, which is covered in silicone. It is applied to the debrided burn. The silicone layer is stripped off at 3 weeks and replaced with an ultra-thin epithelial autograft. Fibroblasts and vascular cells grow in to the integra. It is said to result in less hypertrophic scarring but is certainly not cheap!
- Dermagraft—cultured human foetal fibroblasts in polyglycolic acid mesh. This is a dermal substitute and must be autografted with a thin split-skin graft.
- Cultured epithelial autograft—the recipient's own cells are cultured with bovine serum from a full-thickness skin biopsy. It takes 3 weeks to make a $1m^2$ sheet, which is five cells thick. The graft is very fragile and there is often late graft loss.

In most cases, post-burn reconstruction should be postponed until all wounds have healed. The main priorities are to prevent deformity, restore function, and improve cosmesis. Full-thickness grafts can be harvested from the upper eyelids, naso-labial fold, pre-/post-auricular area, scalp, and supraclavicular fossa. These areas should provide a good colour match for facial skin. Other options include Z-plasty, W-plasty, and tissue expansion. Free flaps are also used, as necessary. Currently, there is much media interest in the possibility of facial transplantation. This obviously raises many ethical concerns and is far from a 'quick fix'.

Psychiatric considerations

These patients often suffer from post-traumatic stress syndrome and may have delusions and hallucinations in the initial stages of their injury. Longer term problems include poor self-esteem, anxiety, and phobias. Because a person's face is highly visible and difficult to camouflage, burn scars are always a difficult reconstructive problem. Most patients require repeated scar revisions and contracture releases. Patient management is complex and should involve a multidisciplinary team.

Chapter 14

Miscellaneous conditions

☣ Airway obstruction

The upper airway is **at risk** when the following findings are present:
- **physical findings of actual or potential obstruction;**
- **laryngeal laryngeal/tracheal injury;**
- **upper tracheal injury;**
- **inability to handle normal secretions;**
- **uncontrolled haemorrhage;**
- **surgical emphysema;**
- **foreign bodies;**
- **adjacent soft tissue injuries;**
- **maxillofacial injury;**
- **reduction in conscious level;**
- **epiglottitis;**
- **alcohol and drugs.**

Obstruction may occur in drowsy patients laying on their backs, e.g. following head injury, drugs, or alcohol. While supine, the relaxed tongue falls back and obstructs the pharynx. Partial obstruction is accompanied by loud snoring, complete obstruction is silent. Agitation should make one think of hypoxia, rather than putting it down to alcohol or drugs.

Fractures of the mandible (usually severe and multiple), can also result in the tongue loosing its support and falling back, especially when the patient is lying supine. With such high-energy injuries, the patient may also have a head injury and, therefore, associated drowsiness can aggravate the loss of airway control.

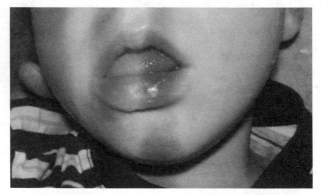

Fig. 14.1 Impending airway obstruction—the child will not lay down, is drooling and has difficulty in swallowing.

☠ Foreign bodies (FBs)

Objects may pass through the aerodigestive tract in one of two ways:
- inhalation—common in the younger age group, who may also wedge small objects in their nasal cavity or the external auditory canal;
- ingestion—again seen in children but often also seen in elderly confused patients or in the psychiatrically disturbed.

☠ Inhaled FBs

Of patients with this condition, 90% are under the age of 8 years: the classic picture being one of a child who develops acute respiratory problems having been previously well. Clinical presentation is very dependent on the nature of the foreign body and the site of impaction:
- larynx—impaction here may rapidly prove fatal due to complete airway obstruction;
- trachea—respiratory compromise with a bilateral wheeze;
- bronchial—unilateral symptoms are seen (wheeze, reduced breath sounds), commonly on the right.

Late presentation includes:
- infection;
- airway collapse/obstruction—due to excessive mucus production or mucosal inflammatory response.

Management
- 'Life-saving' measures may be necessary in critically obstructed patients:
  - **bend patient forward and slap firmly on back several times;**
  - **Heimlich manoeuvre (see p. 437);**
  - **hold infants up by their legs and slap back several times;**
  - **surgical airway—may be necessary as an emergency procedure**.
- Supportive measures, reassurance, antibiotic treatment of established infections.
- Identification of the site of impaction. Radiographs if object is radio-opaque.
- Retrieval—this may involve endoscopic removal or rarely, a thoracic procedure.

① Ingested FBs

Commonly, beads or coins in children, or bones or chunks of meat in adults. Patients often give a good history of swallowing the foreign body. Generally, ingested FBs that impact in the mouth and upper pharynx produce unilateral symptoms (e.g. a fish bone in a tonsil), whereas FBs in the oesophagus usually give symptoms localized to the mid-line. **Neck/back stiffness, tachycardia, dyspnoea, and surgical emphysema (air in the soft tissues) suggest oesophageal perforation**, and should be acted upon immediately as surgical repair may be indicated. This should especially be considered in psychiatric patients who may ingest sharp objects.

Management
Identification of the site of impaction is the key to management. Radiographs may be useful in localization as even radiolucent FBs may show up as subtle soft tissue changes.

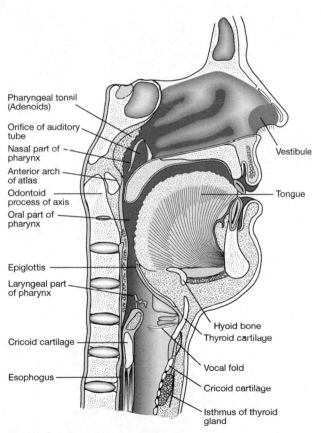

Pharyngeal tonsil
(Adenoids)

Orifice of auditory
tube

Nasal part of
pharynx

Anterior arch
of atlas

Odontoid
process of axis

Oral part of
pharynx

Epiglottis

Laryngeal part
of pharynx

Cricoid cartilage

Esophogus

Vestibule

Tongue

Hyoid bone
Thyroid cartilage

Vocal fold

Cricoid cartilage

Isthmus of thyroid
gland

Fig. 14.2 Basic upper airway anatomy.

- Mouth and pharynx—FBs here are usually easily identified with the aid of good light, tongue depressors, and mouth/laryngeal mirrors—it is then often the case of simply removing the FB with forceps under topical anaesthesia (paediatric cases may require a GA).
- Oesophageal—FBs that have passed through the gastro-oesophageal junction will usually continue their journey to be passed spontaneously. An object impacted in the oesophagus may otherwise have to be endoscopically removed under sedation/GA.

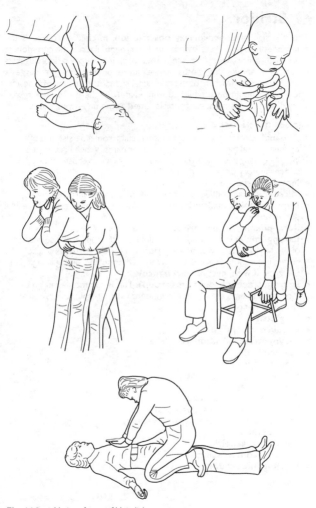

Fig. 14.3 Various forms of Heimlich manoeuvre.

☠ Stridor

This is a sign of **upper-airway obstruction**. In children, croup is the commonest cause of acute stridor, while laryngomalacia is the commonest cause of chronic stridor. As a rule of thumb, an inspiratory stridor suggests obstruction above the glottis, while an expiratory stridor suggests obstruction in the trachea. Both types suggest a glottic or subglottic lesion. The airway should be established immediately, if there is severe respiratory distress. Treatment of stridor is aimed at the underlying cause.

Causes of stridor

- **Choanal atresia**. This rare condition results from a persistence of the bucconasal membrane in the posterior nares. When bilateral it is life-threatening and a well-recognized cause of airway obstruction and respiratory distress in the newborn.
- **Macroglossia.**
- **Micrognathia** resulting in posterior displacement of the tongue.
- **Hypertrophic tonsils/adenoids**. Often the stridor is most noticeable during sleep.
- **Retropharyngeal or peritonsillar abscess**.
- **Laryngomalacia**. This is due to a defect in the supporting structures of the larynx. The airway partially obstructs as the tissues prolapse during inspiration. This is usually worse when supine, crying or agitated.
- **Laryngeal web, cyst, or laryngocele**
- **Laryngotracheobronchitis (croup)**. This is commonly caused by the para-influenza virus, but also influenza virus, respiratory syncytial virus, and rhinoviruses.
- **Epiglottitis.**
- **Vocal cord paralysis.**
- **Laryngotracheal stenosis.**
- **Foreign body.**
- **Cystic hygroma.**
- **Subglottic hemangioma.**
- **Laryngeal papilloma.**
- **Angioneurotic oedema.**
- **Lingual thyroid or thyroglossal cyst.**
- **Laryngospasm (hypocalcemic tetany).**
- **Tracheomalacia.**
- **Bacterial tracheitis.**
- **External compression.**
- **Psychogenic stridor.**

:☼: Epistaxis (non-traumatic)

Patients should have their pulse and blood pressure checked and, if bleeding has been severe, should be investigated for bleeding disorders. **Elderly patients, in particular, are affected more by blood loss** and may develop postural hypotension or syncope. Occasionally intravenous fluids may be required. Patients who have had major nose bleeds should be admitted for observation, bed rest, pain relief, and IV fluids. Following trauma, although technically compound fractures, nasal fractures associated with epistaxis generally do not require antibiotic cover.

① Minor bleeding

This usually settles on its own, or requires only simple first-aid measures (sitting forward and pinching the nose for at least 20 min). If this fails, the vestibule and septum should be examined for bleeding points. These may be **cauterized using silver nitrate sticks** or needle diathermy under topical anaesthesia. Cocaine paste causes vasoconstriction and help to control bleeding; however, care is required as too much is toxic. Xylocaine spray can be used instead. Where the bleeding source cannot be seen, the nose can be **packed using ribbon gauze** impregnated with vaseline or bismuth iodoform paraffin paste (BIPP).

:☼: Major bleeding

More secure packing involves using a soft **Foley catheter**, which is inserted (deflated) through the nose until visible at the back of the throat. The balloon is then inflated and gentle traction applied 'wedging' the balloon between the soft palate and nasopharynx. Ribbon gauze can then be packed anteriorly. Simpler alternatives include commercially available **nasal 'tampons'**. Packs are generally retained for around 48 h following control of haemorrhage. Antibiotics may be required.

In rare instances where there is **torrential haemorrhage**, which cannot be controlled by packing, external carotid artery and anterior ethmoidal artery ligation may be necessary. The anterior ethmoidal artery passes through the orbit and is exposed via a transorbital approaches. Alternatively, ligation can be achieved endoscopically through the nose. These are 'last ditch' attempts, but may be required in those cases of continuing major bleeding resistant to all other treatments.

☼ Urticaria and angioedema

These are hypersensitivity conditions affecting up to 15% of the population at some time. Urticaria affects the skin with transient, oedematous, itchy swellings. Angioedema is similar but involves the subcutaneous tissues and mucous membranes, especially around the face. In the rare syndrome of hereditary angioedema, the respiratory tract may be affected, resulting in **stridor, which can be fatal**. Episodes may be precipitated by drugs, insect stings, specific foods, animals, and pollens, or by cold, heat, sunlight, direct pressure, water, vibration, and exercise. Viruses and parasites are common precipitants in children. Angioedema can be diagnosed, by showing the specific defect of compliment C1 esterase inhibitor in the blood.

Treatment

Antihistamines and steroids are the usual treatment for both acute and chronic angioedema. Potential airway obstruction requires immediate intramuscular adrenalin, repeated if necessary and followed by an antihistamine. A surgical airway may be necessary. Patients who have had such an episode should be given adrenaline with clear instructions and a demonstration of how to inject themselves. In hereditary angioedema donor serum C1esterase inhibitor concentrate is required. Patients may also be treated prophylactically with stanasol or danosol, which raise serum levels of C1 esterase. Tranexamic acid offers a less effective alternative.

! Dizzyness/'vertigo'

See also: The ear.

Disorders of the middle and inner ear can result in loss of balance. They include:
- **acute otitis media;**
- **otitis media with effusion;**
- **chronic suppurative otitis media;**
- **trauma;**
- **labyrinthitis;**
- **Ménière's disease;**
- **otosclerosis;**
- **otosclerotic drugs;**
- **syphilis.**

Other general causes include:
- **vertebrobasilar insufficiency;**
- **postural hypotension and cardiovascular disease;**
- **ageing;**
- **migraine;**
- **transient ischaemic attacks;**
- **head injury;**
- **epilepsy;**
- **hyperventilation**.

ⓘ Sore throat

This is a symptom of many possible causes, although infections cause the majority of them. Common infections include flu, the common cold, infectious mononucleosis, streptococci, or hemophilus.

Viral

Most **viral** sore throats are associated with a congested runny nose, sneezing, and generalized aches and pains. These are highly contagious and usually last about a week. Sore throat can also occur in measles, chicken pox, whooping cough, and croup. Infectious mononucleosis, a severe illness in teenagers, can be transmitted by saliva and is therefore also known as 'kissing disease'. This virus causes massive enlargement of the tonsils and generalized lymphadenopathy. In severe cases it can result in breathing difficulties, jaundice, and fatigue that can last several months. **If suspected avoid amoxycillin**.

Bacterial

Bacterial **sore throats are less common. However,** 'strep throat' can also result in rheumatic fever and nephritis, cause scarlet fever, tonsillitis, pneumonia, sinusitis, and ear infections. It therefore should be treated with antibiotics. Tonsillitis is an infection of the lymphatic tonsils on each side of the back of the throat. Mild cases are common; however, healthy tonsils do not remain infected. Frequent bouts of tonsillitis suggest the infection is not fully eliminated between episodes. The most dangerous throat infection is **epiglottitis**, which untreated can obstruct the airway. This is an emergency condition that requires prompt attention and admission. Usually there is a sudden onset of high fever, toxicity, agitation, stridor, dyspnea, muffled voice, dysphagia, and drooling. Older children may prefer to sit leaning forward with the mouth open and the tongue protruding. There is no spontaneous cough. An oedematous, cherry red epiglottis is the hallmark of this but **do not depress** the tongue to look for it.

Allergic

Allergic **sore throats can be caused by the same allergens** that irritate the nose. Cats, dogs, and house dust are common culprits.

Irritation

During cold weather, dry heat can cause mild sore throats. This often responds to humidification. Pollutants can also irritate the nose and throat, the most common being smoke. Rare causes include **voice overusage (shouting), reflux, and tumours**.

Indications for further treatment or investigations include:
- rash;
- fever;
- severe, prolonged or recurrent sore throats;
- difficulty breathing;
- difficulty swallowing;
- difficulty opening the mouth;

- joint pain;
- earache;
- blood in saliva or phlegm;
- lumps in neck;
- hoarseness lasting over 2 weeks.

⑦ Drugs and dressings commonly used in head and neck surgery

For detailed information regarding each drug refer to any drug prescribing formulary.

Analgesics

Effective pain relief depends on choosing the appropriate drug, anticipating its need, and regular administration rather than waiting for pain to develop. Remember additional measures (e.g. TENS, cryotherapy, and nerve blocks).

Simple analgesics such as paracetamol and aspirin are useful in the treatment of mild pain, and in combination with codeine for moderate visceral pain. They can be given either on their own, or in combination with each other.

Non-steroidal anti-inflammatory drugs (NSAIDs)

These are useful in trauma, infection, and bone pain. They have an analgesic and anti-inflammatory action. NSAIDs can be used in conjunction with other analgesics, such as codeine or morphine. Peri-operative administration enhances post-operative pain relief and, when used in conjunction with morphine, is thought to be opioid-sparing (i.e. pain relief is achieved using a lower dose of morphine).

Moderate to severe pain

This is usually best treated with multimodal therapy and attention to any treatable causes. Opioids act in the central nervous system. In acute pain, consideration must be given to the route, e.g. subcutaneous versus intravenous route; continuous infusion versus patient controlled analgesia.

Neuropathic pain

This type of pain, such as the pain experienced with trigeminal neuralgia, does not generally respond well to opiates. Other types of analgesia are required. These include topical analgesics and centrally-acting drugs. Examples include:
- carbamazepine
- amitriptyline
- dothiepin
- baclofen
- capsaicin (substance P depletor).

Antibiotics

Not all infections require antibiotics. Indications for antibiotics may include:
- evidence of systemic involvement (pyrexia, tachycardia, raised WCC, etc.);
- rapidly spreading infection (e.g. cellulitis);
- infections placing the airway at risk (e.g. Ludwig's angina, epiglottitis);
- deep-seated infections (e.g. frontal, ethmoidal sinusitis);
- deep-seated penetrating injuries (e.g. gunshot);

- 'at risk' patients (e.g. immunocompromised, risk of developing bacterial endocarditis, cavernous sinus thrombosis, cerebral abscess);
- bone infection;
- infected fractures, foreign bodies (e.g. miniplates), and bone graft;
- some abscesses;
- failure of other measures to effectively treat infection.

These are, however, only guidelines. Each case must be treated individually, the decision to use antibiotics being a balance of risks versus benefits. Alternative measures include:

- drainage (surgical, posture, inhalations);
- removal of underlying local cause (tooth, foreign body, graft);
- debridement (mucky wounds);
- local measures (mouthwashes, removal of sutures);
- treatment of systemic factors (diabetes).

In all cases pus or infected tissues should be obtained for culture before antibiotics are started if at all possible. Subsequent sensitivities will guide the final choice of antibiotic. Many antibiotics are available and most units have a protocol for prescribing. If in doubt discussion with a clinical microbiologist is usually very helpful.

Commonly prescribed antibiotics are the penicillins, cephalosporins, and metronidazole. Tetracyclins and fuscidic acid are useful for bone infection. Occasionaly, gentamicin or vancomycin may be necessary but ideally only after consultation with the microbiologist.

Antiseptics

The use of antiseptics in wound care is controversial. In some circumstances experimental evidence has shown that some antiseptics adversely affect wound healing. There is an increasing amount of anecdotal evidence that iodine plays a role in non-healing wounds. Examples include:

- betadine
- proflavin
- chlorhexidine.

Betadine comes in a wide range of products including surgical antiseptics, skin, and wound preparations and mouth washes. Iodine (1%) in aqueous solution is good for wound care. It is also available in ointment, spray form, and impregnated into a dressing, e.g. inadine.

Betadine has been shown to be effective against methicillin-resistant *Staphylococcus aureus* (MRSA). It is also effective against viruses, other bacteria, fungi, and their spores. Because of this, iodine has replaced most topical antibiotics. Patients may become sensitive to iodine and it should only be used short term where there is clinical evidence of infection. It becomes inactive when there is pus or exudate. It should not be used on large wounds, as absorption of iodine may occur. The alcoholic solution should never be used on wounds.

Terra-cortril ointment contains hydrocortisone and oxytetracycline, and is used for the treatment of over-granulation tissue. It should only be used sparingly for a short period, e.g. most units only use it for a maximum of 2 weeks at a time.

Antiseptic dressings

Whitehead's varnish is a mixture of iodoform, benzoin, storax, tolu balsam, and solvent ether. It is commonly used in the treatment of dry socket and for packing mucky/infected cavities. This may be left in place for several months without becoming infected.

Bismuth iodoform paraffin paste (BIPP) applied to ribbon gauze can be used in packing nasal and paranasal cavities.

Anti-emetics

Many types are available in common practice—stemitil, maxalon, etc., and the choice is frequently down to hospital and local practice. Ondansetron is a useful, although expensive, anti-emetic for resistant post-operative vomiting. Granisetron has recently been introduced for intravenous infusion as an alternative and early results suggest it may resemble Odansetron, however, comparative trials are still required.

Dressings

Traditional

For example, cotton wool, gauze, and gamgee. Cotton wool should no longer be used to cleanse wounds, as it can leave tiny fibres in the wound that can trigger the inflammatory phase later in the wound-healing process. Gauze and gamgee are still widely used as a secondary dressing to help to control exudate. However, they should not be used as a primary dressing directly onto a moist wound surface.

Low adherent

For example, mefolin, release, skintact, tricotex, NA dressing, silicone NA, and telfa. These dressings are low adherent—they have little or no absorbency, so a secondary dressing is advisable. Alternatively, they are best used on wounds that have a low exudate. These can be used in conjunction with other agents, such as hydrogels and ointments to help such substances remain in place.

Mepitel consists of a polymide mesh impregnated with a silicone gel. It does not adhere to the wound but is tacky to the touch and so is a good dressing for burns or abrasions. A secondary dressing is required to control any exudate. It can be left in place for up to 10 days, thereby reducing the disturbance of the wound.

Alginate dressings

For example, sorbsan, kaltostat, kaltogel, fibracof, and comfeel alginate. Alginates are dry absorbent dressings made from seaweed, which contain varying amounts of mannuronic and guluronic acid. The dressing absorbs exudate from the wound and becomes a gel. The dressings are absorbent and so are useful for moderately exudating wounds. There are also higher absorbency versions of the dressings, such as sorbsan plus and kaltostat fortex. These dressings should only be used on exudating wounds, never on dry wounds. Alginates are also useful as haemostats. Kaltostat achieves haeomstasis by the exchange of calcium ions for sodium ions in the blood.

Charcoal dressings

For example, actisorb plus, kaltocarb, and lyofoam C. These products contain activated charcoal, which is effective in absorbing chemicals released from fungating and necrotic wounds. This offensive smell is extremely distressing for patients and their carers, especially those who have a malignant wound. Actisorb plus is an activated charcoal cloth with silver enclosed in a nylon porous bag; the silver helps to reduce bacterial growth, which can lead to more odour. Kaltocarb consists of a layer of alginate fibre bonded onto a piece of activated charcoal cloth. Both these dressings can be used as primary dressings.

Foams

For example, allevyn, allevyn adhesive, lyofoam, tielle, spyrosorb, alievyn cavity, and cavicare. Foams are synthetic dressings of hydrophilic polyurthane. They absorb wound exudate and maintain a moist wound-healing environment. They can be used on moderate to heavily exudating wounds, which are healthy and granulating. Since many are waterproof, patients can bathe and do not require a secondary dressing. It is possible for the dressing to be left *in situ* for up to 7 days.

Hydrocolloids

For example, granuflex, comfeel, and tegasorb. These consist of a hydro-colloid base made from gelatin, cellulose, and pectins with a backing of a polyurethane film or foam. They are completely occlusive and provide a moist wound-healing environment. Fluid from the wound is absorbed into the dressing and forms a gel. These dressings can cause over-granulation tissue to develop. Hydrocolloids can be used on necrotic, sloughy, and granulating wounds, and can be left *in situ* for up to 7 days.

Enzyme preparations

For example, varidase. This contains two enzymes: streptokinase and streptodornase. It comes in the form of a powder and is reconstituted with normal saline. Streptokinase breaks down fibrin and fibrinogen, and streptodornase liquifies and aids the removal of DNA derived from the cell nuclei. Varidase is used to debride and clean wounds, especially necrotic eschar. It requires a secondary dressing or a semipermeable membrane to be applied and it will require changing daily.

Hydrogels

For example, intrasite gel, granugel, 2nd skin, and vigilon. These dressings are made up of a copolymer starch and have a high water content. Vigilon and 2nd skin are a sheet hydrogel and contain 98% water. They can be used on a variety of wounds, such as minor burns and abrasions, and can be left *in situ* for 3–4 days. They are applied directly to the wound and require a secondary dressing. Hydrogels can be used on necrotic tissue in order to debride the wound. They should not, however, be used where an anaerobic infection is indicated. They can also be used on sloughy, granulating and epithelializing wounds.

Impregnated dressings

For example, jelonet and inadine. Paraffin gauze such as jelonet is a cotton woven fabric, which is impregnated with soft white paraffin. It is commonly used on minor burns and abrasions but can adhere to granulation tissue causing pain on removal. It is also used as a primary dressing over split-skin grafts in most areas. Inadine is made of rayon mesh impregnated with 10% providone–iodine. The iodine is released directly onto the wound. It can be used on infected wounds, superficial burns, and minor contaminated injuries.

Vapour-permeable films

For example, tagaderm, opsite, flexigrid, and bioclusive. These are sterile, thin, semi-permeable, hypoallergenic, adhesive-coated film dressings. They maintain a moist environment by preventing evaporation of water from the wound.

Beads

For example, debrisan, Iodoflex, and Iodosorb. These products are also known as xerogels and are made up of hydrophilic beads or powder, which absorb exudate and form a gel. They should only be used on exuding wounds and can be used on sloughy necrotic or infected wounds.

Antibacterials

For example, flammazine cream and metrotop gel. Flammazine is a hydrophilic cream, which contains silver sulphadiazine 1% oil in water emulsion. It is a topical, broad-spectrum antibacterial and inhibits the growth of nearly all pathogenic bacteria and fungi *in vitro*. Is particularly effective against pseudomonas and *Staphylococcus aureus*. It is widely used in the treatment of burns to prevent Gram-negative sepsis. Silver ions are gradually released from the cream, so prolonging its antibacterial effect. It can be used to treat an infected wound or where it is essential to prevent infection as in the case of burns patients. An absorbent dressing is required.

Metrotop gel is clear and colourless and contains metronidazole BP 0.8% w/v. It is particularly effective in the control of odour from fungating and malodorous tumours as it is active against anaerobic bacteria.

Local anaesthetics (LA)

These work by temporarily blocking nerve conduction, different drugs varying widely in strength, toxicity, and duration of anaesthesia. Once the solution has been injected into the tissues around the nerve, it is slowly absorbed into the circulation, terminating its action. However, the rate of absorption is also related to toxicity and, therefore, it is essential to make sure that the needle has not been introduced inadvertantly into a blood vessel prior to injection. Self-aspirating syringes, commonly used in dental practice, usually enable this but are not fool-proof. Maximum concentration in the blood occurs around 10–25 min after infiltration and, therefore, observation is required for the first 30 min. Toxicity may involve the central nervous system (confusion, respiratory depression, and convulsions) or cardiovascular system (dysrhythmias, hypotension, and cardiac arrest).

Some LA solutions contain a small amount of adrenaline (epinephrine). This stimulates vasoconstriction, thereby delaying absorbtion and increasing the duration of anaesthesia. Vasoconstriction also helps reduce bleeding during surgery, improving visability. Contrary to popular belief, adrenaline-containing solutions can be used safely on the pinna and nose. Solutions commonly used include:

- lignocaine 2% with adrenaline 1 in 80 000 (lasts up to 3 h);
- prilocaine 3% with octopressin 0.03 units/ml;
- bupivacaine (marcaine) 0.5% (lasts up to 8 h with adrenaline).

Each drug has a maximum safe dose, (mg per kg), which therefore depends on the weight of the patient and the drug used. Anyone giving local anaesthetic drugs must be familiar with these dose limits or refer to the BNF or drug information leaflet.

Mouthwashes

Good oral hygiene is essential for oral wound healing and should be started as soon as possible. Not only must obvious debris be cleared from the mouth, but also microscopic deposits, which rapidly become colonized and contaminated. In the early phases, hygiene is limited by swelling and discomfort, and it is then that mouthwashes are particularly helpful. Mouthwashes, however, are not a substitute for good toothbrushing.

- Chlorhexidine has good bacteriocidal effects. It is particularly helpful in patients at risk of bacterial endocarditis.
- Hot salt water mouthwashes are often advised following meals. They are helpful in keeping the mouth clean, provide some relief of discomfort and are cheap.
- Difflam (benzydamine) may be used to relieve the pain associated with oral ulcers or radiation mucositis.

Saliva substitutes and flouride

Dry mouth is a common problem, which can occur with no apparant cause or in association with salivary gland disease, e.g. Sjögren's syndrome. It can be particularly severe following radiotherapy to the salivary glands and oral mucosa as part of the treatment of some head and neck cancers. Saliva substitutes are available as sprays or aerosols, which simulate these mucoproteins and help with chewing, swallowing, and releif of discomfort. Examples include glandosane, saliva orthana.

Glossary

#: Fracture.

A&E: Accident and emergency.

ABBE FLAP: A pedicled flap used in lip reconstruction. A wedge of the lower lip, attached at corner by its blood supply is rotated into the defect in the upper lip. This uses the principle of replacing like with like. Up to one-third of the lower lip can be used in this way, the resulting defect is closed primarily.

ABG: Arterial blood gases.

ADNEXAL: Skin organs, e.g. hair follicles, sweat glands.

AEROCELE: A collection of air in a body cavity, e.g. intra-cranial air.

AETIOLOGICAL: refers to known or suspected factors in disease or trauma, e.g. smoking and lung cancer, alcohol and assaults.

ALGIA: PAin arising from, e.g. arthralgia = painful joint, neuralgia = pain arising from a nerve.

ANGIOGENESIS: Development of new blood vessels.

ANKYLOSIS: Abnormal fusion across a joint. Can be bony or fibrous.

ANTIMONGALOID SLANT: Increased downward slant of the corners of the eyes (palpebral fissure). Normally the outer corner is just slightly higher than the inner corner.

ANTROSTOMY: An artificial opening made into the maxillary antrum, either through the mouth or nose, for access or drainage.

ATLS: Advanced trauma life support.

ARDS: Adult respiratory distress syndrome.

ARTHRIDITIES: A group of inflammatory disorders involving joints.

AVM: Arteriovenous malformation.

AVPU: Refers to the rapid neurological assessment in trauma: Alert, responds to Voice, Pain, Unresponsive.

BICORTICAL SCREWS: These are screws that, when placed, pass through and engage both inner and outer cortices of bone. These are used predominantly in the mandible, which is thick enough to support them.

BLEEDING DIATHESES: Disorders resulting in an increased bleeding tendency.

ß BLOCKERS: A group of drugs acting on the cardiorespiratory systems. One important effect is to slow the heart down and reduce its ability to mount a tachycardia.

B12: One of the B group of vitamins.

BOLUS: A small quantity, e.g. food bolus or fluid bolus.

BRONCHOSCOPY: Direct visualization of the respiratory tract using a flexible or rigid optical scope.

BULLAE: A large fluid-filled blister.

CALCULUS: A calcified mass, e.g. renal, salivary gland or gallstones.

CALDWELL-LUC: A surgical procedure in which an opening is made in the maxillary antrum.

CAPILLARY REFILL: A clinical observation in which pressing on a finger-nail results in blanching of the nail-bed, which restores to its pink colour on release. It is a gross assessment of tissue perfusion. This should take less than 2 s.

CLAUDICATION: Severe pain in a muscle following exercise—implies ischaemia. Can be seen in the leg and chewing muscles

COMMENSALS: Micro-organisms found normally in humans (skin/oral commensals).

COMMINUTED: A fracture in which there are more than two fragments. Implies a significant injury.

CONING: Seen in head injuries. Very high intra-cranial pressure forces the brain stem (conus) through the foramen magnum.

CONTRA-COUP INJURY: Commonly seen in brain injury, the shift of the brain following a blow to the head results in a second blow against the inside of the skull. Injury is, therefore, seen at the other end or opposite side.

CONTRALATERAL: The opposite side, e.g. pupil, limb.

CN: Cranial nerve (12 exist).

CREPITUS: Grating sensation felt between the fragments of a fracture.

CRICOTHYROID MEMBRANE: A fibrous membrane passing between the thyroid cartilage (above) and the cricoid cartilage (below).

CRYSTALLOID: Intravenous fluid composed of water and electrolytes, sometimes with dextrose (e.g. normal saline, dextrose/saline, hartmanns solution, ringers lactate).

CSF: Cerebral spinal fluid: lines, protects and supports the brain and spinal cord.

CVA: Cerebrovascular accident: a stroke.

CVP: Central venous pressure: the pressure within the superior vena cava. An indirect measure of the hearts pumping ability

CYANOSIS: Blue discoloration of the skin, lips, and mouth due to low levels of oxygenated blood.

DDAVP: 1-deamino, 8 D-arginine vasopressin. A synthetic analogue of vasopressin. This alters coagulation by effects on vascular endothelium and platelets.

DEBRIDE: To surgically clean and remove dead tissue.

DEHISCE: Wound breakdown.

DIASTASIS: Abnormal separation of a suture

DYNIA: 'Pain of', e.g. glossodynia.

DYSAESTHESIAS: Disturbance of sensation (often uncomfortable).

DYSPHAGIA: Difficulty in swallowing.

DYSPHASIA: Difficulty in expression.

DYSPHONIA: Difficulty in voice production.

EAM: External auditory meatus.

ECTOMY: Removal of, e.g. appendicectomy.

EICOSANOIDS: These are a class of lipids that include the prostaglandins, thromboxanes, and leukotrienes. They exert specific physiological effects on target cells, like hormones. However, eicosanoids are distinct from most hormones in that they act locally, near their sites of synthesis.

ELECTIVE: Routine.

ENDOCRINOPATHY: Disorders of the endocrine glands.

END ORGAN ISCHAEMIA: Ischaemia of tissues or an organ which depends on a single artery/arteriole for its blood supply.

ENTROPIAN: Inversion of the lower eyelid, i.e. the eyelashes lay against the eyeball.

ENTONOX: Gas composed of 50% nitrous oxide and 50% oxygen. Very useful for analgesia.

EPISTAXIS: Nose bleed.

EPULIS: Pyogenic granuloma.

ERYTHEMA: Red appearance of tissues (usually skin) due to inflammation.

ESCHAROTOMY: Division of burnt, contracted skin (to release tension).

ESR: Erythocyte sedimentation rate.

EXOPHYTIC: Cauliflower or warty-like growth

EXOPHTHALMOS: Bulging appearance of the eyes seen in overactive thyroid disorders.

EXTREMIS: On the point of a cardiorespiratory arrest.

FASCIA: Fibrous layers separating organs and structures.

FAUCES: Refers to the muscular folds passing down from the soft palate to the tongue, usually representing the junction between the oral cavity and the pharynx.

FB: Foreign body.

FND: Focal neurological deficit.

FOLEY CATHETERS: Urinary catheters.

FREE FLAPS: Tissue transferred from one site to another (same patient) dependent on a single artery and vein for its blood supply (e.g. radial forearm, parascapular). Requires microvascular anastamosis.

GA: General anaesthetic.

GI TRACT: Gastro-intestinal tract.

GLOSSODYNIA: Painful tongue.

GLOTTIC: Opening to the larynx.

GP: General practitioner or gutta percha (a filling material used in dentistry)

GUNNING SPLINTS: Plastic splints used to support mandibular fractures. Very much like dentures, but without the teeth. They are secured (wired/screwed) to the top and bottom jaws and then fixed together. The patient's own dentures can be used if applicable.

HAEMATOCRIT: Refers to the 'thickness' or viscosity of blood, due to the concentration of red cells.

HAMARTOMATOUS: Like a hamartoma. (A non-cancerous growth, which is made up of tissues normally found in the area that it is in, but in an unusual mixture. This type of growth results from a developmental anomaly of embryonic cells).

HOMOGENOUS: Uniform in consistency.

HSV: Herpes simplex virus.

HYPERBARIC OXYGEN: Oxygen breathed at *pressures* greater than in the atmosphere: patient needs to be placed in a pressure chamber.

HYPOGLOBUS: Displacement of the eye down, seen as a difference in the pupillary heights. Often seen in 'blow-out' fractures of the orbit.

IATROGENIC: As a result of treatment.

ID NERVE: Inferior dental (aka inferior alveolar) nerve.

IDIOPATHIC: Unknown cause.

IMF: Intermaxillary fixation, i.e. the jaws are held together (with elastics or wire).

INDURATION: Palpable thickening of tissues, implies chronic infection, scarring or malignancy.

INR: International normalised ration: a measure of the clotting ability of blood.

IN SITU: In/on the patient.

IPSILATERAL: The same side.

-ITIS: Inflammation of (e.g. appendicitis).

KARTAGENER'S SYNDROME: The trio of sinusitis, bronchitis and situs inversus (reversal of the position of all organs in the chest and abdomen with the heart and stomach on the right, the liver on the left).

KERATOCONJUNCTIVITIS SICCA: A syndrome resulting in dry eyes due to reduced tear production. May be seen in Sjögren's syndrome.

LA: Local anaesthetic.

LAG SCREW: Fixation technique in which tightening the screw compresses the bone fragments together.

LEUKOPLAKIA: 'White patch'.

LFTs: Liver-function tests.

LIGATED: Closing a tube (usually blood vessel) with a suture.

LIGHT REFLEX (EARDRUM) The eardrum normally appears light-grey in colour or a glistening pearly-white. The small bones of the middle ear usually push on it like tent poles. This results in a cone of light (light reflex) reflecting off the surface. May be lost in infection.

LINGUAL FRENUM: The midline fold of mucosa passing from the tongue to the floor of mouth: responsible for tongue-tie

LP: Lumber puncture.

LUXATED: Dislocated. A term used when a tooth has been displaced from its socket.

MACULES: Flat skin lesions.

MICROLEAKAGE: Leakage of fluid and bacteria at a microscopic level.

MILIEU: Local environment.

MMF: Maxillomandibular fixation (aka IMF).

MRSA: Methicillin-resistant *Staphylococcal aureus*

MUA: Manipulation under anaesthetic.

MYXOEDEMATOUS: Clinical findings seen in reduced thyroid activity.

NAI: Non-accidental injury.

NARES: External opening of the nose (nostrils).

NASO-LACRIMAL DACROCYSTITIS: Infection of the sac that drains tears out of the eye. Typically, there is pain, redness and swelling over the inner aspect of the lower eyelid associated with excessive tearing, It is sometimes associated with fever and severe swelling around the lower lid.

NOCICEPTIVE: Painful

NSAIDS: Non-steroidal anti-inflammatory drugs.

NYSTAGMUS: Abnormal gyratory movement of the eyes, e.g. horizontal or rotatory.

OBTURATION: To fill a defect with an artificial material, e.g. following maxillectomy.

OPHTHALMOPLEGIA: Paralysis or weakness of one or more of the muscles that control eye movement. The condition can be caused by any of several neurological disorders.

ORIF: 'Open Reduction and Internal Fixation'.

OSTEOSYNTHESIS: Generally refers to the fixation of bones (especially fractures) using plates and screws.

OSTIA: Opening into a cavity (e.g. maxillary).

OTOMY: To create an opening into (e.g. laparotomy, craniotomy).

OXYGEN DISSOCIATION CURVE: The oxygen dissociation curve is a graph that shows the percentage saturation of haemoglobin at various partial pressures of oxygen.

PATHOGNOMONIC: Clinical findings imply diagnosis with certainty.

PATHOLOGICAL FRACTURE: Fracture occurring in weakened bone (e.g. infection, tumour, osteoporosis).

PIRIFORM APERTURE: Bony opening of the nasal cavity.

PO2/PCO2: Partial pressure of oxygen/carbon dioxide.

POP: Plaster of Paris.

PRE-AURICULAR: Just in front of the ear.

PRION: Abnormal forms of a membrane protein (which is normally found on the surface of neurons), now known to be infectious particles. Involved in CJD, BSE, Kuru and Scrapie.

PRODROME: Early symptoms and signs that a patient experiences before the full blown syndrome of an illness becomes evident (e.g. vague aches and tired feeling patients sometime experience the day before coming down with a case of the flu or other viral illness).

PROPTOSED: Bulging of the eye.

PSEUDOTELECANTHUS: Illusory appearance in which the inner corners of the eyes seem to be too far apart.

PTOSIS: Drooping of especially upper eyelid.

PVS: Persistent vegetative state.

RAYNAUD'S: Raynaud's *disease* is a condition caused by constriction and spasms of small arteries, primarily in the hands, after exposure to cold. The cause is unknown. Raynaud's *phenomenon* causes similar symptoms, but it is the result of connective tissue disease or exposure to certain chemicals.

RBS: Random blood sugar.

RETROGRADE INTUBATION: A technique in which a guide wire is passed through the cricothyroid membrane and out through the mouth or nose. An endotracheal tube is then inserted over this into the trachea and the wire withdrawn.

RHABDOMYOLYSIS: The breakdown of skeletal muscle.

RHINITIS: Inflammation of nasal mucosa.

RHOMBERG'S TEST FOR EQUILIBRIUM: Assesses the ability of the vestibular apparatus to help maintain standing balance. Ask patient to stand up with feet together and arms at side. When stable have them close eyes; slight swaying may occur. Positive Romberg's: loss of balance that occurs when closing eyes.

RUBBER DAM: Rubber sheet used in dentistry to isolate and keep dry a tooth.

SAPONIFICATION: The reaction of a base with a fatty ester to form soap.

SCC: Squamous cell carcinoma.

SEPTA: Fibrous or bony partitions.

SEQUESTRUM: A fragment of dead bone.

SIALADENITIS: Inflammation of salivary tissue.

SIALOCELE: A cyst full of saliva.

SJÖGREN'S: A chronic autoimmune disease involving moisture-producing glands. The hallmark symptoms are dry eyes and dry mouth, but it is a systemic disease.

SMR: Submucosal resection (of the nasal septum).

SOMATOSENSORY: The somatosensory system includes multiple types of sensation from the body: light touch, pain, pressure, temperature, and joint and muscle position sense (also called proprioception). However, these modalities are lumped into three different pathways in the spinal cord and have different targets in the brain.

SOMATIZATION: The expression of psychological problems as physical symptoms.

STENOSIS: Abnormal narrowing of.

STENTS: Devices placed to keep tubes patent.

STRESS SHIELDING: The loss of bone that occurs adjacent to a prosthesis (e.g. following ORIF) when stress is diverted from the area.

STRIDOR: Inspiratory noise: represents obstruction.

SUB: Below.

SUPRA: Above.

SUPRA-TARSAL GROOVE: Deep grove above upper eyelid.

SURGICEL: Synthetic mesh used in haemostasis.

SYSSARCOSIS: Tissue between two bones or muscles to enable them to pass over each other (e.g. buccal fat pad).

THIRD MOLAR: '8s': Wisdom teeth.

TRACHEOTOMY: Artificial opening in the trachea.

TRISMUS: Limitation of mouth opening due to muscle spasm.

URTI: Upper respiratory tract infection.

USS: Ultrasound scan.

VERRUCAL: Warty like.

VESICULAR: Small fluid-filled vesicles.

WCC: White cell count.

XANTHOCHROMIA: Red cloudiness of cerebrospinal fluid. Indicates blood in CSF as following subarachnoid hemorrhage (SAH).

XERO: Dryness of.

XEROSTOMIA: Dry mouth.

Index